Field Research Methods in Agriculture

Andrea Onofri

Field Research Methods in Agriculture

An Introduction with R

Springer

Andrea Onofri
Department of Agricultural, Food and Environmental Sciences
University of Perugia
Perugia, Italy

ISBN 978-3-032-08198-8 ISBN 978-3-032-08199-5 (eBook)
https://doi.org/10.1007/978-3-032-08199-5

This Springer imprint is published by the registered company Springer Nature Switzerland AG
The registered company address is: Gewerbestrasse 11, 6330 Cham, Switzerland

To Miriana, Martina, and Riccardo:
Thank you for your love, your patience, and all the evenings and weekends you so generously lent me to write this book.
To Umberto, Gabriella, and Alberto:
For showing me the joy of having interests and the value of always pursuing them.

Preface

Field research is one of the key elements of scientific progress in agriculture and applied biology, as it serves as the "bridge" between laboratory experiments conducted under highly controlled conditions and on-farm tests with purely demonstrative purposes. Similarly to laboratory research, field research is based on scientifically sound protocols and provides reliable answers to research questions; similarly to on-farm tests, field research takes place in "real-life" conditions so that the results are directly transferable to farmers and growers. The need to use near-to-commercial-scale field equipment and the need to comply with several sources of random variability, such as fertility gradients, pest attacks, and other more or less dangerous intrusions, has favored the establishment of a peculiar body of methods, concerning both the design of experiments and the analyses of results. All these peculiar methods are rarely found altogether in a single, short introductory book that is both easy to read for practitioners and students in the agricultural and biological sciences and contains practical hints on the use of statistical software.

This book aims at filling that gap, focusing on field research and, particularly, on small-plot experiments, which are the fundamental engine of progress in agriculture and represent the primary tool to evaluate and compare, e.g., innovative genotypes, agronomic practices, pesticides, and other plant protection methods, as well as their side effects on the farming systems.

How This Book Is Organized

In this book, I adopted a "learning-by-doing" approach, incorporating several examples and case studies, while keeping theory and mathematics at a minimum level. However, I did not want to remove all hand calculations: they represent the best way to understand the fundamentals of statistical methods and, eventually, master them. Examples are conceived as much as possible as stand-alone entities, so that the proposed approaches can be followed and reproduced. This practical approach emphasizes the real-world applications of the techniques discussed.

This book begins by covering the design of experiments (Chaps. 1 and 2) and the three fundamental traits of research (control, replication, and randomization), which make the difference between valid and invalid data. It also covers the main elements of scientific research and the techniques by which experimental treatments can be randomly allocated to the experimental units (completely randomized designs, block designs, split-plot designs, and so on).

Chapter 3 is devoted to the fundamentals of descriptive statistics, presenting several simple statistics for quantitative data, including the mean, median, variance, standard deviation, and the Pearson correlation coefficient. Chapter 4 makes the point that data analyses for field experiments can be viewed as a model fitting process by which the cause-effect relationships under study can be described and explored. Several simple linear models are introduced, and guidance is provided on how we can easily fit them to the experimental data to draw reliable conclusions.

Starting from the premise that every good model should be able to tackle stochastic effects (experimental "errors"), Chap. 5 introduces the Gaussian density function and shows how we can use it to assign a probability to the possible outcomes of an experiment and to simulate its results, by using Monte Carlo methods. Chapters 6 and 7 focus on the most essential inferential tools, i.e., confidence intervals and P-values. Chapter 8 presents several techniques to ensure that the fitted model provides an accurate description of the experimental data and that the basic assumptions for inferences and hypothesis testing are met. Chapter 9 illustrates how linear and nonlinear combinations of model parameters permit to address the most relevant research questions.

Finally, Chaps. 10–12 present and discuss several case studies based on real datasets collected in field experiments. With these case studies, additional classes of linear and nonlinear models are introduced, and their potential usefulness in agricultural research is highlighted.

Who Should Read This Book

This book is designed for a 6 ECTS introductory course in biometry (approximately 54 hours of teaching), and it is suitable for master's or PhD students in agriculture and biology. It will also be helpful as a self-study text for practitioners, experimenters, or researchers who wish to obtain introductory information about biometry and R before starting a job related to field research in agriculture. Intended for beginners, this book assumes no prior knowledge of statistics or programming.

Statistical Software

Statistical software is fundamental for data analysis, providing a set of modern tools and efficient algorithms that are necessary for all users. In this book, we will use the

R statistical software within the RStudio environment. The reasons for this choice are multiple: it is one of the most commonly used languages for data analysis and statistical computing, it is freeware (which is not irrelevant for students), and it is also fun to work with. Beginners or those who need a refresher will find an introductory appendix at the end of this book. Before studying this book, readers will need to install the packages listed in Appendix A.13.

Supporting Material

This book is associated with an R package (`statforbiology`) and a website (follow the link to www.statforbiology.com), which are free to use and licensed under the Creative Commons Attribution-NonCommercial-NoDerivs 3.0 License. The website features several additional case studies, with new ones being added continuously. Corrections and updates are incorporated regularly, as R is a rapidly evolving language. I can be contacted by email at `andrea.onofri@unipg.it` and would greatly appreciate receiving comments and being informed of errors. I will post the updates and corrections on the accompanying website.

Perugia, Italy
June, 2025

Andrea Onofri

Acknowledgement I want to mention my colleague and friend Dario Sacco (University of Torino, Italy). We started working together on this book project, and he was very eager to contribute to the first two chapters in an earlier Italian version. Unfortunately, he had no luck and suddenly died far too early. This book is heavily based on the lengthy discussions we had during the statistics courses of the Italian Society of Agronomy, and the final result would have been much better if it had benefited from the continuing support and contributions from Dario.

I also want to thank my Colleagues at the Department of Agricultural, Food, and Environmental Sciences (University of Perugia, Italy): it has been a long road together, and I am happy we walked it together. In particular, I would like to thank Dino Alberati, Egidio Ciriciofolo, Gino Covarelli, Marcello Guiducci, Euro Pannacci, and Francesco Tei, from whom I have learned most of the subtleties of the research work.

This book owes much to the countless questions, confusions, and concerns shared by my students. In striving to support their learning journey, I found the motivation to write more clearly, think more deeply, and explain more simply.

I am also grateful to several people who have read this book or parts of it and, with their comments, have contributed to better clarity. In particular, I would like to thank Marcin Kozak (College of Media and Social Communication, University of Information Technology and Management in Rzeszow, Poland), Alessia Perego (Department of Agricultural and Environmental Sciences, University of Milan, Italy), Hans-Peter Piepho (Institute of Crop Science, Biostatistics Unit, University of Hohenheim, Germany), Christian Ritz (National Institute of Public Health, University of Southern Denmark, Copenhagen, Denmark), and Annamaria Stellacci (Department of Soil, Plant and Food Sciences, University of Bari, Italy) for their helpful comments. Of course, any remaining mistakes are solely my responsibility.

Last but not least, I am deeply indebted to the R Core development team for the availability of the R language and environment, as well as for their efforts to maintain and preserve its freeware nature. I also want to mention that this book and its associated website are written in `RMarkdown`, using the `bookdown` and `blogdown` packages, which are three valuable additions to the R project, for which I am very much indebted.

Contents

Acronyms

ANOVA	Analysis of Variance
CI	Confidence Interval
CRD	Completely Randomized Design
DF	Degrees of Freedom
EDA	Exploratory Data Analyses
LM	Linear Model
LMM	Linear Mixed Model
RCBD	Randomized Complete Block Design
SD	Standard Deviation
SE	Standard Error
SEM	Standard Error of a Mean
SED	Standard Error of a Difference
SS	Sum of Squares

In this book, we will also use the term "dataframe" to refer to the R "data.frame" object, i.e., a tabular data structure with rows and columns.

Chapter 1
Science, Data, and Experiments

A witty saying proves nothing
—Voltaire

Abstract Scientific experiments play a crucial role in acquiring reliable knowledge about the natural world and its phenomena. Still, they must be appropriately designed so that the resulting data are precise and accurate. This chapter focuses on the main components of an experiment (e.g., the hypothesis, treatments, their allocation to experimental units, and variables). It presents the three fundamental techniques to obtain valid data: control, true replication, and randomization. Reasons to support the adoption of these three techniques are discussed, and several examples of valid and invalid experiments are provided, enabling readers to build a solid foundation for scientifically sound research in agriculture.

In the age of "information overload," we have plenty of knowledge at our fingertips; we can "google" for a topic or ask ChatGPT, and plenty of information fills our computer screen. However, an important question remains unanswered: which information is reliable? We know from experience that the web is full of personal views, opinions, and beliefs or, even worse, fake news; we have nothing against opinions (although we would rather avoid fake news), but we need to be able to distinguish between subjective opinions and objective facts. We can refer to the body of reliable and objective knowledge by using the term "science," in contrast to "nonscience" or "pseudoscience"; the question is "how can we draw the line between science and pseudoscience?"

A theory, in itself, is not necessarily science. It may be well substantiated, and it can incorporate good laws and/or equations; it may come from either a brilliant intuition or meticulous research work; it may come from an ordinary man or a very authoritative scientist; it does not matter: Theories do not necessarily represent objective facts, and they need to be proved.

The method by which we proceed to establish scientific facts is usually attributed to Galileo Galilei (1564–1642); it can be summarized as a sequence of steps, as shown in Fig. 1.1, where we identify three key elements:

A. Onofri, *Field Research Methods in Agriculture*,
https://doi.org/10.1007/978-3-032-08199-5_1

1. The data that need to be produced in support of preexisting theories (hypotheses)
2. The experiment to produce reliable data
3. The iterative nature, where a supported hypothesis holds its validity until new data disprove it and/or support an alternative hypothesis

1.1 Data, Errors, and Truth

"In God we trust, all the others bring data." This famous aphorism is commonly attributed to W. Edwards Deming (although such attribution does not appear to have strong support; see Hastie et al. 2009), and it serves as a good starting point for understanding what science is. As seen in Fig. 1.1, science cannot exist without data; however, we must also recognize that not all data are good enough to reliably support the acceptance or rejection of a scientific hypothesis.

Indeed, data may be bad because they may not represent the truth; that is, they may indicate that a plant is 1.85 m tall when, in fact, it is not or they may suggest that a seed is dormant when, in fact, it is dead. Bad data can be produced because the techniques for measuring, counting, or recording phenomena are not suitable for their intended purposes. This problem is relatively common in the social sciences, where it has a tremendous impact on political or economic decisions (Sturge 2022). In agriculture and biology, phenomena are most often (but not always) objectively measured by using rigorous and well-defined methods; however, researchers must deal with the so-called **experimental error**, which is an intrinsic and unavoidable component of every field experiment. This final word "error" should not mislead us: It does not necessarily mean that someone is doing something wrong; on the contrary, despite the application of a rigorous and correct research protocol, the results may contain several intrinsic sources of uncertainty, such as:

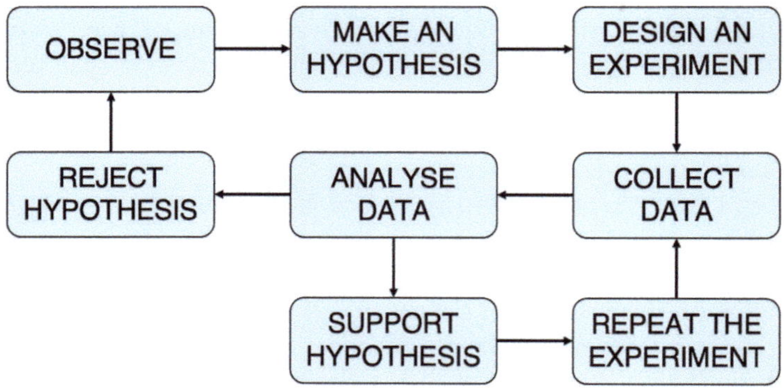

Fig. 1.1 The steps of the scientific method

1. Measurement errors
2. Sampling errors

Measurement errors can be due to (i) uncalibrated instruments, (ii) incorrect measurement/classification protocols, (iii) failures of the measuring devices, (iv) scoring/reading/writing errors and other inaccuracies relating to the experimenter's work, and (v) irregularities in the object being measured (e.g., the diameter of a melon is not simple to record, because that fruit is not exactly spherical).

Apart from measurement errors at the individual "object" level, there are other, less obvious, sources of uncertainty relating to the fact that, most often, we do not study a single object (e.g., a plant), but we study a group of objects (e.g., a crop), and, thus, we need to make multiple measurements. Even if we managed to avoid all errors for every single measurement (which is nearly impossible), we should nonetheless cope with a certain degree of subject-to-subject variability and consequently use a statistic, such as the mean, to summarize the results. Whenever the group under study is too numerous to measure all individuals, we are obliged to consider a small representative sample, and we can never be sure that such a sample fully matches the corresponding characteristics of the whole population (e.g., the mean of the sample does not coincide with the mean of the population under study). What would have happened if we had selected another sample? Sampling errors are unavoidable, and they represent an intrinsic component of most research data in agriculture and biology.

The experimental errors impact the quality of data and, particularly, in terms of **precision** and **accuracy** (Fig. 1.2). Data are precise when they exhibit slight variation across repeated measurements. At the same time, they are accurate when they are close to the "true" value. From these definitions, it follows that precision

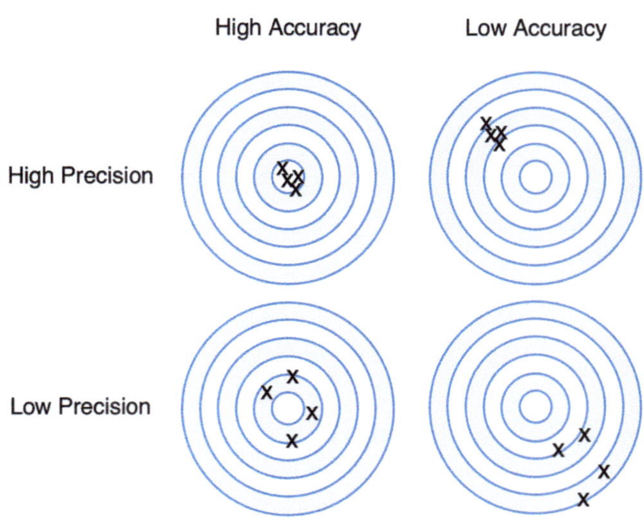

Fig. 1.2 Differences between accuracy and precision

is important, but accuracy is fundamental: Inaccurate data (*biased* data) can lead to erroneous conclusions.

To understand the extent to which experimental errors may impact precision and accuracy, it is helpful to distinguish between systematic and random errors. **Systematic errors** tend to occur repeatedly with similar extents and signs; the typical example is an uncalibrated scale that always adds 20 g to the real weight: It does not matter how many times we repeat the measurement; our result will be an overestimation of the real weight, and, thus, it will be inaccurate. Apart from uncalibrated instruments, other typical sources of systematic errors include incorrect measurement protocols, improper sampling methods, or, in general, any external elements that act repeatedly and consistently on every measurement process.

Conversely, **random errors** relate to unknown, unpredictable, and episodic events and tend to occur with random extents and random signs. These errors are dangerous because they produce highly variable data (low precision). However, their random nature produces underestimations or overestimations with equal probability, so performing multiple measurements should help preserve accuracy.

Scientific progress requires that the most rigorous and reliable methods be employed to remove any reasonable doubts about the quality of research data. However, some types of errors (e.g., sampling errors) can never be totally avoided and can even occur without being noticed, so it is never possible to be sure that research data correspond to the absolute truth unless we set an iterative process of reevaluation and confirmatory research, by which good theories can find their way to success, while wrong theories are, more or less quickly, abandoned.

1.2 The Design of Experiments

Data are typically collected through a scientific experiment (Fig. 1.1), in which we observe the responses of various "subjects" (e.g., plants, plots, fields) to a set of experimental stimuli. The elements that concur to define whether an experiment is good or bad are:

1. The hypothesis
2. The experimental treatments
3. The experimental units
4. The allocation of treatments to units
5. The response variable(s)

1.2.1 Hypothesis and Objectives

A well-defined hypothesis is a fundamental component of good experiments; indeed, we need to ask the right question if we want to obtain a sensible answer.

The hypothesis is a predictive statement about the outcome of a biological system, and it is usually based on literature information or previous research. A well-defined hypothesis naturally leads to the definition of the experimenter's objectives and, ultimately, to the definition of materials and methods. Expectedly, unclear objectives may lead to inefficient research, wherein unnecessary data are collected while other essential data are neglected.

The prevailing approach to setting a hypothesis has often been based on the **falsification principle**, as defined by Karl Popper (1902–1994); he argued that it is not possible to demonstrate that a theory is true because we can never exclude the possibility that future observations might falsify it. A famous example is that it is not possible to demonstrate that "all swans are white" because we would need to observe all swans, which is impossible. On the contrary, it is possible to demonstrate that the previous statement is false by simply observing one "non-white" swan.

Even before Popper, Ronald Fisher had emphasized that we can never prove a theory, but we can only falsify it; he suggested that, instead of testing the actual hypothesis we are interested in, we should test its "negation" ("null hypothesis"). For example, suppose we are interested in demonstrating that genotypes A and B give different yields. In that case, we should start with the hypothesis that the yields of A and B are not different from each other and organize an experiment to falsify it. Fisher provided a heuristic rule to decide when the null can be rejected and a statistic to measure the strength of the evidence against the null (see Chap. 7); a few years later, Jerzy Neyman (1894–1981) and Egon Pearson (1895–1980) proposed the adoption of an alternative hypothesis, which must be true if the null is false. In our example, the alternative hypothesis would be that the yields of A and B are not the same. If the null hypothesis is rejected, such an alternative is held as true until some other experiment falsifies it.

Although some of the above concepts have been vigorously debated (see, e.g., Quinn and Keough 2002), the idea that the role of experiments is to reject hypotheses is fundamental for traditional hypothesis testing.

1.2.2 The Experimental Treatments

Once the hypotheses and objectives have been established, the definition of the experimental protocol is a logical consequence. In particular, based on the hypotheses, we usually select the **experimental treatments** or **experimental factors**, i.e., a set of related "stimuli" for which responses need to be assessed; for example, if we intend to compare genotypes A, B, and C, we will make an experiment that includes the genotype factor with three levels. If we have an experiment with only one factor with a unique level, we usually refer to it as a *mensurative experiment*. Otherwise, we refer to it as a *comparative experiment*, which is the most common situation in field research.

When we have two (or more) experimental factors, we can conduct either separate experiments or a **(multi)factorial experiment**, wherein we combine the levels of the two (or more) factors. This second solution is more interesting, as it allows us to assess possible interaction effects between the factors (see Chap. 4).

Factorial experiments can be planned in two different ways: They can be **crossed** or **nested**. In a crossed design, we have all possible combinations between the levels of all factors; for example, if we want to compare three sunflower genotypes (A, B, and C) at two different nitrogen rates (N1 and N2), a crossed factorial experiment should include all the six combinations A-N1, A-N2, B-N1, B-N2, C-N1, and C-N2. Otherwise, in a nested design, the levels of one factor are different, depending on the level of the other factor; for example, if we want to assess which species, between maize and grain-sorghum, is more suitable for organic farming, we might like to include several genotypes so that our final judgment is not specific to the genotype that was included in the experiment. The selected genotypes will differ for each species, and the experiment will employ a nested factorial design.

Very often, comparative experiments need a suitable *check* level, which is used as the reference against which all other treatments are evaluated.[1] We can include either:

1. An untreated check or
2. A check treated with a placebo or
3. A check treated with ordinary practices

For example, in a genotype experiment, we typically include a reference genotype that is very widely grown on all nearby farms. For herbicide experiments, we always include an untreated check, which is used to assess the composition of weed flora and quantify the weed control efficacy of all herbicides under investigation. Furthermore, we can also include a weed-free check (usually hand-weeded) as the reference to evaluate possible symptoms of herbicide phytotoxicity to the crop. In toxicology, the untreated check may be replaced by a check treated with a placebo, i.e., a compound containing the same components as the experimental treatment except for the active ingredient. The placebo is usually necessary when:

1. The experimental subject (usually a human) perceives its condition and reacts to the expectation about the efficacy of the chemical under investigation.
2. The commercial formulation, apart from the active ingredient, contains other components, such as adjuvants, surfactants, and other substances, which may exhibit some biological effects.

1.2.3 The Experimental Units

The experimental unit is the physical entity to which the treatment is allocated, such as a field, a small piece of land (referred to as a *plot*), a plant, an animal, or a pot.

[1] The "check" is often named "control," but we will not use this term here to avoid possible confusion with the "control of errors," as discussed in the next section, 1.3.1.

It is helpful to distinguish between the **experimental unit** which is subjected to the allocation of the experimental treatments (also referred to as the **randomization unit**) and the **observational unit**, which is subjected to measurements or observations. In some cases, these two types of units coincide, such as, when we allocate the treatment to a field plot and measure the yield of the entire plot. In other cases, randomization and observational units are physically different, such as when we allocate the treatment to one plot and measure several plants within that plot. Later in this book, we will see that a clear distinction between experimental units and observational units is a prerequisite for a valid data analysis process.

The experimental units are typically selected from a broader population of interest. For example, we choose plots from a field, plants from a crop, or animals from a herd. A sample should be representative and homogeneous, although these may be two contrasting characteristics. Indeed, if we select very homogeneous individuals, we run the risk of obtaining a sample that no longer represents the entire population but only a subset of it. For example, if our sample consisted of adult male bovines in good health, it may not necessarily represent a population that also included females, young animals, and those with diseases. Sampling a population of interest properly may be a daunting task, especially in the social sciences. Several sampling protocols have been defined (e.g., random sampling, systematic sampling, stratified sampling, clustered sampling, convenience sampling, quota sampling, and others), which are far beyond the scope of this book (see Daniel 2011).

In some cases, the process of sampling is less obvious, but that does not mean that there is no sampling. For example, in manipulative laboratory experiments, the experimental units are specifically prepared for each assay, such as the pots for an herbicide assay or the Petri dishes for a germination assay. Even if there is no real selection process, these units should be regarded as sampled from the broader population of pots or Petri dishes that we could have prepared.

1.2.4 The Allocation of Treatments

The allocation of treatments to experimental units is typically performed through a manipulation process, such as sowing different genotypes, spraying various herbicides, or using different sowing densities in different plots (**manipulative experiments**). It may, sometimes, be appropriate to conceal specific details of the allocation process; for example, in medical research, subjects might be better left unaware of which treatment they have received (**single-blind experiments**) to avoid possible unconscious effects. In agriculture, when performing visual and sensory assessments, it is usually required that the researcher is unaware about which treatment was allocated to each unit to maintain the objectivity of such evaluations. Experiments in which neither the subjects nor the researcher are aware of the treatments are called **double-blind experiments**.

There may be cases where it is either impossible, inconvenient, unethical, or even illegal to manipulate the subjects to allocate the treatments; in these cases, the experiment will have to consist of observing units that are "naturally" treated (observational study, see, e.g., Mann 2003). For example, if we want to assess the efficacy of seatbelts, it would be illegal to design an experiment where people are sent out with or without fastened seatbelts; what we can do, in this case, is only to record retrospectively the outcome of previous accidents. This book focuses on small plot experiments, which are typically manipulative. However, it is worth noting that observational studies are also important in several disciplines, such as the social sciences and medicine, although they are often assumed to yield a lower level of evidence compared to well-conducted manipulative experiments (Burns et al. 2011).

1.2.5 The Variables

The final product of an experiment is a set of data (dataset) composed of a collection of variables describing the experimental units about their traits (one variable per trait). We usually distinguish (i) response variables, (ii) predictor variables, and (iii) accessory variables.

The response variables describe the response of units to the experimental treatments (e.g., yield, weight, height, etc.). In contrast, the predictor variables describe the experimental stimulus allocated to each unit (e.g., tillage method, fertilization rate, genotype, etc.). In some cases, we also record other accessory variables (or covariates), which measure potential confounding effects. For example, suppose we intend to study the yield of some trees, depending on how they were fertilized. In that case, the effect of tree age can act as a confounder; therefore, we can record the age as an accessory variable to be used during data analysis as a covariate.

All variables (response, predictor, and accessory variables) can be classified as:

1. Nominal
2. Ordinal
3. Count/ratio or
4. Continuous

Nominal variables are produced by assigning the subjects to one of a set of categories, such as dead/alive, germinated/ungerminated, red/blue/green, and so on. The categories can be two: (*binomial variable*) or more (*multinomial variable*); they should not have any intrinsic ordering and should be mutually exclusive in the sense that one individual can only belong to one of those categories.

Ordinal variables are similar to nominal variables, but the categories are intrinsically ordered. For example, we could ask a farmer to express his appreciation for a specific agronomic practice by using five categories in increasing order of appreciation such as VERY LOW, LOW, AVERAGE, HIGH, and VERY HIGH.

Nominal and ordinal variables are often referred to (e.g., in the R software) as "factors" and "ordered factors," respectively. Even though specific methods of analysis for these variables exist (see Agresti 2002), very often they are expressed in grouped form, by counting the number of individuals in each class and, possibly, transforming these counts into proportions or percentages. For example, disease incidence data are obtained by classifying several plants per plot as either diseased or healthy and then grouping this data into counts of diseased plants per plot or, more frequently, into the percentage or proportion of diseased plants per plot.

The process of grouping nominal or ordinal data produces **count or ratio variables** that consist of discrete data in the sense that they can only take specific values (i.e., there is some "space" between two consecutive values). Count variables can also be produced whenever the observational units are characterized by some countable property, such as the number of weeds per unit surface, or the number of lateral tillers in wheat plants, or the number of fruits on a tree.

Continuous variables, such as weight, height, yield, and time, can take any values within an interval as long as the resolution of the measuring instrument is sufficiently high for practical purposes. These variables also include some kinds of ratio and percentage data, such as concentrations expressed as percentages or humidity contents in soil.

In some instances, the experimental variables cannot be easily classified into one of the above groups, as is often the case with data from sensory assessments. A typical example in weed science is when weed control ability and selectivity of herbicides is visually scored on a scale, e.g., from 0 to 100%. The resulting variable may seem ordinal (we assign one of a set of ordered categories), although the underlying scale is more or less continuous. Apart from weed science and, in general, plant protection, sensory assessments are relatively common in several disciplines, because they are low cost and high speed, although the operators require specific training and experience.

1.3 Valid/Invalid Experiments

Now that we have defined the main components of an experiment, we can identify the distinguishing characteristics of a valid experiment. In this respect, a fundamental contribution was made by the English scientist Ronald A. Fisher (1890–1962) in his famous book "The Design of Experiments" (Fisher 1937). In that book, he mentioned three fundamental characteristics that are: (i) control, (ii) replication, and (iii) randomization.

1.3.1 Control

The term "control" is very often mentioned in Fisher's book, and the most convincing definition is given at the beginning of Chap. 6: "*'Control' consists of establishing controlled conditions in which all factors except one can be held constant*." We can slightly widen this definition by saying that there should be no difference between the experimental units apart from those factors that are under investigation (the so-called *ceteris paribus* assumption).

As an example, let us imagine that we have found an innovative fertilizer and we want to compare it with a traditional one: A well-controlled experiment would consist of using both treated and untreated plots that are next to each other, with the same environmental conditions, same soil, same genotype, and same everything else, apart from the fertilizer, which will be different. In these conditions, any observed differences in response between the two plots shall be reasonably attributed to the fertilizer.

Apart from isolating the effect under study, a good control is also exerted by using the most excellent care to minimize the impact of all potential sources of experimental error. This may seem obvious, but putting it into practice may be overwhelming. Indeed, different types of experiments will require different techniques, and the best way to master those techniques is "learning by doing," preferably under the supervision of an expert technician. I will only underline three general aspects:

1. Methodological rigor
2. Accurate selection of experimental units
3. Avoiding intrusions

Methodological rigor refers to the soundness and precision of a study, encompassing planning, data collection, analysis, and reporting. It is evident that, e.g., if we intend to study the degradation of a herbicide at 20 °C, we need an oven that can keep that temperature constant, the herbicide needs to be thoroughly mixed with the soil at the exact concentration, and we need to use a well-calibrated instrument and a correct protocol of chemical analyses.

The accurate selection of homogeneous experimental units is also fundamental to minimize errors and maximize precision, although we should not forget that the sampled individuals should be representative of the whole population about which conclusions are sought. For instance, if we want to assess the effect of a particular diet, we could select cows of the same age, weight, and sex so that the diet effect is isolated from all other possible confounding effects. If we do so, we will likely obtain very high precision, but our results will not permit sound generalizations to the entire population of cows, which also contains individuals of different ages, weights, and sexes.

Last but not least, it is necessary to mention the so-called intrusions, i.e., all external events that occur and negatively impact on the experiment (e.g., drought, fungal attacks, and aphid infestations). Sometimes, these events are simply unpredictable, and we will see that replication and randomization (the other two principles of experimental design) are primarily intended to avoid that such intrusions produce systematic errors in our results. At other times, these events are not totally unpredictable, and they must be anticipated and mitigated by taking appropriate action (so-called demonic intrusions; see Hurlbert 1984).

1.3.2 Replication

In the previous paragraph, we have laid the basis of a comparative experiment, wherein the experimental units must be placed in the same conditions, except for the allocation of a different experimental treatment. Of course, *no one would now dream of testing the response to a treatment by comparing two plots, one treated and the other one untreated* (Fisher and Wishart, 1930; cited in Hurlbert 1984).

In every valid experiment, we need to replicate each treatment in more than one experimental unit for the following principal reasons:

1. To demonstrate that the effect is replicable in the same conditions
2. To calculate the mean of replications, that is, a reliable estimate of the real value under measurement in the absence of systematic errors
3. To assess the precision of the experiment by measuring the variability among replicates

The key issue regarding replication is that to be valid, replicates must be truly independent; that is, they must have independently received the whole manipulation process to allocate the treatment. True replicates must be clearly distinguished from pseudo-replicates, which have received, altogether, at least part of such manipulation process (Fig. 1.3).

Some typical examples of pseudo-replication are:

1. Spraying a pot with five plants and measuring separately the weight of each plant
2. Treating one soil sample with a herbicide and making four measurements of concentration on four subsamples of the same soil

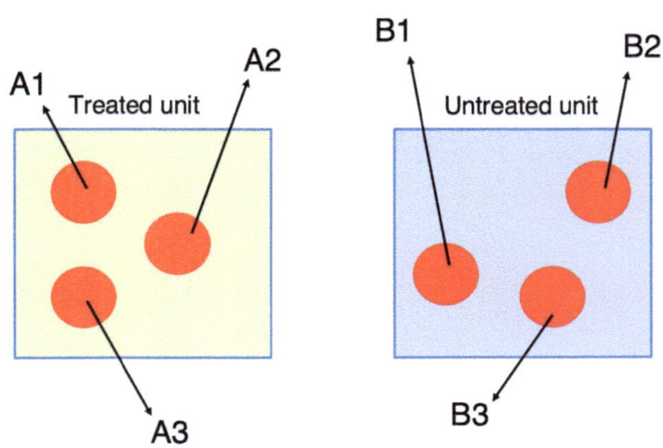

Fig. 1.3 Schematic example of an invalid experiment where pseudo-replication is committed. The two squares represent two plots to which two treatments were allocated. Three subsamples were harvested in each plot, but these subsamples do not represent true replicates because they were not independently treated

3. Collecting one soil sample from a field plot and repeating four times the same chemical analysis

In all the above cases, each treatment is applied only to one unit (pot or soil sample), and there are no true replicates, regardless of how often the unit is subsampled. If a random error is committed during the manipulation process, it propagates to all pseudo-replicates and becomes a very serious systematic error.

Apart from some specific circumstances, the general rule is that valid experiments require true replicates, while pseudo-replicates can only be used in addition to true replicates. For example, it is correct to independently spray four pots with five plants (the randomization units) and separately measure the weights of those plants (the observational units), obtaining an experiment with four true replicates and five sub-replicates per replicate. In this case, however, true replicates and pseudo-replicates carry different information and should never be confounded in the data analysis stage. In other words, we should never regard such an experiment as if it had 20 true replicates (Morrison and Morris 2000). You will learn by experience that there might be exceptions to these rules, but, at this moment, it is better to sound rather prescriptive: The lack of true replication usually leads to the rejection of manuscripts submitted to scientific Journals.

1.3.3 Randomization

Control and true replication, in themselves, do not guarantee that the experiment is valid. Indeed, some innate characteristics of experimental units or external intrusions might systematically influence all replicates of a single treatment so that the effect of such intrusions is confounded with the effect of the experimental treatment (we usually refer to this as **confounding**). For example, think that we have a field with eight plots along a positive gradient of fertility, as shown in Fig. 1.4; if we treat the plots from 1 to 4 with fertilizer A and the plots from 5 to 8 with fertilizer B, the innate difference between the plots might be confounded with the treatment effect.

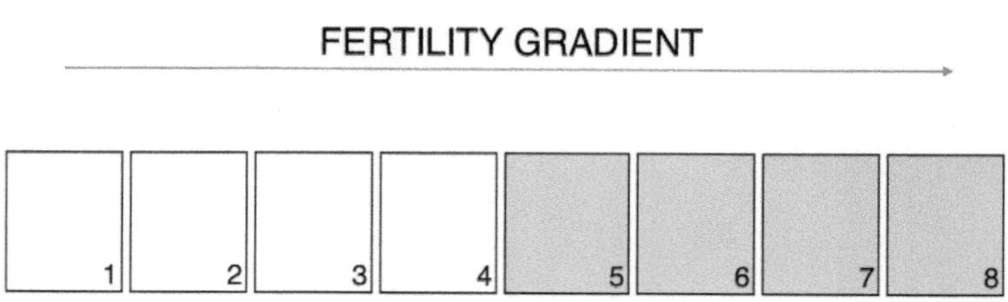

Fig. 1.4 Example of lack of randomization: The two colors identify two different experimental treatments. In such a situation, there is a high risk of confounding the innate difference in fertility with the effect of the experimental treatment

Randomization is typically performed in manipulative experiments by randomly allocating treatments to experimental units. In the case of field experiments, randomization can also relate to random spatial and temporal dispersion (the interspersion of the experimental treatments), as discussed in the next chapter. With observational experiments, where treatments are not allocated by a manipulation process, randomization is achieved through the random selection of individuals.

As the result of using proper randomization, all experimental units are equally likely to receive any possible disturbance/intrusion so that the probability of systematic errors and confounding effects are minimized.[2]

1.3.4 Confirmatory Experiments

Even if we are completely sure that an experiment is perfectly valid, we can never exclude the possibility that some unforeseen systematic error has slipped through and distorted the observed results. For this reason, confirmatory experiments are usually regarded as strictly necessary in all types of research.

In field research, confirmatory experiments usually take place in different environmental conditions (different seasons or sites), and, consequently, the fact that they do not fully confirm the original results is not necessarily seen as the negation of their validity, but it is seen as the evidence that the original results might only be valid in some specific circumstances, motivating the search for a more general theory.

Confirmatory experiments give the learning process a fundamentally iterative nature, where previous hypotheses may be falsified and, consequently, abandoned in favor of new hypotheses. Along this path, it is necessary to decide what we should do when two hypotheses prove to be equally good; in this case, we can apply the so-called **Occam's razor**, which is a principle of parsimony devised by the English friar and philosopher William of Occam (1287–1347). It is usually introduced with the Latin aphorism: "*Entia non sunt multiplicanda praeter necessitatem*" (entities must not be multiplied beyond necessity), and it may be interpreted as follows: If an experiment supports the idea that two competing hypotheses are equally good, we need to select the simplest one. The application of this principle is handy, as it encourages us to focus on the essential aspects of a biological problem that are fully supported by the data, thereby eliminating all unnecessary complications. We will apply this principle also in this book, for example, to select one from a list of competing models (see Chap. 11).

---

[2] Confounding may result from a disturbance that affects all replicates of the same experimental treatment, which is made highly unlikely by the randomization process.

1.3.5 Invalid Experiments

In my experience as a reviewer/editor of scientific journals, the most frequent problems with submitted manuscripts are:

1. There are pseudo-replicates, but no true replicates.
2. True replicates and pseudo-replicates are mistaken.
3. There is no randomization.
4. Randomization was constrained, but the constraint has not been accounted for in statistical analyses (see the next chapter).

Experiments that lack either proper control or replication or randomization are regarded as invalid, and, in principle, they are not capable of producing good data. Among the three possible violations, lack of good control is less concerning because it often results in imprecise data and decreased power. Hence, the experiment ends up being inconclusive and eliminates itself. On the contrary, lack of replication and careless randomization can be very dangerous because the effect of systematic errors can be wrongly interpreted as the effects of experimental treatments (Fig. 1.4). Other deviations may be less critical (mistaking true- and pseudo-replicates or failing to account for constraints to complete randomization), and they can be solved by appropriately reanalyzing the results.

1.4 Questions and Exercises

1. What are the fundamental traits of a valid experiment? List and discuss briefly.
2. What was Galileo's research method? Describe briefly.
3. Discuss the differences between random and systematic errors. Which is more concerning for an experimenter? Give examples.
4. What is the main difference between true replicates and pseudo-replicates? Give examples.
5. What do we intend with the term "confounding"? What is the result of confounding in a scientific experiment? Give examples.
6. What is the difference between precision and accuracy? Give examples.
7. What do we intend with the term "replication"? Describe and discuss. How many replicates do we usually use in research?
8. What do we intend with the term "randomization"? Describe and discuss.
9. What do we intend with the term "control," i.e., one of the fundamental traits of valid experiments? Discuss the main measures to exert good control in designed experiments.
10. What is a "check," and why might we like to add it among the other treatment levels?
11. What are the differences between mensurative, observational and manipulative experiments? Give examples.

12. What main types of variables can we encounter in research studies? List and describe briefly; give examples.
13. What is the difference between crossed and nested factorial experiments? Give examples.

References

Agresti A (2002) Categorical Data Analysis. Wiley Series in Probability and Statistics, 2nd edn. Wiley-Interscience, New York

Burns PB, Rohrich RJ, Chung KC (2011) The levels of evidence and their role in evidence-based medicine. Plastic Reconstr Surgery 128(1):305–310. https://doi.org/10.1097/PRS.0b013e318219c171. http://journals.lww.com/00006534-201107000-00046

Daniel J (2011) Sampling Essentials: Practical Guidelines for Making Sampling Choices. SAGE, Thousand Oaks

Fisher R (1937) The Design of Experiments, 2nd edn. Oliver and Boyd, Edinburgh

Hastie T, Tibshirani R, Friedman J (2009) The Elements of Statistical Learning. Springer Series in Statistics. Springer Science + Business Media, New York

Hurlbert SH (1984) Pseudoreplication and the design of ecological experiments. Ecol Monogr 54(2):187–211

Mann CJ (2003) Observational research methods. Research design II: cohort, cross sectional, and case-control studies. Emerg Med J 20(1):54–60. https://doi.org/10.1136/emj.20.1.54. https://emj.bmj.com/lookup/doi/10.1136/emj.20.1.54

Morrison DA, Morris EC (2000) Pseudoreplication in experimental designs for the manipulation of seed germination treatments. Austral Ecol 25:292–296

Quinn GP, Keough MJ (2002) Experimental Design and Data Analysis for Biologists. Cambridge University Press, Cambridge

Sturge G (2022) Bad Data: How Governments, Politicians and the Rest of Us Get Misled by Numbers. Bridge Street Press, London. https://books.google.it/books?id=BxDQzgEACAAJ

Chapter 2
The Design of Field Experiments

Nature will best respond to a logical and carefully thought out questionnaire

—Ronald Fisher

Abstract Experimental design deals with the methods for planning and conducting valid experiments. Designing field experiments requires a set of correct decisions, such as the selection of treatments, the number of replicates, the size and shape of plots, and the techniques for allocating treatments to experimental units, among others. Although there cannot be a unique and consistent protocol across all disciplines in agriculture, some general hints are given in this chapter. In particular, the main layouts for the allocation of the experimental treatments (e.g., completely randomized, complete blocks, Latin square, split-plot, and strip-plot) are presented, and their advantages and limitations are discussed.

In the previous chapter, we saw that every valid experiment should adhere to three fundamental principles: control, replication, and randomization. You may wonder "how do we put such principles into practice for field experiments in agriculture research?" The body of methods to plan and conduct scientifically sound experiments is named "Experimental Design"; although there is no unique and consistent protocol across all disciplines, it is nonetheless possible to provide some general hints that apply to all field experiments in agriculture. Preliminarily, it is helpful to distinguish between:

1. Small plot research trials
2. Demonstrative on-farm trials

Small plot research trials are set up in the field, but the experimental units are small enough to keep a very high degree of control for most confounding factors and sources of experimental error. Sowing, fertilizing, spraying, harvesting, and other practices are typically performed using specialized or modified machinery that is adapted to work on small surfaces yet reproduces close-to-real management conditions. Due to high level of control, the results of small plot experiments are

A. Onofri, *Field Research Methods in Agriculture*,
https://doi.org/10.1007/978-3-032-08199-5_2

usually very precise and realistic; however, the growing conditions can be highly favorable to the crop resulting in yield levels that are 10–30% higher than those in real farm conditions.

On the other hand, on-farm trials represent the final stage of research, and they are typically conducted to validate or demonstrate the efficacy of new practices and technologies at the farm level, under realistic management conditions, using the equipment and resources that local farmers would typically have available.

2.1 Treatments and Replicates

Let us start from the premise that an accurate literature search and some preliminary work have suggested reasonable research hypotheses and objectives, leading to a clear definition of the experimental treatments to be included in the experiment. For small plot experiments, the number of such treatments often goes from 2 to 20; however, some research projects, such as breeding programs in the early stages, may require the inclusion of a much higher number of treatments (accessions).

The number of true replicates[1] is of paramount importance, and, in the field, it usually ranges from 3 to 5; a lower number is not to be recommended because the experiment becomes very inefficient, and it may be wise to suggest that also three is rather a low number due to the high weight of possible outliers in the calculation of means and other statistical indices. A higher number of replicates might be beneficial in theory, but it is rarely adopted in practice, due to the high time and cost requirements associated with it.

For demonstrative trials, the number of treatments under comparison is low, and most often one new management practice (e.g., crop management, crop protection, plant nutrition, and plant growth regulator) is compared to a local/farmer "check." Such a pair (the new management practice and the check) is a replicate, and usually, we should have a minimum of three (four is better) replicates.

For both small plot trials and demonstrative trials, the required number of experimental units is equal to the product of the number of treatments by the number of replicates.

2.2 Selecting the Field

Once we have an idea of the type of experiment we want to perform and the number of plots, selecting an appropriate field is one of the fundamental keys to success. A field must be:

[1] Please go back to Chap. 1 if this term does not sound familiar to you.

1. Close enough to roads, laboratories, and other facilities, which will permit a timely execution of samplings and measurements
2. As homogeneous as possible in terms of soil type, drainage, slope, previous crop, and other characteristics (see also Chap. 1)
3. Of known and suitable history

The history of the field is of paramount importance because it determines, for example, the level of fertility and the presence or absence of pests, pathogens, and weed species. For example, if we need to perform an N-fertilization experiment, we would rather avoid a field that hosted alfalfa or other legume crops in the previous season due to the possible excess of residual nitrogen content in the soil. Likewise, if we need to perform an herbicide experiment, we would rather avoid a field that hosted another herbicide experiment in the previous season, as the seed shed in the untreated controls and other plots treated with low-efficacy herbicides might have created nonuniform weed infestation levels.

In some cases, it is advisable to take preliminary actions to improve the suitability of a field for certain types of experiments and minimize the environmental variability. For example, it is possible to (i) grow an oat catch crop to remove excess soil nitrogen, (ii) grow alfalfa or other forage crops to suppress weed growth, or (iii) perform deep plowing to reduce the weed seed bank in the uppermost soil layer. Another practice often used in small plot trials to favor the establishment of a homogeneous stand is sowing at overly high densities and then thinning out to the optimal density a few days after crop emergence.

2.3 Plot Size and Shape

In the case of demonstrative experiments, the experimental unit is a big, very long and rectangular, plot in the form of a **strip**, large enough to use the common farming machinery (such as plow, planter, sprayer, and combine harvester) in one or more passes. Sometimes, the plot can also coincide with a single field so that the experiment consists of several fields, one beside the other. For example, Fig. 2.1 illustrates a demonstrative experiment with four fields, each containing two strips, and the two treatments are randomly allocated to the two strips within each field.

In the case of small plot experiments, plots are of rectangular shape, with a width equal to a multiple of the width of the available machinery for sowing and harvesting (Fig. 2.2). The length is selected accordingly so that the surface area is big enough to accommodate a sufficiently high number of plants, such as, at least, 20–40 m^2 for low-density crops (e.g., maize) and 10–20 m^2 for high-density crops (e.g., wheat or alfalfa). Smaller plots may not produce representative results, but unless we plan on-farm experiments, larger plots can also be disadvantageous, as they may not permit a sufficient degree of control. If we have a large field at our disposal, we prefer to increase the number of replicates instead of increasing the size of the plots.

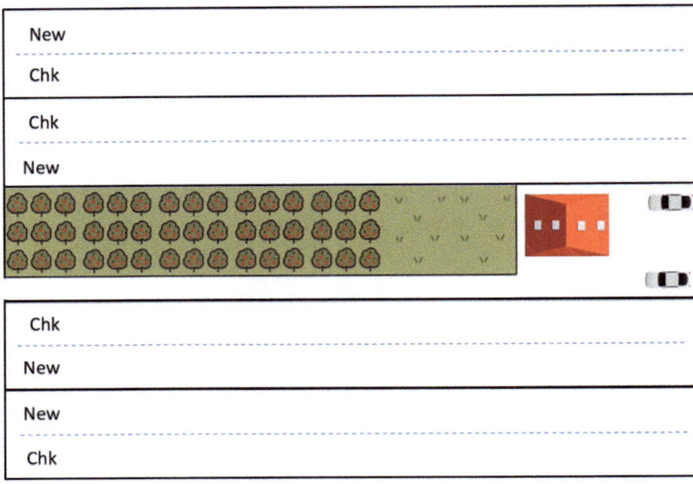

Fig. 2.1 The possible layout of an on-farm trial, with four fields, two strips per field, and a different treatment per strip (New: innovative treatment; Chk: check)

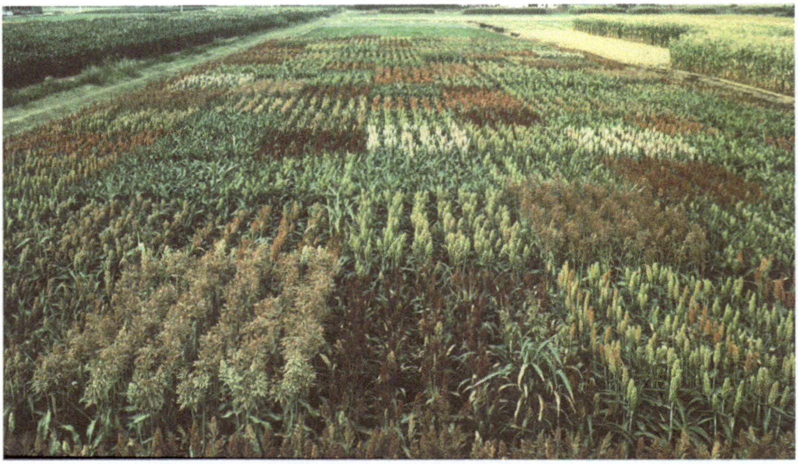

Fig. 2.2 A small plot experiment in the field (Ph. D. Alberati)

When selecting plot shape and size, we should consider the presence of **border effects**, which represent a relevant source of variability. Indeed, plants growing along the plot edges are not in the same conditions as those in the middle of each plot; for example, they might be more vigorous and productive due to the lack of competition on one side. Alternatively, they may be affected by, for example, the carryover effects of fertilizers and herbicides across neighboring plots. Border effects need to be minimized by restricting all measurements to the central rows of each plot, while the plants along the edges are omitted. This way, the surface area for harvest and other measurements (useful plot area) is smaller than the total plot surface area, which should be taken into account while designing the experiment.

The useful plot area may be further restricted in some circumstances, such as when taking destructive measurements of crop or weed weight at a given moment of the crop cycle on a small subplot within each plot. For these cases, the validity of the experiment should be assessed considering the real sampled surface rather than the total plot surface.

2.3.1 *The Field Map*

Once the number and characteristics of the plots have been determined, the next step is to draw the so-called *field map*. An example is reported in Fig. 2.3, relating to an experiment on wheat with eight treatments and four replicates (32 plots, in total); the plots are laid out in a 4×8 grid, and they have a rectangular shape with a length of 8 m and a width of 2 m so that their surface area is equal to 16 m^2. To minimize border effects, 24 additional plots are accommodated along the external perimeter, and they are grown under similar conditions to all other plots inside the experiment. An arrow pointing north or some other reference is added to the map to clarify the orientation of the experiment for researchers and visitors. A univocal numbering/coding system clearly identifies all plots.

2.4 The Experimental Layout

As mentioned earlier, field experiments are manipulative, and we need to decide the criterion to allocate the treatments to the different plots. Depending on such a criterion, we distinguish several types of experimental layouts, which are presented in the following sections.

2.4.1 *Completely Randomized Design (CRD)*

With this design, treatments are allocated to plots in a completely randomized fashion, as shown, for example, in Fig. 2.4, where four replicates of eight treatments (the letters from A to H) were allocated to the 4×8 grid in Fig. 2.3.

Such an approach is straightforward, although it has the disadvantage that every possible systematic source of heterogeneity goes unnoticed. For example, let us imagine that, for some reason, the first three plot columns in Fig. 2.4 (plots 1, 2, 3, 9, 10, 11, 17, 18, 19, 25, 26, and 27) are less fertile than all the other columns or

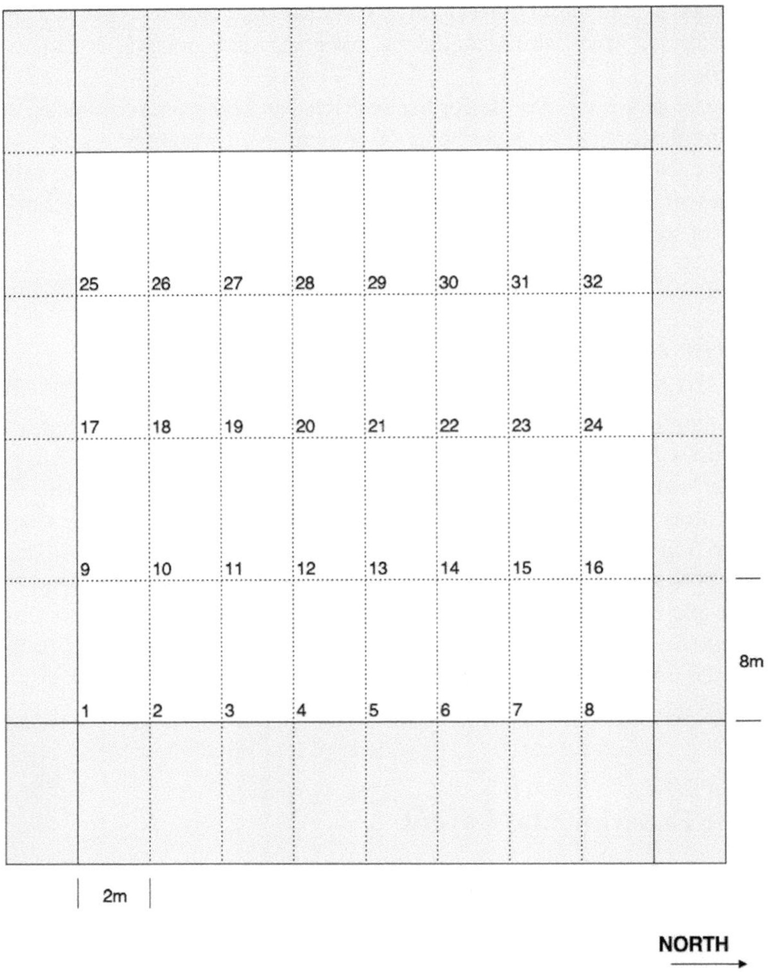

Fig. 2.3 Example of a field map for an experiment with 32 plots. A set of plots is added around the experiment (in gray) to minimize border effects. It is assumed that the crop is sown in rows along a west-east direction, and the width of the plots corresponds to the width of the sowing/harvesting/spraying machinery

they are subjected to some systematic intrusion, such as a pest attack. In this case, treatment G is penalized, because three of the four replicates are located in the least fertile part, while treatment H is favored, because only one replicate is in the least fertile part.

For this reason, CRDs are very common in laboratory or greenhouse experiments or wherever environmental conditions are highly uniform, whereas they are relatively uncommon in field experiments.

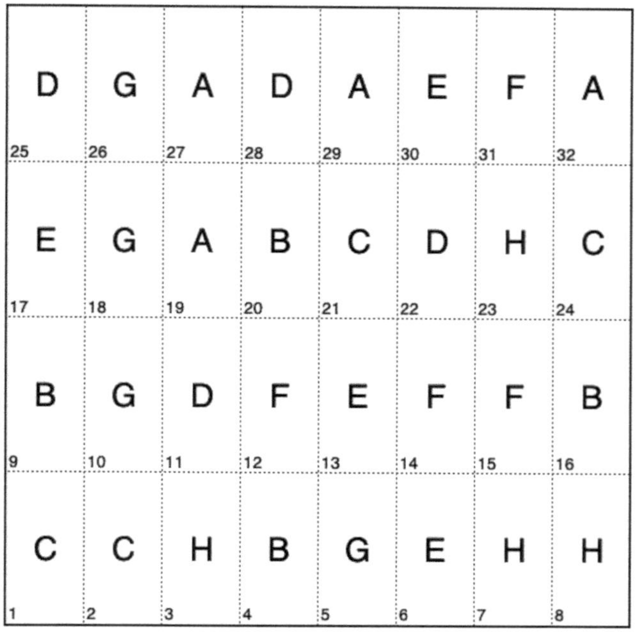

Fig. 2.4 Example of a completely randomized design, for an experiment with eight treatments (the letters from A to H) and four replicates

2.4.2 *Randomized Complete Block Design (RCBD)*

In RCBDs, the experimental units are divided into homogeneous groups with as many subjects as there are treatments to be allocated. For field experiments, plots are grouped according to some possible fertility gradients; for example, should we expect a bottom-to-top fertility gradient for the plots in Fig. 2.3, we could divide the experiment into four blocks with one row each (eight plots per block and block 1 would, e.g., contain plots 1–8). Subsequently, we could randomly allocate the eight treatments to the plots in each block, ensuring one replicate per block, and, thus, no treatment would be penalized or favored (Fig. 2.5).

Blocks are usually accommodated along the main fertility gradient so that the plots in each block occur in the same position of the gradient. For example, if we have a left-to-right fertility gradient and we are to design an experiment in a 4×8 grid, as shown in Fig. 2.3, we could take four vertical blocks with two columns each (block 1 would, e.g., contain plots 1, 2, 9, 10, 17, 18, 25, and 26; Fig. 2.6, left). However, with this layout, the plots within each block would not all be in the same position of the gradient, which would increase the level of variability within each block. An alternative arrangement to accommodate a left-to-right fertility gradient would be to lay out the experiment on an 8×4 grid, with four vertical blocks of one

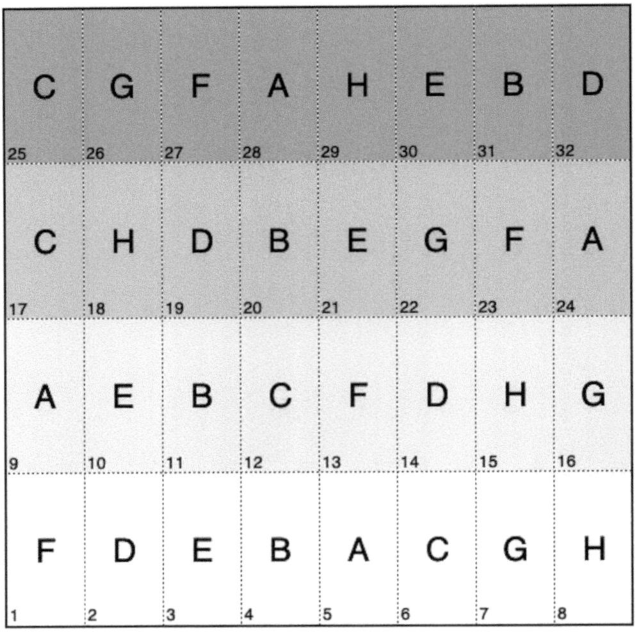

Fig. 2.5 Example of a completely randomized block design with four blocks (in different shades of gray) accounting for a bottom-to-top fertility gradient

column each (Fig. 2.6, right). However, with such an arrangement, the experiment becomes very long (64 m), and the risk of including nonuniform field parts may become higher.

The RCBD is the most common design for field experiments. Still, it can also be used for other types of experiments, where the experimental units can be grouped according to some innate property, such as age, sex, or proximity. It is a very efficient design, and it is preferred over a CRD whenever the units can be clearly distinguished in different groups.

2.4.3 *Latin Square Design*

RCBDs do not account for the existence of two fertility gradients, and in such conditions, it may be possible to use the so-called Latin square design. An example is shown in Fig. 2.7 for an experiment with four treatments and four replicates (16 plots in total); both the rows and the columns serve as blocking variables, and the treatments are allocated so that they can be found in all rows and all columns.

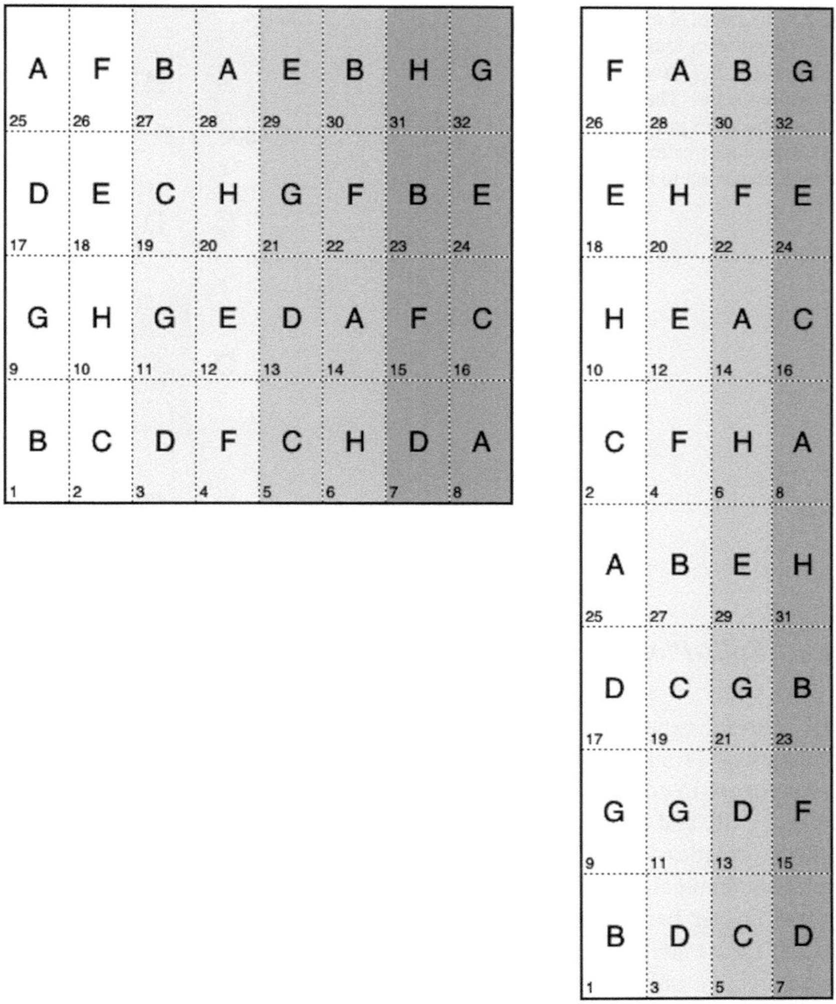

Fig. 2.6 Two possible layouts to accommodate a left-to-right fertility gradient (see the text for more details)

Latin square designs take their name from the fact that the number of replicates is equal to the number of treatments, the number of rows, and the number of columns so that the field map consists of a square grid. They are not only useful for field experiments but can also be applied to all types of experiments whenever we suspect that the experimental units can be grouped according to two innate properties. However, the experiments must be relatively small, with fewer than 4–5 treatment levels, to avoid the number of replicates becoming unacceptably high.

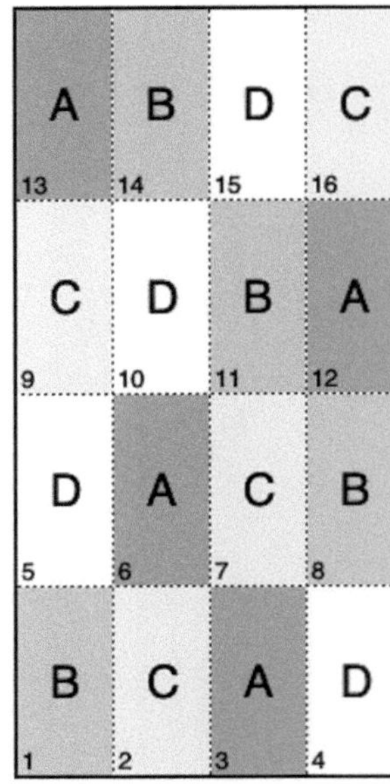

Fig. 2.7 Example of a Latin square design with four treatments (A, B, C, and D) and four replicates. The different shades of gray help identify the four treatments and their allocation to the plots

2.4.4 Split-Plot and Strip-Plot Designs

With factorial experiments, we can use a CRD or an RCBD by allocating the combinations of all factor levels to the different plots. For example, think about an experiment to compare three types of tillage (minimum tillage = MIN, shallow plowing = SP, and deep plowing = DP) and two types of chemical weed control methods (broadcast = TOT and in-furrow = PART). With four replicates, the six treatment combinations (MIN-TOT, SP-TOT, DP-TOT, MIN-PART, SP-PART, and DP-PART) can be allocated to 24 plots, according to an RCBD, as shown in Fig. 2.8. Please note that we need large plots and ample space between them to operate tractors and tillage machinery effectively. On the contrary, the allocation of herbicide treatments could be done on smaller plots.

To reduce the size of the experiment, we could consider using large plots (**main-plots**) to allocate tillage treatments and splitting these main-plots into **subplots**, to allocate weed control treatments (**split-plot** design). The example is illustrated in Fig. 2.9, where the allocation of tillage treatments to the 12 main-plots is done according to a Randomized Complete Block Design (RCBD). In contrast, the two weed control treatments are randomly allocated to the two subplots, within each main-plot. With this arrangement, the size of the experiment is smaller than that shown in Fig. 2.8, which is an advantage in terms of controlling random errors more effectively.

An important consequence of split-plot designs is that every main-plot represents a replicate for all subplot factor levels. Indeed, if we examine Fig. 2.9, we see that there are four replicates for each tillage level, but there are 12 replicated subplots

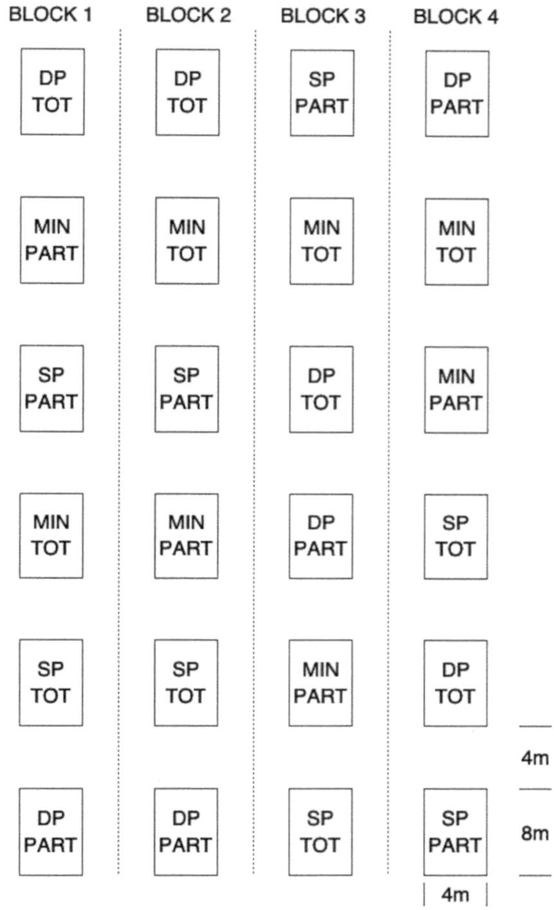

Fig. 2.8 Field map for a factorial experiment with two factors, i.e., tillage with three levels (minimum tillage = MIN, shallow plowing = SP, and deep plowing = DP) and weed control, with two levels (broadcast = TOT and in-furrow = PART). The experiment is laid out as an RCBD, and the allocation of the tillage factor necessitates large plots and ample space between them

for each weed control level. Therefore, the comparison between the means of the subplot factor and between the interaction means is made with higher precision than the comparison between the means of the main-plot factor.

A useful variant of the split-plot is used when the treatments are allocated in strips (**strip-plot** designs), as shown in Fig. 2.10, which represents the layout of an experiment where four crop species were sown 40 days after two herbicide treatments to determine possible phytotoxicity effects due to the presence of herbicide residues beyond the no-observable effect level (recropping experiment). Each block is organized into three rows and four columns; the crop species were randomly allocated to the columns, and the herbicide treatments (including the untreated control) were randomly allocated to the rows. The combinations are, consequently, allocated to the subplots. In this design, we have three types of plots: row-plots, column-plots, and subplots with the advantage that the allocation of treatments can be done rapidly and promptly.

Fig. 2.9 The map refers to the same experiment as in the previous figure (three tillage and two weed control methods) but laid out as a split-plot, where different shades of gray identify the two subplots in each main-plot

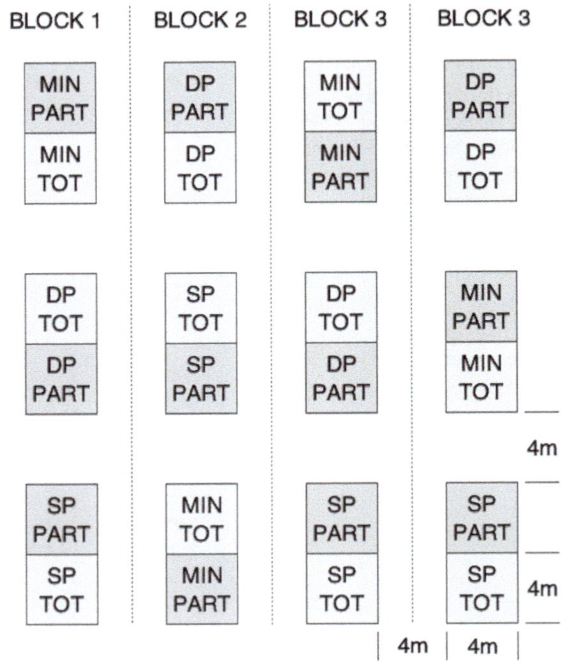

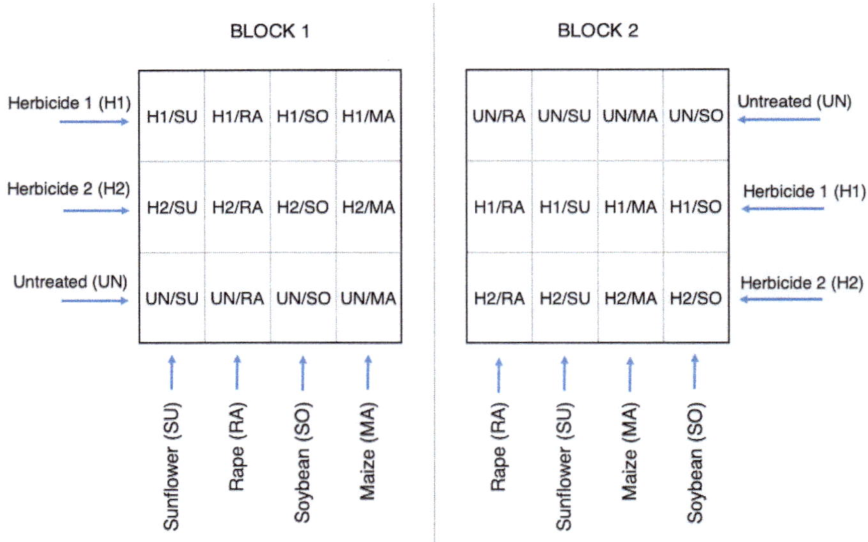

Fig. 2.10 Map of a recropping experiment, where four crops are sown either on untreated soil or on soil that was previously treated with two herbicides. The experiment is laid out as a strip-plot in two blocks

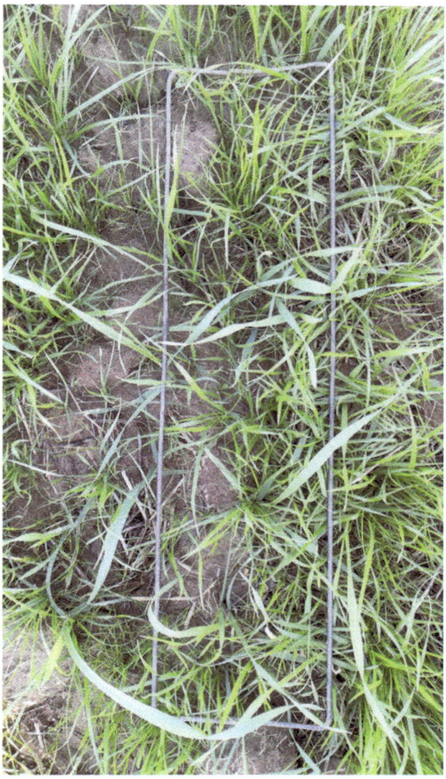

Fig. 2.11 Example of a quadrat for weed samplings (Ph. Euro Pannacci). Typically two or more quadrats are used within each field plot, and they represent subsamples

2.4.5 Subsampling Design

Pseudo-replicates cannot replace true replicates, but they can be associated with true replicates in the so-called subsampling design. For example, for the determination of weed abundances, several quadrats can be used for counts or biomass determinations in each plot (Colbach et al. 2000), as shown in Fig. 2.11. As mentioned in Chap. 1, taking subsamples from a valid experiment with true replicates is a good practice. Still, we need to be careful not to put sub-replicates (subsamples) on equal footing with true replicates during the data analysis stage because the variability of true replicates and the variability of subsamples within each replicate may differ and convey different information. For example, in experiments involving chemical determinations, it is customary to take several subsamples from, e.g., the grain yield of each plot, and submit those subsamples to different measurements; in this case, the variability of true replicates is a reliable estimate of the whole experimental error, while the variability of subsamples is usually smaller, and it is only a reliable estimate of the errors committed during the stage of chemical analyses.

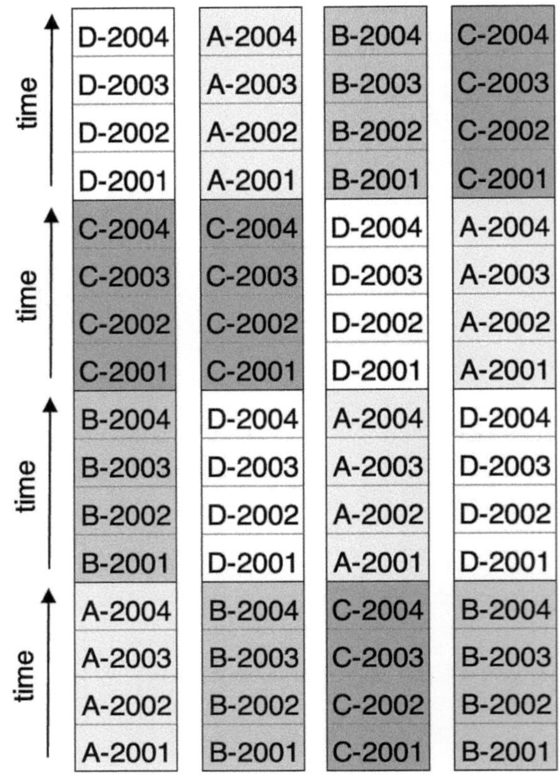

Fig. 2.12 A genotype experiment in alfalfa (with genotypes A, B, C, and D, identified by different shades of gray) laid out as an RCBD, with repeated yield measures taken across 4 years. To highlight the similarity between this design and a split-plot design, it is imagined that the plots extend over space, although they, in reality, extend over time (split-plot in time). It is to be noted that the repeated factor (year) is not randomized to subplots, as its levels can only be in systematic order (from 2001 to 2004)

2.4.6 Repeated Measures Design

A repeated measures design is similar to a split-plot design in the sense that we have (at least) two factors: The first one is allocated to the plots, while the second one (repeated factor) consists of taking multiple measurements in each plot, in different times (e.g., phenological phases, seasons, years, etc.) or different positions (e.g., depths, plant organs, canopy positions, etc.). The difference with the split-plot is that while the subplot factor is allocated to the subplot in each main-plot in randomized order, the repeated factor (e.g., time) is not and, usually, cannot be randomized, but its levels need to be allocated in systematic order (e.g., according to the time scale). When the repeated factor is the time, a repeated measures design is often referred to as a **split-plot in time** (Fig. 2.12).

2.5 Examples of Dubious/Wrong Designs

The experimental layouts presented in the previous section are formally correct and are commonly used in field research for agriculture and biology. However, to comply with the requirements dictated by the availability of labor, time, and money, a certain degree of flexibility is often adopted with randomization. In this respect, a reasonable recommendation is always to design experiments that are formally correct unless experience and common sense suggest that some slight simplifications can produce increased feasibility and decreased costs with no loss in precision and accuracy, which is a rare event.

2.5.1 *Example 2.1*

To measure the residual concentration of two herbicides in soil 20 Days After the Treatment (DAT), a valid experiment should be planned using true replicates, which are independently and randomly treated with the two herbicides, as shown in M1 (CRD) or M2 (RCBD) in Fig. 2.13. The design can be further improved by taking multiple subsamples in each plot and/or submitting each sample or subsample to multiple chemical determinations (subsampling design). Sometimes, the above design is simplified, for example, by (i) spraying two field plots (one plot per herbicide), collecting one soil sample per plot and, for each sample, making three chemical determinations, (ii) spraying two field plots (one plot per herbicide), collecting four soil samples per plot and, for each sample, making one chemical determination, and (iii) spraying two field plots (one plot per herbicide), collecting four soil samples per plot and, for each sample, making three chemical determinations. According to randomization theory, none of these simplifications is valid because pseudo-replication is committed; in the case of (i) the situation is similar to that shown in M3 in Fig. 2.13: There are no replicates, and the three chemical determinations can only give an account of possible errors during the stage of chemical analyses, while all the other potential sources of random errors are neglected (with loose language, these pseudo-replicates are often named "technical" replicates, as opposed to "biological" replicates). In the cases of (ii) and (iii), the situation is similar to M4 in Fig. 2.13: We have biological replicates (the three soil subsamples), but the treatments are not allocated independently to them, no matter how many chemical determinations are performed.

2.5.2 *Example 2.2*

To compare the early growth of 16 genotypes of a field crop, a pot experiment was designed in a climatic chamber, using different shelves as blocks, to account

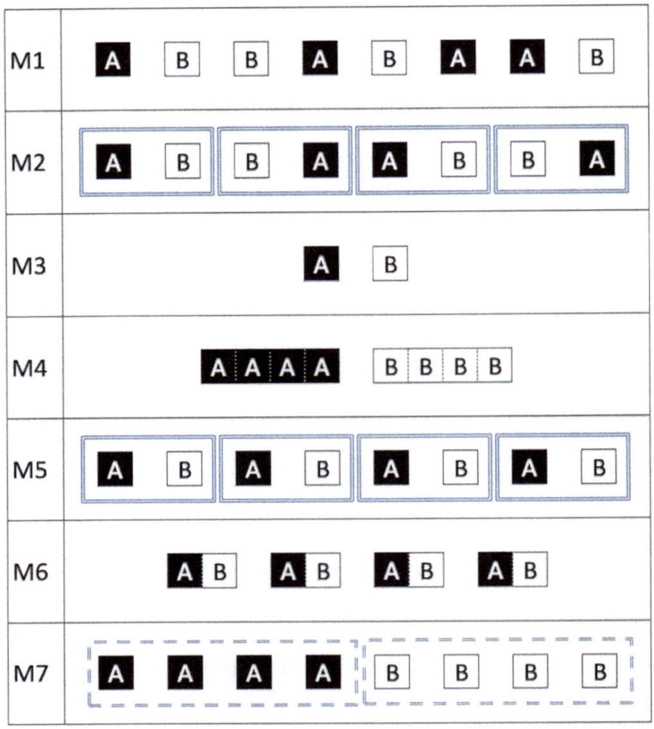

Fig. 2.13 Two experimental treatments (A and B) are compared with several types of layouts that are not necessarily correct (from Hurlbert, 1984; modified). M1: CRD with four true replicates per treatment; M2: RCBD with four complete blocks, identified by double lines; M3: A and B are compared in two plots next to each other (no replicates); M4: A and B are compared in two plots next to each other, and several subsamples are taken from each plot (pseudo-replication); M5: RCBD with systematic allocation of treatments within each block (A is always to the left of B); M6: paired measurements, where A and B are observed in the same unit in different times (e.g., before and after the treatment); and M7 represents an experiment where the two treatments are not interspersed, but they are grouped in two locations (segregation). See the examples in the text for more details

for possible variations between shelves. Within each shelf, the 16 genotypes were accommodated in a randomized order (RCBD). Such a design is often simplified by placing the genotypes on each shelf in systematic order, following the same left-to-right sequence, which is motivated by a more effective visual appraisal of the differences between the treatment levels. Such a systematic arrangement is similar to the one depicted in M5 in Fig. 2.13, and it is discouraged, both for experiments conducted in controlled conditions and, above all, for field experiments, because any possible left-to-right environmental gradient might be confounded with the treatment effect.

2.5.3 Example 2.3

We intend to study how the position of branches affects the photosynthesis of a tree species; to this aim, a CRD trial could be planned by considering eight trees and measuring the photosynthesis in low branches for four randomly selected trees and in high branches for the other trees (as in M1, Fig. 2.13). This design can be simplified by considering four trees, and for each of these, measuring photosynthesis in both low branches and high branches, following a typical repeated measures design (paired measurements: see M6 in Fig. 2.13), which is advantageous for better control of experimental errors.

2.5.4 Example 2.4

We intend to compare two irrigation systems (sprinkler and localized) using four fields in each of two nearby farms. A correct way to lay out such an experiment is to use, in each farm, an RCBD with two blocks of two fields each (RCBD repeated in two locations). A considerable simplification could be achieved by using the four fields in the first farm to allocate the sprinkler irrigation treatment and the four fields of the other farm to allocate the localized irrigation treatment B, as shown in M7 in Fig. 2.13. However, this simplification would produce an invalid design because the two treatments would not be interspersed (Hurlbert 1984), and the "irrigation effect" would be entirely confounded with the "farm effect" (location effect); in other words, any differences between the two farms, either preexisting (e.g., agronomic history, soil type, or environment) or produced by any kinds of intrusions (e.g., a pest attack in one of the two locations), could be wrongly attributed to the irrigation effect.

In general, the lack of interspersion (segregation) is a case of wrong randomization. It arises when we introduce a spatial or temporal separation between the levels of the experimental treatments, making the design suitable only for testing location effects rather than treatment effects. For example, if we want to assess the difference in performance for a genotype at two sites, growing this genotype in four fields at one site and in four fields at the other site would be regarded as fully appropriate.

2.5.5 Example 2.5

We intend to compare two irrigation systems (sprinkler and localized) by using eight rows of an orchard, and we design such an experiment by random allocation of the two treatment levels to the eight rows (four replicates per level). In this situation, it would be rather common to simplify the experiment by assigning one irrigation type to the first four contiguous rows and the second irrigation type to the other four rows, which introduces a spatial segregation between the two treatment levels, as observed in Example 2.4. In principle, such a simplification would be wrong (lack of interspersion), and the experiment should be regarded as invalid. In practice, the consequences of such segregation should be far less serious than in the previous example because the two blocks of four rows are very close to each other, and the occurrence of confounding "location" effects can be regarded as unlikely. Although this type of segregation is regarded as acceptable in some disciplines, it is advisable to avoid it whenever possible, as the interspersion of treatments is a crucial safeguard against spurious results.

2.6 Further Developments

The experimental layouts presented in this chapter are the most common in field experiments, even though several other possibilities exist to comply with the specific needs of every discipline and, in particular, to reduce the size of blocks and the intra-block variability for experiments with a very high number of treatments. In this respect, balanced incomplete block designs or other types of incomplete block designs (e.g., row-column, partially balanced, and lattice designs) may prove helpful in some instances. They are described, for example, in Kuehl (2000), Le Clerg et al. (1962), and Cochran and Cox (1950). Especially for these complex designs, the aid of a computing system, such as the R package `agricolae`, can be beneficial in performing appropriate randomizations (de Mendiburu 2023).

It is also necessary to mention some relatively recent approaches to account for the variability of soil in small plot experiments, such as the "spatial designs" (Richter et al. 2014) and the "nearest neighbor method" (Mohanty 2001); these approaches are not covered in this introductory book.

Finally, it is also important to remind that the results of field experiments always need to be confirmed in other years or locations. For these multi-environment projects, the experimental design (treatments and replicates) is usually the same, but randomization must always be independently performed in subsequent years, locations, or runs.

2.7 Questions and Exercises

1. List and discuss the main traits of field plots (shape, size, number, etc.).
2. What is the border effect, and how is it usually minimized?
3. Discuss the differences between CRDs, RCBDs, and Latin square designs concerning their role in agricultural research.
4. What is a split-plot experiment, and how is it laid out?
5. What is a strip-plot experiment, and how is it laid out?

6. Discuss the possible methods to design an experiment with two experimental factors.
7. You have been requested to design a breeding experiment with 16 wheat genotypes coded by using letters of the Roman alphabet. The aim is to determine which genotype is the best in a given environment. Write the experimental protocol, where you specify all the main elements of your project (subjects, variables, replicates, experimental design), and draw the field map. Consider a field measuring 400 m in length, 20 m in width and with the longer side aligned north-south. Sowing is carried out longitudinally, along the north-south axis, with a 2.5 m wide machine. The field is uniform along its longitudinal axis, although there is a significant transversal fertility gradient.
8. Describe the protocol of an experiment to determine the effect of sowing date (autumn and spring) on seven faba bean genotypes. Include all possible elements to assess whether the experiment is valid, describe the type of design, and include the field map, showing all relevant information (including plot sizes and orientation in space). Consider the same field and sowing macine as described in Exercise 7, but now assume that the available space is 100 m long and 30 m wide. Motivate all choices.
9. Describe the protocol of an experiment to determine the effect of nitrogen dose (four levels) on two wheat genotypes. Include all possible elements to assess whether the experiment is valid, describe the type of design, and include the field map, showing all relevant information (including plot sizes and orientation in space). Consider a field of 50 m in length and 30 m in width, with its longer side aligned east-west. Sowing is carried out longitudinally, along the east-west axis, with a 2 m wide machine. There is a relevant longitudinal (not transversal) fertility gradient. Motivate all your choices.

References

Cochran WG, Cox GM (1950) Experimental Design. Wiley, Hoboken

Colbach N, Dessaint F, Forcella F (2000) Evaluating of field-scale sampling methods for the estimation of mean plant densities of weeds. Weed Res 40:411–430

de Mendiburu F (2023) Agricolae: Statistical Procedures for Agricultural Research. https://CRAN.R-project.org/package=agricolae, r package version 1.3-0

Hurlbert SH (1984) Pseudoreplication and the design of ecological experiments. Ecol Monogr 54(2):187–211

Kuehl RO (2000) Design of Experiments: Statistical Principles of Research Design and Analysis. Duxbury Press, Pacific Grove

Le Clerg EL, Leonard WH, Clark AG (1962) Field Plot Technique. Burgess Publishing Company, Minneapolis

Mohanty RG (2001) Papadakis nearest neighbor analysis of yield in agricultural experiments. In: Conference on Applied Statistics in Agriculture. https://doi.org/10.4148/2475-7772.1216. https://newprairiepress.org/agstatconference/2001/proceedings/6

Richter C, Kroschewski B, Piepho HP, Spilke J (2014) Treatment comparisons in agricultural field trials accounting for spatial correlation. J Agricul Sci 153:1–21. https://doi.org/10.1017/S0021859614000823. http://www.journals.cambridge.org/abstract_S0021859614000823

Chapter 3
Describing the Observations

Statistics is the grammar of science
—K. Pearson

Abstract The outcome of every field experiment is a dataset consisting of a set of measures or scores taken on several experimental subjects about one or more properties (e.g., height, weight, concentration, sex, and color). The first task of data analysis is usually to describe such datasets by using the most appropriate statistics. This chapter considers continuous data, counts, and proportions. It introduces the main statistics of central tendency (mean and median), spread (range, interquartile range, deviance, variance, standard deviation, and coefficient of variation), and joint variation (Pearson's correlation coefficient). The use of R for descriptive statistics is demonstrated, and four types of descriptive graphs (barplots, boxplots, histograms, and scatterplots) are introduced, along with the R coding to produce them.

Every field experiment yields a dataset, which contains all variables recorded during the experiment, in relation to all the experimental units. The first task of data analysis is to describe those variables by using the most appropriate statistics. This chapter represents a brief introduction to descriptive statistics, while more detailed information can be found, e.g., in Holcomb (2017); it considers continuous data, counts, and proportions, while it is assumed that nominal and ordinal data are converted into counts or proportions before analyses (e.g., the count/proportion of diseased plants per plot), which is the most common practice in field research.

For quantitative data, we need to describe (i) location, (ii) spread, and (iii) shape. The location of a variable describes where the values are positioned along the measurement scale, while the spread indicates how close the values are to one another. The shape describes whether the values are symmetrically distributed around the central value or skewed to the right or left. In this chapter, only the statistics of location and spread will be considered, as the statistics of shape are not commonly used in agriculture and biology although they are not unimportant.

A. Onofri, *Field Research Methods in Agriculture*,
https://doi.org/10.1007/978-3-032-08199-5_3

3.1 Statistics of Location

The most widely known statistic of location is the **mean**, which is obtained as the sum of data divided by the number of values:

$$\mu = \frac{\sum_{i=1}^{n} x_i}{n} \tag{3.1}$$

The mean can be regarded as the central value in terms of Euclidean distances, in the sense that, by definition, the sum of the Euclidean distances between each value and the group mean is always zero, implying that the values above the mean and those below the mean, on average, are equally distant from the mean itself. However, suppose we sort the values in decreasing or increasing order; in this case, the mean is not necessarily in a central position, in the sense that the number of values above the mean may not be the same as the number of values below the mean. For example, if we examine a sorted list of values composed of 1, 4, 7, 9, and 10, the mean is 6.2, and the number of values below the mean is lower than the number of values above the mean. If we change the highest value from 10 to 100, the new mean is shifted upward to 24.2 and is higher than all the values except one.

Another relevant statistic of location, which by definition represents the “central value” in every sorted variable, is the so-called **median**. It is easily calculated by sorting the values in increasing order and, if the number of values is odd, taking the value in the $(n + 1)/2$ position (n is the number of values) while, if the number of values is even, taking the two values in the $n/2$ and $n/2 + 1$ positions and averaging them. For example, if we consider the same values as before (1, 4, 7, 9, and 10), the median remains 7, even if the highest value is changed to 100. In practice, the median is entirely independent of the highest or lowest values in a variable, and for this reason, it is more **robust** than the mean with respect to the so-called **outliers**.

3.2 Statistics of Spread

Knowing the location of a variable is not enough for our purpose, as we miss a relevant piece of information: How close are the values to the mean? The simplest statistic to express the spread is the **range**, which is the difference between the highest and lowest values. However, the range is a very rough indicator, as it is susceptible to outliers.

Another statistic of spread is the **interquartile range**, which is the interval defined by the 25th and 75th percentiles. In general, the **percentiles** are the values below which a given percentage of observations fall. More specifically, the 25th percentile is the value below which 25% of the observations fall and the 75th percentile is the value below which 75% of the observations fall (you may have understood that the median corresponds to the 50th percentile). The interval between the 25th and 75th percentiles, consequently, contains 50% of all the observed values, and, therefore, it is a good statistic of spread. Like the median, the 25th and 75th percentiles are relatively unaffected by outliers. Hence, the interquartile range is used as a statistic of spread in the presence of a few outliers and is most often associated with the median as a statistic of location.

Another statistic of spread is the sum of squared differences between the observed values and the group mean, which is simply referred to as the **sum of squares (SS)**:

$$SS = \sum_{i=1}^{n} (x_i - \mu)^2 \tag{3.2}$$

In a model fitting perspective (see Chap. 4), the mean is the expected value, and the difference between the observed and expected values in Eq. (3.2) is referred to as the **residuals** so that we also speak about the residual sum of squares.

A high SS value corresponds to a high spread, although we can also have a high SS with a low spread and a large number of values. Therefore, the SS should not be used to compare the spread of two groups with different sizes. Another problem with the SS is that the measurement unit is equal to the square of the measurement unit for the mean. For example, if the original variable is measured in centimeters (cm), the SS is measured in square centimeters (cm^2), which is not very clear.

A second important measure of spread is the **variance**, which is usually obtained by dividing the SS by the number of observations minus one:

$$\sigma^2 = \frac{SS}{n-1} \tag{3.3}$$

The variance is also known as the **mean square**, and you may wonder why we do not divide the SS by the number of observations instead of subtracting one from this number. Indeed, both expressions are possible to obtain, respectively, the so-called population variance (SS/n) and sample variance [$SS/(n-1)$], and the latter is preferable whenever the group of measurements represents a sample from a broader population, which is the most common case in field research. In this situation, we need to decrease the amount at the denominator by one unit to account for the fact that we do not know the real population mean (μ), and we have to replace it with the sample mean (see Sokal and Rohlf 1981, see Chapter 6; additional information is also available in the companion blog[1]).

The variance can be used to compare the spread of two groups with different sizes, but the measurement unit remains squared with respect to the original variable.

The most important measure of spread is the **standard deviation**, that is, the square root of the variance:

$$\sigma = \sqrt{\sigma^2} \tag{3.4}$$

[1] Go to https://www.statforbiology.com/2018/stat_general_variancesamplepop/.

The measurement unit is the same as the data. For this reason, the standard deviation is usually associated with the mean to return the interval $l = \mu \pm \sigma$, which is often used to describe the **absolute uncertainty** of replicated measurements.

Sometimes, the standard deviation is expressed as a percentage of the mean (**coefficient of variability**), which is used to describe the **relative uncertainty** of measurement instruments:

$$CV = \frac{\sigma}{\mu} \times 100 \tag{3.5}$$

3.3 Populations and Samples

To avoid confusion, the mean, variance, and standard deviation in the previous sections were represented by Greek letters and refer to a population of individuals representing the entire group we are interested in and want to draw conclusions about. Most often, the group of experimental subjects represents a sample from a broader population, and its size is smaller than that of the original population. For the sample, the descriptive statistics are often represented by Latin letters, to highlight the fact that these statistics are different from the corresponding statistics of the population from which the sample was obtained. We will revisit this aspect in Chap. 6 when discussing the topic of inference.

3.3.1 Example 3.1: Descriptive Statistics by Hand

Let us consider four maize plants with heights of 178 cm, 175 cm, 158 cm, and 153 cm, respectively. Considering that this is a sample from a wider population, the mean height is

$$m = \frac{178 + 175 + 158 + 153}{4} = 166$$

The SS is calculated by using Eq. (3.2) and plugging in the sample mean m:

$$SS = (178 - 166)^2 + (175 - 166)^2 + (158 - 166)^2 + (153 - 166)^2 = 458$$

The sample variance and standard deviation are calculated as, respectively,

$$s^2 = \frac{458}{3} = 152.67$$

$$s = \sqrt{152.67} = 12.36$$

3.4 The Propagation of Errors

If we have two amounts A and B with standard deviations equal to, respectively, σ_A and σ_B and two constant values p and q, the *law of propagation of errors* permits to calculate the standard deviation for any linear combinations of the type $C = pA + qB$. In particular, when the two amounts A and B are independently obtained, it is:

$$\sigma_C = \sqrt{p^2\sigma_A^2 + q^2\sigma_B^2} \tag{3.6}$$

Those who are interested can find more details about the law of propagation of errors on the blog associated with this book.[2]

3.4.1 *Example 3.2: Standard Deviation for the Sum*

We have independently determined the sucrose and fructose content in a specific growth substrate, which are, respectively, equal to 22 ± 2 mg/g and 14 ± 3 mg/g. What are the total sugar content and its standard deviation? The solution can be easily derived by summing the two contents ($22 + 14 = 36$ mg/g) and calculating the standard deviation as $\sqrt{2^2 + 3^2} = 3.6$.

3.4.2 *Example 3.3: Standard Deviation for the Mean*

For the case of the previous Example 3.2, what is the average concentration of the two sugars, with its standard deviation? We can easily calculate the average concentration as

$$Av = \frac{22 + 14}{2} = \frac{1}{2} \times 22 + \frac{1}{2} \times 14 = 18$$

while the standard deviation is

$$\sigma_{Av} = \sqrt{\left(\frac{1}{2}\right)^2 2^2 + \left(\frac{1}{2}\right)^2 3^2} = 1.803$$

[2] Go to https://www.statforbiology.com/2024/stat_general_errorpropagation/.

3.5 Joint Variation

Suppose we have recorded two or more quantitative traits on each subject. In this case, we might be interested in assessing whether, for each pair of variables, when one variable changes, the other also changes (**joint variation**). The *Pearson correlation coefficient* is a measure of joint variation, and it is equal to the codeviance of the two variables divided by the square root of the product of their deviances:

$$r = \frac{\sum_{i=1}^{n}(x_i - \mu_x)(y_i - \mu_y)}{\sqrt{\sum_{i=1}^{n}(x_i - \mu_x)^2 \sum_{i=1}^{n}(y_i - \mu_y)^2}} \tag{3.7}$$

If we have a sample, we need to plug in Eq. (3.7) the sample statistics m_x and m_y in place of the population statistics μ_x and μ_y. The codeviance (at the numerator in Eq. (3.7)) consists of the sum across individuals of the products between the residuals for the two variables. It is positive when, for most individuals, the two residuals have the same signs, which means that greater values of one variable correspond to greater values of the other variable ("positive" joint variation). At the same time, the codeviance is negative when, for most individuals, the two residuals have opposite signs ("negative" joint variation). A codeviance close to 0 means that the signs of the two residuals are mostly independent (no joint variation).

The codeviance has no predefined plateau, and it is normalized by dividing it by the product of the two deviances so that the r coefficient ranges from $+1$ to -1: A value of $+1$ implies that when x increases, y increases by a proportional amount so that the points on a scatterplot lie on a straight line with a positive slope. On the other hand, a value of -1 implies that when x increases, y decreases by a proportional amount, so that the points on a scatterplot lie on a straight line, with a negative slope. A value of 0 indicates that there is no joint variability. In contrast, intermediate values indicate a more or less high degree of joint variability, although the points on a scatterplot do not exactly lie on a straight line (Fig. 3.1).

3.5.1 Example 3.4: Correlation

Let us consider that we have measured the oil content in sunflower seeds using two different methods (A and B) and want to determine the degree of concordance between the two measurements by using the correlation coefficient. The observed data are presented in columns A and B of Table 3.1.

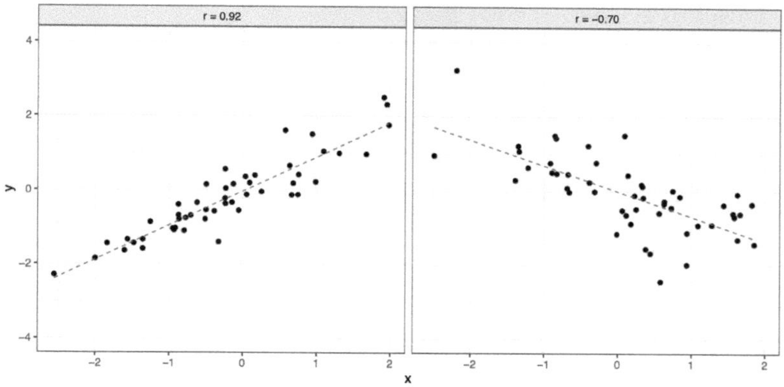

Fig. 3.1 Examples of positive (left) and negative (right) correlation

Table 3.1 Hand calculations for the correlation coefficient (Example 3.4)

A	B	z_A	z_B	z_A^2	z_B^2	$z_A \times z_B$
45	44	−1.222	−1.444	1.494	2.086	1.765
47	44	0.778	−1.444	0.605	2.086	−1.123
49	49	2.778	3.556	7.716	12.642	9.877
51	53	4.778	7.556	22.827	57.086	36.099
44	48	−2.222	2.556	4.938	6.531	−5.679
37	34	−9.222	−11.444	85.049	130.975	105.543
48	47	1.778	1.556	3.160	2.420	2.765
42	39	−4.222	−6.444	17.827	41.531	27.210
53	51	6.778	5.556	45.938	30.864	37.654

To calculate the correlation coefficient, we need to organize our calculations as follows:

1. Calculate the residuals for A (z_A)
2. Calculate the residuals for B (z_B)
3. Calculate the SS and codeviance

First, we calculate the two means, which are 46.22 and 45.44, respectively. Second, we can calculate the residuals for both variables, as shown in Table 3.1.

From the residuals, we can calculate the SS, which are 189.55 and 286.22, respectively, and the codeviance, which is 214.11. Accordingly, the correlation coefficient is

$$r = \frac{214.11}{\sqrt{189.55 \times 286.22}} = 0.919$$

It is close to 1, so there is quite a good agreement between the two methods.

3.6 Descriptive Stats with R

Before reading this part, please ensure that you have some basic knowledge of the R environment, or refer to Appendix A in this book for a brief introduction. Furthermore, make sure you have installed all packages listed in Appendix A.13.

Another essential prerequisite is that you should be aware of the correct format in which research data should be prepared for data analysis. In general, a dataset should be in a "tidy" format, **with one row per observation and one column per variable, while the first row is reserved for the names of variables**. While other data formats may be more suitable for visualization, the "tidy" format serves as the starting point for most statistical analyses with software tools, and it can be easily transformed into other formats whenever necessary (Wickham 2014).

In R, the descriptive statistics are calculated by the respective functions: `mean()`, `median()`, `var()`, and `sd()`, passing the data vector as the first argument. The percentiles are calculated using the `quantile()` function, which takes the data vector and the selected probabilities as fractions in a vector, specified through the `probs` argument. To calculate the residual sum of squares in R, we can use Eq. (3.2); however, an alternative method will be presented in the next chapter. We can easily obtain the correlation coefficient using the `cor()` function and passing the two vectors as arguments.

3.6.1 *Example 3.5: Describing a Dataset with R*

Let us consider the dataset "heights," which is available in the `statforbiology` package and contains the heights and yields of 20 maize plants, belonging to four different genotypes, as measured in an experiment laid out as a CRD, with a different number of replicates per genotype (unbalanced data). The main descriptive statistics for height are calculated in Code Box 3.1.

Code Box 3.1

```
# Example 3.5
# Calculating descriptive statistics with R

# Load the data and package
library(statforbiology)
dataset <- getAgroData("heights")
head(dataset)
##   id var height yield
## 1  1   N    172 11.54
## 2  2   S    154 14.80
## 3  3   V    150 10.77
```

```
## 4  4   V     188 12.03
## 5  5   C     162 13.53
## 6  6   N     145 11.44

# Mean and median
mean(dataset$height)
## [1] 164
median(dataset$height)
## [1] 162.5

# Variance and standard deviation
var(dataset$height)
## [1] 213.1579
sd(dataset$height)
## [1] 14.59993

# Coefficient of variability
sd(dataset$height)/mean(dataset$height) * 100
## [1] 8.902395

# Quantiles
quantile(dataset$height, probs = c(0.25, 0.75))
##    25%    75%
## 152.75 174.25

# Sum of squares
sum( (dataset$height - mean(dataset$height))^2 )
## [1] 4050
```

The correlation between height and yield is calculated in Code Box 3.2. In this box, the `with()` function is used to evaluate a function within the dataframe that is passed as the first argument, which permits to avoid using the extractor $ for both variables.

Code Box 3.2

```
# Example 3.5 [continuation]

# Correlation with R
with(dataset, cor(height, yield))
## [1] 0.4150642
# cor(dataset$height, dataset$yield) # Equivalent expression
```

3.7 Groupwise Statistics

A field experiment typically produces replicated data for different treatment groups, such as different genotypes or fertilizers. With base R, we can calculate the descriptive statistics for each group using the `tapply()` function, which takes three arguments: the vector of observations, the vector of groups, and the function to be calculated in a groupwise fashion. The vector of groups indexes the observations according to the group to which they belong, and we can use the argument `FUN` to pass any other R function, such as `median()` or `sd()`.

We can use the above method to calculate summary statistics (means and standard deviations) for the four genotypes in the "height" dataset and store them into the "descStat" dataframe, for later use (Code Box 3.3).

It is worth mentioning that these groupwise operations can also be efficiently performed using the `dplyr` package (Wickham et al. 2023).

Code Box 3.3

```
# Example 3.5 [continuation]

# Calculating group-wise statistics with base R

# Groupwise means
mu.height <- with(dataset, tapply(height, var, FUN = mean))
mu.height
##       C      N      S      V
## 165.00 164.00 160.00 165.25
#
# Groupwise standard deviations
sigma.height <- with(dataset, tapply(height, var, sd))
sigma.height
##        C        N        S        V
## 14.36431 16.19877 12.16553 19.51709
#
# A dataframe for the results
descStat <- data.frame(group = names(mu.height),
                       mu = mu.height,
                       sigma = sigma.height,
                       row.names = 1:4)
descStat
##   group     mu    sigma
## 1     C 165.00 14.36431
```

```
## 2      N 164.00 16.19877
## 3      S 160.00 12.16553
## 4      V 165.25 19.51709
```

3.8 Graphical Representations

Descriptive statistics can be presented by using tables or, even better, graphs. Visualization is a vast topic, and it is covered by, e.g., Wickham (2016); Soage (2024); Holtz (2024), although several other books and websites are available.[3] This chapter gives some basic introduction about the four most common types of plots, which we can be easily produced by using the `ggplot2` package:

1. Barplots
2. Boxplots
3. Histograms
4. Scatterplots

A **barplot** is used to visualize the relationship between a numeric variable and a nominal variable. Each class of the nominal variable corresponds to a bar, and the height of that bar is proportional to the value of the numeric variable for that class.

When the number of replicates is high (e.g., >15), the relationship between a nominal variable and a quantitative variable can also be represented by a **boxplot** (Box-Whisker plot), where each group is represented by a box, with the 75th percentile as the uppermost side and the 25th percentile as the lowermost side. At the same time, a line is drawn to indicate the median (50th percentile). Two vertical bars (whiskers) start from the 25th and 75th percentile and extend, respectively, to the maximum and minimum values. In R, data points beyond 1.5 times the interquartile range are regarded as outliers and are plotted individually, while the length of the whisker is limited to 1.5 times the interquartile range.

Another type of chart is the **histogram**, which is similar to a barplot but used to represent the probability density in each of a series of intervals (bins). The density is the relative frequency of subjects in each interval divided by the width of the interval so that the area of each bar represents the probability mass in each interval. The use of histograms is not very frequent in field research, but we will encounter them a few times in this book.

Last but not least, one of the most used graphs is the **scatterplot**, which represents the relationship between two numeric variables by showing, for each individual, a symbol drawn at the position dictated by the observed values for the two variables, used as the coordinates.

[3] For example, the websites "R Charts" at r-charts.com and "The R graph gallery" at r-graph–gallery.com.

3.8.1 Example 3.6: A Barplot with R

A barplot is suitable for representing the "descStat" dataframe that we have just created in Code Box 3.3. To make such a graph with `ggplot2`, we first need to create an instance of the plot (first line of code) and then add layers (`geom_col` and `geom_errorbar`), which must be mapped to the necessary information for plotting (Code Box 3.4).

The first layer (`geom_col`) produces the bars, which are mapped to the vector `mu` in `descStat` to determine the heights of the bars for each level in the `group` variable. The second layer (`geom_errorbar`) augments the barplot with error bars to represent the standard deviations ($\mu \pm \sigma$). Ultimately, the `theme_bw()` theme is used, but other themes are available to suit everyone's preferences. The resulting plot is shown in Fig. 3.2.

Code Box 3.4

```
# Example 3.6

# A barplot with ggplot2
# (the descStat dataframe was obtained in Code box 3.3)

library(ggplot2)
ggplot(data = descStat) +
  geom_col(mapping = aes(y = mu, x = group), width = 0.45,
           color = "black", fill = "lightgrey") +
  geom_errorbar(mapping = aes(ymin = mu - sigma,
                              ymax = mu + sigma, x = group),
                width = 0.05) +
  scale_y_continuous(limits = c(0, 200),
                     name = "Height (cm)") +
  scale_x_discrete(name = "Genotype") +
  theme_bw()
```

3.8.2 Example 3.7: A Boxplot with R

Let us consider the "WeedCounts" dataset, relating to the counts of plants for three weed species in 20 random quadrats in one field of central Italy (Code Box 3.5). As the number of counts for each species is pretty high, this dataset can be represented by a boxplot, with the coding reported in Code Box 3.5; in the case of *Chenopodium album* (CHEAL), the maximum value is 16, and it is regarded as an outlier and represented as a full black circle (Fig. 3.3)

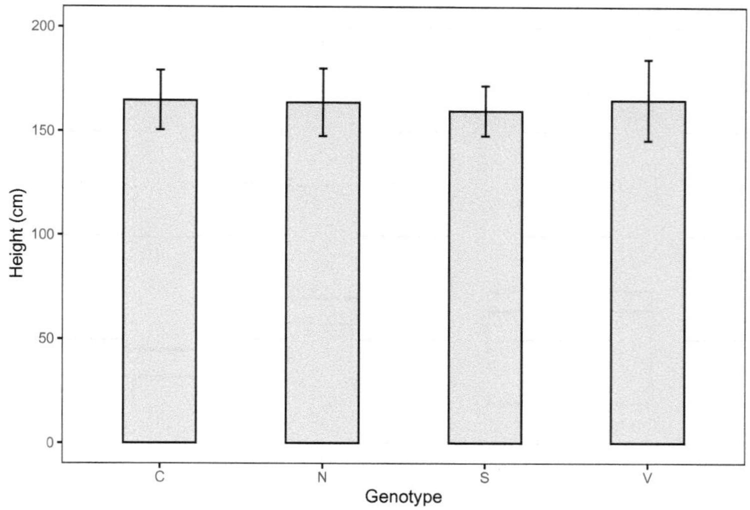

Fig. 3.2 Example of a simple barplot in R (Code Box 3.4)

Code Box 3.5

```
# Example 3.7

# A boxplot with ggplot2
library(statforbiology)
dataset <- getAgroData("WeedCounts")

ggplot(data = dataset) +
  geom_boxplot(mapping =aes(x = Species, y = Count)) +
  scale_y_continuous(name = "Count per square meter") +
  scale_x_discrete(name = "") +
  theme_bw()
```

3.8.3 Example 3.8: A Histogram with R

The dataset "Rainfall22" reports the daily rainfall levels (in millimeters) in central Italy for 2022. This variable comprises a very high number of observations, and calculating simple descriptive statistics, such as the mean and standard deviation, is useful, but it is not enough to grasp the essential traits of rainfall at that site and year.

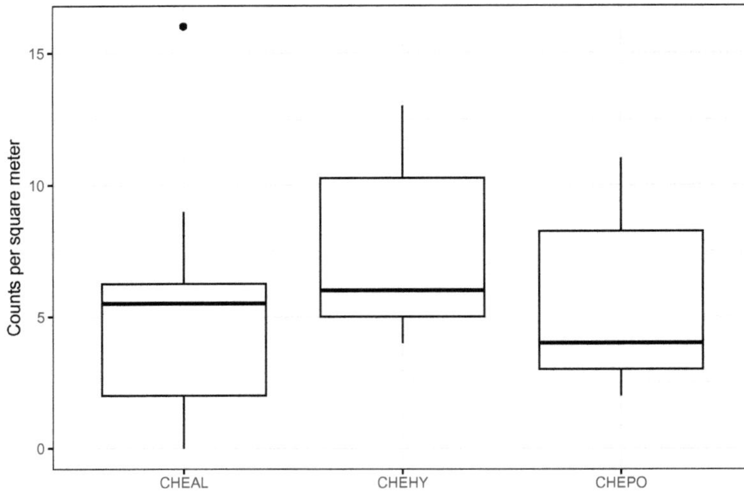

Fig. 3.3 A simple boxplot with R; the three groups represent three weed species (CHEAL: *Chenopodium album*, CHEHY: *C. hybridum*, and CHEPO: *C. polyspermum*) that were counted in 20 quadrats each in a field of central Italy (Code Box 3.5)

Therefore, it is interesting to build a distribution of frequencies by considering six rain classes (0.1–2.4 mm: very light rain, 2.5–7.5 mm: light rain, 7.6–35.5: moderate rain, 35.6–64.4: rather heavy rain, 64.5–124.4: heavy rain, and >124.5 mm: very heavy rain) and assigning each rain to the appropriate class (this operation is usually called **binning** or **bucketing**).

With R, this is accomplished by using the `cut()` function, and passing the vector of rains and a vector containing the margins of the intervals. These latter are, by default, left-open and right-closed (Code Box 3.6). Next, we can use the function `table()` to count the number of rains in each bin (**absolute frequency**) and divide this number by the total number of rainfall events (**relative frequency**). According to the frequentist definition of probability (i.e., the number of favorable events divided by the number of total events), this relative frequency corresponds to the probability of each class of rain (Code Box 3.6).

Code Box 3.6

```
# Example 3.8

# Frequencies and probabilities

# Read the data and package
library(statforbiology)
dataset <- getAgroData("Rainfall22")
```

```
dataset <- dataset[dataset$PRP > 0, ] # Remove the days with
  no rain

# Set the margins of classes
margins <- c(0, 2.4, 7.5, 35.5, 64.4, 124.4, Inf)

# Calculate the frequencies in each class
binned <- cut(dataset$PRP, breaks = margins)
frequencies <- table(binned)
frequencies
##     (0,2.4]    (2.4,7.5]  (7.5,35.5] (35.5,64.4]   (64.4,124]
##          52           21          31            2            0
##    (124,Inf]
##           0

# Probabilities of each class of rain
probab <- frequencies/length(binned)
probab
##     (0,2.4]    (2.4,7.5]  (7.5,35.5] (35.5,64.4]   (64.4,124]
## 0.49056604  0.19811321  0.29245283  0.01886792  0.00000000
##    (124,Inf]
## 0.00000000
```

Representing these probabilities with a barplot might be misleading because the different widths of intervals would be neglected. We may note that the probability in the second bin (0.198) is lower than the probability in the third bin (0.292), but it is "concentrated" in a very small interval. In other words, there are a lot of events in the third interval just because such an interval is wide. Still, it is reasonable to expect that the probability of a 20 mm rain (third interval) is lower than the probability of a 5 mm rain (second interval). In technical terms, we say that the probability mass is more dense in the second interval with respect to the third. Thus, we can calculate the density by dividing the probability in each interval by the width of the interval (Code Box 3.7)

Code Box 3.7

```
# Example 3.8 [continuation]

# Calculation of densities

widths <- diff(margins)
probab/widths
```

```
##       (0,2.4]     (2.4,7.5]    (7.5,35.5]  (35.5,64.4]
## 0.2044025157 0.0388457270 0.0104447439 0.0006528694
##    (64.4,124]     (124,Inf]
## 0.0000000000 0.0000000000
```

We can use these densities to draw a histogram composed of a set of rectangles, with heights equal to the density in each interval and widths equal to the width of the interval so that the area represents the probability mass in each interval. These calculations are performed automatically in R by passing the margins of the intervals (bins) to the `geom_histogram()` layer, as shown in Code Box 3.8. The resulting histogram is shown in Fig. 3.4.

Code Box 3.8

```
# Example 3.8 [continuation]

# A histogram with ggplot
#
ggplot(data = dataset) +
  geom_histogram(mapping = aes(x = PRP,
                         y = after_stat(density)),
                 breaks = margins, fill = "white",
                 col = "black") +
  scale_x_continuous(name = "Rainfall class",
                     breaks = seq(0, 200, by = 10),
                     limits = c(0, 100)) +
  theme_bw()
```

3.8.4 *Example 3.9: A Scatterplot with R*

A scatterplot can be created using the `geom_point()` layer in `ggplot2`. As an example of its usage, we can plot the relationship between height and yield in the "`heights`" data (Code Box 3.7; Fig. 3.5).

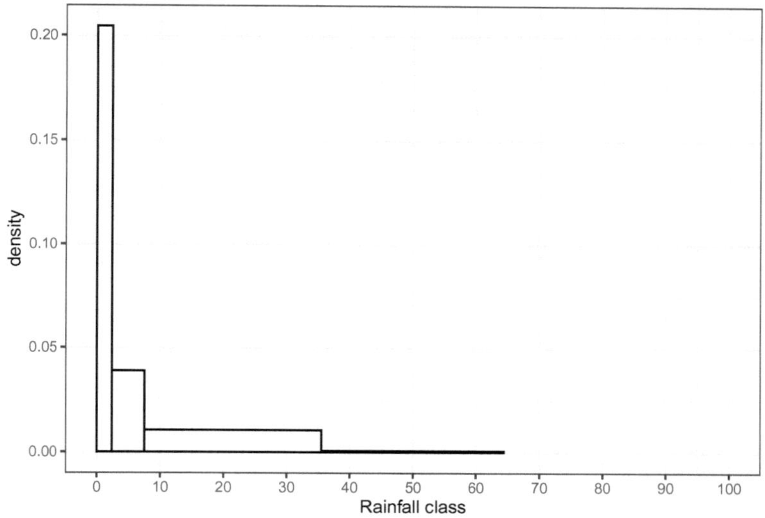

Fig. 3.4 A histogram representing the probability of rainfall events in several classes, as observed in central Italy, in 2022. The height of bars is the density, while the area represents the probability in the whole interval

Code Box 3.9

```
# Example 3.9

# A scatterplot with ggplot

# Load data and package
library(statforbiology)
dataset <- getAgroData("heights")

ggplot(data = dataset) +
  geom_point(mapping = aes(x = height, y = yield),
             cex = 2.5, col = "blue") +
  scale_x_continuous(name = "Height (cm)") +
  scale_y_continuous(name = "Yield (t/ha)") +
  theme_bw()
```

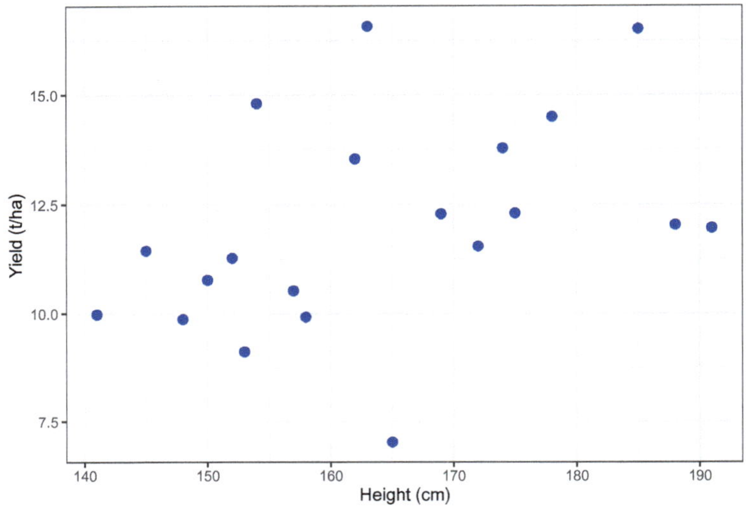

Fig. 3.5 Scatterplot showing the relationship between two numeric variables

3.9 Questions and Exercises

1. List and discuss the main statistics of central tendency for quantitative variables.
2. Describe and discuss briefly the coefficient of correlation of Pearson.
3. A chemical analysis was performed in triplicate, with the following results: 125, 169, and 142 ng/g. Calculate the mean, the sum of squares, the mean square, the standard deviation, and the coefficient of variation. What is one of the correct ways to display the result?
4. A scientist has measured the height and the diameter of four trees. The results are reported below. Calculate the coefficient of correlation, and determine the degree of joint variation between the two variables.

```
# Data for the exercise
Height <- c(2.3, 2.7, 3.1, 3.5)
Diameter <- c(0.46, 0.51, 0.59, 0.64)
```

5. Consider the `rimsulfuron` dataset in `statforbiology`, which results from a field experiment comparing 14 herbicides and two untreated checks, with four replicates per treatment. The response variables are maize yield and weed coverage. Describe the dataset, and show the results on a barplot, including some measure of variability. Check whether yield correlates to weed coverage and comment on the results.
6. Three random samples harvested from an alfalfa field showed that the yield at the first cut (in May) was 8 t DM ha^{-1} with a standard deviation of 0.7 t ha^{-1}. Three other independent random samples showed that the yield at the second cut (July) was 5 t DM ha^{-1} with a standard deviation of 0.4 t ha^{-1}. Calculate the total and average yield with the respective standard deviations.

References

Holcomb Z (2017) Fundamentals of Descriptive Statistics. Routledge (Taylor and Francis Group), Milton Park

Holtz Y (2024) The r graph gallery. https://r-graph-gallery.com/index.html

Soage J (2024) R charts. https://r-charts.com

Sokal RR, Rohlf FJ (1981) Biometry. W.H. Freeman and Company, New York

Wickham H (2014) Tidy data. J Stat Softw 59(10). https://doi.org/10.18637/jss.v059.i10. http://www.jstatsoft.org/v59/i10/

Wickham H (2016) Ggplot2. Elegant Graphics for Data Analysis. Use R!. Springer International Publishing, Cham. https://doi.org/10.1007/978-3-319-24277-4. http://link.springer.com/10.1007/978-3-319-24277-4

Wickham H, François R, Henry L, Müller K, Vaughan D (2023) dplyr: A Grammar of Data Manipulation. https://CRAN.R-project.org/package=dplyr, r package version 1.1.4

Chapter 4
Cause-Effect Relationships

> *If there is anything in the world which I do firmly believe in, it is the universal validity of the law of causation*
>
> —T. Huxley

Abstract Causation is one of the most critical types of relationship among experimental variables and is often the primary focus of scientific experiments. In this chapter, model fitting is introduced as a method for examining cause-effect relationships in experimental data, using techniques such as the least squares method and variance partitioning (ANOVA). The chapter provides a brief overview of statistical models and their components and presents several commonly used models in agriculture, such as simple linear regression models, one-way and two-way ANOVA models, illustrated through simple yet realistic examples. Additionally, suggestions for handling unbalanced data are provided to prevent misinterpretation in routine research in agriculture.

The most important relationship between variables is **causation**; it occurs whenever one variable (usually called "predictor") causes a change in another variable (usually called "response"); for example, a variation in the genotype level may cause a change in the yield of maize, or, likewise, a variation in fertilization dose may cause a change in protein content of winter wheat grains.

Establishing the existence and extent of a causal relationship between two (or more) variables is often regarded as a primary objective of research. According to the English philosopher John Stuart Mill (1806–1867), three main criteria need to be fulfilled (Shadish et al. 2002):

1. The cause must precede the effect.
2. The cause and effect must be related to each other.
3. Any other alternative explanation can be ruled out.

From those criteria, we ought to conclude that the sole existence of a strong association, as measured, for example, by a Pearson correlation coefficient close to

A. Onofri, *Field Research Methods in Agriculture*,
https://doi.org/10.1007/978-3-032-08199-5_4

1 or -1, is not, in itself, proof of causation because it only implies that two variables change jointly (*correlation does not mean causation*; see, e.g., Zaniletti et al. 2023).

Controlled, replicated, and randomized experiments are particularly tailored to establish cause-effect relationships, as they consist of measuring the response of subjects after the application of a specific stimulus, while "everything else," apart from that stimulus, is kept constant (i.e., the so-called *ceteris paribus* assumption; see Chap. 1). Consequently, it is relevant to explore statistical methods for assessing whether a specific dataset supports the hypothesis of a cause-effect relationship between the variables under study.

4.1 Statistical Models

Cause-effect relationships can be efficiently described using **mathematical models**, i.e., equations that simulate the outcome of a set of predictors. Building models to describe the outcomes of natural systems has become a widespread practice, resulting in models with varying complexity, ranging from simple empirical equations (see Ratkowsky 1990) to complex mechanistic multi-scale models (see Gherman et al. 2023). In agriculture, accounts of available models to describe the behavior of farming or cropping systems can be found, e.g., in Pasley et al. (2023) or in Gavasso-Rita et al. (2024).

This book primarily covers simple empirical models that are most often used to describe cause-effect relationships in controlled experiments, where the number of predictors and, consequently, the degree of complexity have been minimized. These models are referred to as **statistical models**, due to the presence of a "stochastic component," which accounts for all stochastic effects that were not allocated by the experimenter but arose as consequences of possible sources of random errors, as described in Chaps. 1 and 2.

4.2 Model Components

A general deterministic cause-effect model is

$$Y_E = f(X, \theta) \tag{4.1}$$

This model expresses the fundamental idea that the expected outcome Y_E is obtained as the result of the predictor(s) X, according to the function f, based on one or more parameters θ.

The expected response Y_E can take several forms, i.e., it can be either a quantity or a count or a ratio or a quality. Additionally, the expected response can be represented by a single variable (univariate response) or by several variables (multivariate response). This book only covers the simplest situation of one quantitative response variable; however, with some prudence, the proposed techniques can also be applied to counts and ratios.

The set of predictors (X) is represented by one or more quantitative or nominal variables that are supposed to be in a cause-effect relationship with the expect response. In some instances, the predictor is represented by a dose so that we can legitimately talk about a "dose-response" model (e.g., a model for the response of a weed to the increasing dose of an herbicide substance), which is reminiscent of the work of Paracelsus (1493–1541) and his famous dictum "*What is there that is not poison? All things are poison, and nothing is without poison. Solely the dose determines that a thing is not a poison.*"

The third element of a model is the cause-effect function f, which is typically a linear or a nonlinear equation. This function is selected either based on the biological mechanism of the process under investigation or, more often, in a purely empirical manner by examining the responses and choosing a suitable curve shape. Every equation f is based on one or more parameters, i.e., constant values represented by Greek or Roman letters; for example, a generic straight line is defined by the equation $f(X) = \beta_0 + \beta_1 \cdot X$, with the two parameters $\theta = [\beta_0, \beta_1]$.

In practice, reality is more complex than our expectations, and due to experimental errors and other effects of a purely random nature, we never observe the expected outcome Y_E, but we observe $Y_O \neq Y_E$. Therefore, we need to augment the model by adding the stochastic component ε:

$$Y_O = f(X, \theta) + \varepsilon \tag{4.2}$$

The ε value is the so-called residual, i.e., the discrepancy between the model prediction (i.e., indeed, unobservable) and what we observe:

$$\varepsilon = Y_O - Y_E \tag{4.3}$$

In an experiment with n experimental units, we have n residuals, with a mean of 0 and a residual sum of squares equal to

$$RSS = \sum_{i=1}^{n} \left(Y_{O_i} - Y_{E_i}\right)^2 \tag{4.4}$$

The standard deviation of model residuals is referred to as the Root Mean Squared Error (RMSE) or σ, and it is typically obtained as $RMSE = \sqrt{SS/(N-P)}$, where N is the number of observations and P is the number of estimated parameters. Roughly speaking, **the RMSE measures how "bad" the model is: The higher the value, the worse the ability of the model to describe the cause-effect relationship under study**.

4.3 Working with a Model

Working with a model in field research typically consists of:

1. Defining a reasonable model to describe the cause-effect relationship under study. Such a model will initially be posed in general terms and based on a set of unknown parameter values, i.e., θ in Eq. (4.2) and σ.
2. Using the dataset to assign precise values to all the unknown parameters so that the model is fully specified (**model fitting** or, in some applications, **model calibration**).
3. Evaluating whether the fitted model provides an accurate description of the experimental data (**model evaluation**); if so, we can conclude that the data support the model and, consequently, the cause-effect relationship that such a model represents.
4. Comparing the model with other suitable models to rule out alternative explanations for the data at hand (**model comparison**).

4.4 Model Fitting

Model fitting is usually performed by the "least squares" algorithm, which consists of selecting the parameter values that minimize the RSS in Eq. (4.4). Although, in a few cases, unbiased solutions can be easily found by hand calculations, a general solution is provided by the `lm()` function in R, which directly minimizes the least squares function using matrix algebra. The R function uses the following syntax:

```
mod <- lm(Y ~ X, data = dataset)
```

The first argument is the equation we want to fit: On its left side, we have to specify the name of the response variable, the "tilde" means "is a function of" and replaces the "=" sign, while on the right side, we have to specify the name of the predictor(s); we do not need to specify the stochastic term ε, which is included by default. As the second argument, if necessary, we provide the name of the dataset where the variables are stored.

4.4.1 Example 4.1: Fitting the "Model of the Mean"

The **model of the mean** is the simplest in the sense that there is no predictor, and, thus, there is no cause-effect relationship. It is used for mensurative experiments and, in general, as the reference against which to evaluate all the more complex models; for this reason, it is often referred to as the **null model**.

Suppose we conducted a mensurative experiment where we collected three water samples from a well to measure the concentration of a xenobiotic substance.

The results are 116, 119, and 125 mg/L, and we want to report the estimated concentration in the well.

We have no predictors, and therefore, we can assume that the observations are generated according to the following model:

$$Y_i = \mu + \varepsilon_i \tag{4.5}$$

In Eq. (4.5), the ith observation is equal to some predetermined value (μ) apart from the random errors ε_i, which are specific to each observation. With this model, the expected value is equal for all observations, and it is the overall mean μ, which, by definition, provides the lowest sum of squared residuals from all the observations in the group.

Consequently, the estimation of model parameters can be easily performed by using the simple approach outlined in Chap. 3 (i.e., $\mu = 120$ and $\sigma = 4.58$); however, it is interesting to see how the same problem can be cast in the model fitting platform (Code Box 4.1). Please note that since we have no predictors, we use "1" as the right side of the model equation, which, according to matrix algebra for linear models, results in the mean of the observations (intercept) being estimated.

As anticipated, using the least squares algorithm for such a simple problem is not recommended; however, it may be helpful as an introduction to the model fitting technique.

Code Box 4.1

```
# Example 4.1
# Fitting the model of the mean

Y <- c(116, 119, 125)
mod <- lm(Y ~ 1)

# Parameter estimate
coef(mod)
## (Intercept)
##         120

# Expected values
fitted(mod)
##   1   2   3
## 120 120 120

# Residuals
residuals(mod)
##  1  2  3
## -4 -1  5
```

```
# Residual Sum of Squares (RSS)
deviance(mod)
## [1] 42

# Standard deviation of residuals (RMSE)
summary(mod)$sigma
## [1] 4.582576
```

4.4.2 Example 4.2: Fitting a Simple Linear Regression Model

To describe the causal effect of a quantitative predictor on a quantitative response, we can use a simple linear regression model, which is strongly related to simple correlation (see Chap. 3), but, in this case, a distinction is made between the cause and the effect, and the direction of the relationship is clearly defined.

Let us consider an experiment in maize, where the weed coverage (in percentage) was determined early in the crop cycle, along with the yield (in tons per hectare) at the end of the crop cycle. The observed data are available as "WeedCover" in the `statforbiology` package; for this experiment, it is possible to expect a cause-effect relationship, where the weed coverage is the predictor (X_i) and the yield is the response (Y_i), according to the linear function (straight line):

$$Y_i = \beta_0 + \beta_1 X_i + \varepsilon_i \tag{4.6}$$

The two parameters β_0 and β_1 represent, respectively, the intercept (yield level without weeds) and slope (change of yield for a one-unit increase in weed coverage). To estimate these two parameters, we can use the `lm()` function (Code Box 4.2), which produces the results shown in Fig. 4.1. Please note that the intercept is fitted by default for all models, and it does not need to be specified.

Fitted values are obtained as model predictions (e.g., $Y_1 = 10.66 - 0.06 \times 105.35 = 4.3$, apart from rounding errors), and the residuals are differences from model predictions and observations (e.g., $2.98 - 4.3 = -1.32$, apart from rounding errors).

Code Box 4.2

```
# Example 4.2
# Fitting a simple linear regression model

# Loading the packages and data
library(statforbiology)
dataset <- getAgroData("WeedCover")
head(dataset)
```

```
##   WeedCover Yield
## 1    105.35  2.98
## 2     27.50  8.89
## 3     68.80  4.70
## 4     23.80  9.66
## 5     12.70  8.30
## 6     42.70  9.53

# Fitting the model
mod <- lm(Yield ~ WeedCover, data = dataset)

# Inspecting the estimates
coef(mod)
## (Intercept)   WeedCover
## 10.65979798 -0.06033652

# Fitted values
fitted(mod)
##        1        2        3        4        5        6
## 4.303346 9.000544 6.508646 9.223789 9.893524 8.083429
##        7        8        9       10       11       12
## 8.759198 8.379078 9.519438 8.499751 7.974823 9.971962
##       13       14       15       16
## 8.753164 5.356218 2.580738 2.422355

# Residuals
residuals(mod)
##          1          2          3          4          5
## -1.3233458 -0.1105437 -1.8086455  0.4362112 -1.5935242
##          6          7          8          9         10
##  1.4465714  0.3908023  1.4109224 -0.5994378  0.3302494
##         11         12         13         14         15
##  1.7151771 -0.5819617 -0.2931640 -0.1662180 -0.4007382
##         16
##  1.1476452

# RSS
deviance(mod)
## [[1] 17.34042

# RMSE
summary(mod)$sigma
## [1] 1.112925
```

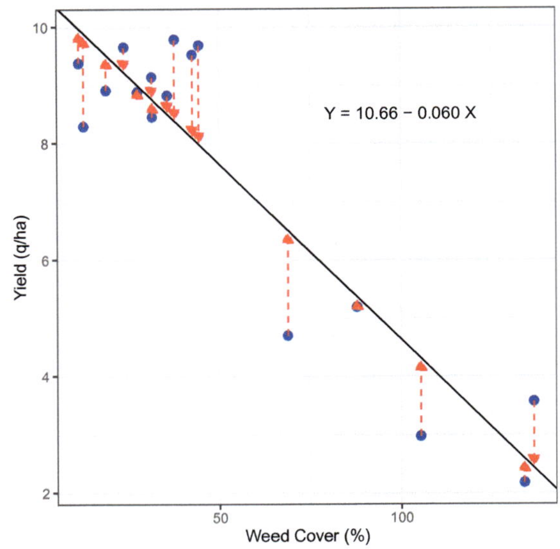

Fig. 4.1 Example 4.2: The least square estimate is represented by the straight line that passes as close as possible to the observed data points

4.4.3 Example 4.3: Fitting a One-Way ANOVA Model

Models containing nominal predictors consist of a set of equations that only predict the outcomes for the predictor levels included in the experiment. With loose language, these models are often referred to as ANOVA models, as the primary interest typically lies in comparing the means of treatment groups by using the ANOVA method, which will be described later in this chapter.

Fitting ANOVA models requires the so-called dummy coding, although modern statistical applications, such as R, handle this coding on our behalf. However, we need to transform the predictor variable into a factor explicitly; otherwise we may fit the wrong model, primarily when the predictor uses a numerical coding. In R, such a transformation is performed by using the `factor()` function (Code Box 4.3).

Let us consider a field experiment to compare the yield of four oat genotypes (designated as A, B, C, and D) using a completely randomized design with three replicates. The dataset is available as “Oat1L” in the `statforbiology` package and is shown in Table 4.1.

A linear model for this example is

$$Y_i = \mu_j + \varepsilon_i \tag{4.7}$$

This model extends the model of the mean in Eq. (4.5) and states that the observed yield in the ith plot equals the mean of the treatment group to which that plot belongs, plus the stochastic effects ε_i, which are specific to each plot and have a mean of 0 and a standard deviation of σ.

The above model is most often coded in another form that includes the intercept term, as in Eq. (4.6):

Table 4.1 Sample data for a field experiment with four oat genotypes (A, B, C, and D) in a completely randomized design with three replicates

Genotype	Yield
A	4.50
A	4.65
A	4.59
B	3.70
B	3.38
B	3.58
C	4.17
C	3.94
C	4.14
D	4.76
D	4.48
D	4.55

$$Y_{ij} = \mu + \alpha_j + \varepsilon_{ij} \tag{4.8}$$

In this equation, the yield in the ith replicate of the jth treatment level is obtained as the sum of the "baseline" intercept value μ, plus the treatment effect α_j depending on genotype j, plus the stochastic effects ε_{ij}.

To understand the biological meaning of μ and α_j, we can consider the first observation $Y_{11} = 4.5$; we need to estimate three values (μ, α_1, and ε_{11}) that sum to 4.5. There are an infinite number of such triplets, and therefore, the estimation problem is undetermined unless we put constraints on some model parameters, corresponding to different **model parameterizations**. A very common constraint is $\alpha_1 = 0$ (**treatment constraint**):

$$\begin{cases} \mu_1 = \mu + \alpha_1 = \mu + 0 \\ \mu_2 = \mu + \alpha_2 \\ \mu_3 = \mu + \alpha_3 \\ \mu_4 = \mu + \alpha_4 \end{cases} \tag{4.9}$$

With such a constraint, μ is the mean of the first treatment level (in R, by default, it is the **first in alphabetical order**), while α_2, α_3, and α_4 are the differences between, respectively, the means of the second, third, and fourth treatment levels and the mean of the first one.

Another possible constraint is $\sum \alpha_j = 0$ (**sum-to-zero** constraint). If we take the previous equation and sum all members, we get

$$\mu_1 + \mu_2 + \mu_3 + \mu_4 = 4\mu + \sum \alpha_j \tag{4.10}$$

Imposing the sum-to-zero constraint, we get to

$$\mu_1 + \mu_2 + \mu_3 + \mu_4 = 4\mu \tag{4.11}$$

and then to

$$\mu = \frac{\mu_1 + \mu_2 + \mu_3 + \mu_4}{4} \tag{4.12}$$

In other words, with the sum-to-zero parameterization, μ is the overall mean, while the α_j values represent the differences between the treatment means and the overall mean (**treatment effects**). The last parameter is not estimated, but it is constrained to be the opposite of the sum of the previous three [$\alpha_4 = -(\alpha_1 + \alpha_2 + \alpha_3)$].

The selection of the parameterization is up to the user; **in R, the treatment constraint is adopted by default**, although the other parameterizations can be easily implemented, by using the appropriate coding (Code Box 4.3).

Code Box 4.3 illustrates the coding for this model; the expected values for all observations are independent of the selected parameterization, and for balanced data (the same number of replicates for all treatment groups), they correspond to the mean of the group to which each observation belongs (Code Box 4.3).

Code Box 4.3

```
# Example 4.3
# Fitting a model with one nominal predictor
# (One-way ANOVA)

# Loading the packages and data
library(statforbiology)
dataset <- getAgroData("Oat1L")
dataset$Genotype <- factor(dataset$Genotype)
   # The previous line is optional

# Fitting the model with treatment constraint (default)
mod <- lm(Yield ~ Genotype, data = dataset)

# Estimated parameters
coef(mod)
## (Intercept)   GenotypeB   GenotypeC   GenotypeD
##  4.58000000 -1.02666667 -0.49666667  0.01666667

# Expected values
fitted(mod)
##        1        2        3        4        5        6
## 4.580000 4.580000 4.580000 3.553333 3.553333 3.553333
##        7        8        9       10       11       12
## 4.083333 4.083333 4.083333 4.596667 4.596667 4.596667
```

```
# Residuals
residuals(mod)
##           1           2           3           4           5
## -0.08000000  0.07000000  0.01000000  0.14666667 -0.17333333
##           6           7           8           9          10
##  0.02666667  0.08666667 -0.14333333  0.05666667  0.16333333
##          11          12
## -0.11666667 -0.04666667

# Deviance of residuals
deviance(mod)
## [1] 0.1374

# Standard deviation of residuals
summary(mod)$sigma
## [1] 0.1310534

# Fitting the same model with the sum-to-zero constraint
mod2 <- lm(Yield ~ Genotype, data = dataset,
           contrasts = list(Genotype = "contr.sum"))
coef(mod2)
## (Intercept)   Genotype1   Genotype2   Genotype3
##   4.2033333   0.3766667  -0.6500000  -0.1200000

# Fitting the same model by removing the intercept (Eq. 4.7)
mod3 <- lm(Yield ~ Genotype - 1, data = dataset)
coef(mod3)
## GenotypeA GenotypeB GenotypeC GenotypeD
##  4.580000  3.553333  4.083333  4.596667
```

Once the model is fully specified, we have the ingredients to predict the 12 experimental observations by summing $\mu + \alpha_j + \varepsilon_{ij}$; for example, for the first observation, belonging to the first genotype, we have

$$y_{11} = 4.5 = 4.58 + 0 - 0.080 \tag{4.13}$$

For the fourth observation, belonging to the second genotype, we have

$$y_{21} = 3.7 = 4.58 - 1.027 + 0.147 \tag{4.14}$$

For the sake of completeness, Code Box 4.3 shows how we can implement the sum-to-zero constraint by setting the argument "contrasts" and passing a list of factors associated with the "contr.sum" string (i.e., `contrasts = list(Genotype = "contr.sum")` in Code Box 4.3). As mentioned before, with this parameterization, the effect of the fourth genotype is constrained, and therefore, it is not estimated and is not displayed.

To fit Eq. (4.7), we can remove the intercept by using "-1" on the right side of the model expression, as shown in Code Box 4.3.

Several other methods exist to change the parameterization, either globally (for the entire R session) or at the factor level; further information can be found, e.g., in Faraway (2025).

4.5 Variance Partitioning

In Example 4.3, the cause-effect relationship between genotype and yield was described through a model containing a single predictor. We may wonder how "strong" such a relationship is, or, in other words, how good is the description of the data provided by the model. A relevant statistic is the RMSE (σ), which is straightforward to interpret: The lower this value, the better the ability of the model to describe the cause-effect relationship under study. In this case, the RMSE is equal to 0.131, which appears to be pretty low, considering that the overall mean of the data is 4.203.

Another statistic of interest is the RRMSE (Relative Root Mean Square of Error), which is analogous to the coefficient of variation and is obtained by dividing the RMSE by the mean of the observed values. In this example, the RRMSE is $0.131/4.203 = 0.031$, indicating that the residual error variability is 3.1% of the overall mean (a relatively good fit, indeed).

To improve our understanding of the relevance of cause-effect relationships, we can use a technique named "ANalysis Of VAriance" (ANOVA), which was initially devised by Ronald Fisher during the 30 s of the twentieth century and has nowadays been enhanced and cast in the platform of model fitting.

The basic principle of ANOVA is that, for the data obtained in every experiment, it is always possible to define two alternative models:

1. The model under study (full model)
2. A reduced model obtained from the previous one by removing one of the predictors

In the case of Example 4.3, the full model (in R coding) is

```
Yield ~ Genotype
```

Otherwise, the reduced model corresponds to the model of the mean:

```
Yield ~ 1
```

The result of removing the predictor is that the RSS increases, indicating that the reduced model is worse than the full model. The difference between the RSS for the reduced model and the RSS for the full model is taken as the sum of squares for the effect under investigation.

4.5.1 *Example 4.3: Variance Partitioning*

We apply this basic principle to the data from Example 4.3. First, we obtain the residual sum of squares (RSS) for the full model (Code Box 4.4).

Code Box 4.4

```
# Example 4.3 [continuation]
# RSS for the full model

RSS.full <- deviance(mod)
RSS.full
## [1] 0.1374
```

Next, the reduced model is fitted, and the RSS for this model is also determined. The RSS for the full model is subtracted from the RSS for the reduced model, and the resulting difference is the SS for the genotype effect (Code Box 4.5).

Code Box 4.5

```
# Example 4.3 [continuation]
# Sum of squares for the genotype effect

# Fitting null model
modnull <- lm(Yield ~ 1, data = dataset)

# RSS for the null model
RSS.null <- deviance(modnull)
RSS.null
## [1] 2.337867

# Contribution of genotype effect
SS_g <- RSS.null - RSS.full
SS_g
## [1] 2.200467
```

The RSS for the null model can be regarded as the total sum of squares for yield, in the sense that it is a statistic measuring total data variation (see Chap. 3). Thus, we have just decomposed the total sum of squares of yield ($SS_{tot} = 2.338$) into two parts: one due to the causal effect of the experimental treatment ($SS_g = 2.200$) and the other due to all other unknown effects of a random nature ($RSS = 0.138$). Our intuition is that **the cause-effect relationship between the genotype and yield is relevant whenever the variability produced by the genotype effect on yield is higher than the variability produced by all the other effects of a random nature**.

Unfortunately, we cannot directly compare SS_g and RSS, as these two sums of squares are based on a different number of Degrees of Freedom (DF). We need to ask ourselves "what is the number of DF for SS_g and RSS?" Indeed, SS_g was calculated using only three different α values (α_1 was constrained to be 0), so it has 3 DF (in general, the number of DF for the treatment sum of squares equals the number of its levels minus one). On the other hand, the RSS was calculated from the differences between each value and the respective group mean, and, therefore, these differences were constrained to sum to zero within each group. Hence, there are 2 DF per group, and the total number of DF is 8. In more general terms, for experiments with one nominal predictor, the number of DF for the RSS is $p \times (k - 1)$ (where p is the number of levels of the nominal predictor and k is the number of replicates, assuming that this is constant across treatments). Even more generally, the number of DF for the RSS is $N - P$, where N is the number of observations and P is the number of estimated parameters (in this case, $12 - 4 = 8$). We can calculate the corresponding variances (mean squares in Code Box 4.6):

Code Box 4.6

```
# Example 4.3 [continuation]
# Mean squares

# Mean square for the treatment effect
MS_g <- SS_g/3
MS_g
## [1] 0.7334889

# Residual mean square
MS_e <- RSS.full/8
MS_e
## [1] 0.017175
```

These two variances (treatment and residual) can be directly compared by using the so-called F-ratio:

$$F = \frac{MS_g}{RMS} = \frac{0.7335}{0.0172} = 42.71 \tag{4.15}$$

The F-ratio derives its name from Fisher, who invented it. The results indicate that the variability imposed by the experimental treatment is more than 42 times higher than the variability due to random noise, which supports the idea that the causal effect of genotype on yield is highly relevant. In general terms, the higher the F-ratio, the stronger the causation. We can summarize these results in the so-called ANOVA table, which is easily obtained by using the `anova()` function in R (Code Box 4.7).

Code Box 4.7

```
# Example 4.3 [continuation]
# Variance partitioning with R

anova(mod)
## Analysis of Variance Table
##
## Response: Yield
##           Df Sum Sq Mean Sq F value    Pr(>F)
## Genotype   3 2.2005 0.73349  42.707 2.866e-05 ***
## Residuals  8 0.1374 0.01717
```

The value at the extreme right is the so-called P-value (2.87×10^{-05}), which serves as an inferential indicator, and will be explained in Chap. 7. For now, it will suffice to say that when the P-value is lower than 0.05, we conclude that the treatment effect (in this case, the genotype effect) is *statistically significant*.

4.6 Models with Blocking Factors

For the experiments designed in blocks, apart from the treatment factor(s) under study, there is a grouping factor (i.e., the blocks) that poses a constraint on complete randomization. Grouping factors need to be included in models, even though the researcher may have no specific interest in their impact. Such an inclusion is required to perform valid inferences and draw reliable conclusions, as will be explained in Chap. 8 and 12.

4.6.1 Example 4.4: Fitting a Model to the Data from an RCBD

Let us reconsider the data from Example 4.3 (Table 4.1) and imagine that the experiment was designed in blocks, with the three replicates of each genotype obtained in blocks 1, 2, and 3, respectively. In this case, the causal relationship needs to be different because the yield levels (quantitative response) depend on two variables, i.e., the genotype and the block, according to the following linear model:

$$Y_{ij} = \mu + \gamma_i + \alpha_j + \varepsilon_{ij} \tag{4.16}$$

where Y_{ij} is the yield for the plot in the ith block and with the jth genotype, μ is the intercept, γ_i is the effect of the ith block, α_j is the effect of the jth genotype, and ε is the residual plot error, with a standard deviation equal to σ. As we did for the one-way ANOVA model in Example 4.3, we need to impose constraints on the α and γ values so that the model parameters are estimable. If we impose that $\alpha_1 = 0$ and $\gamma_1 = 0$ (treatment constraint), the intercept μ is the expected value for the first genotype in the first block. Consequently, there are three genotype parameters and two block parameters to estimate in addition to μ and σ.

The model fitting can be performed with R by transforming the block variable into a factor and adding the block effect to the model, as shown in Code Box 4.8.

Code Box 4.8

```
# Example 4.4
# Data analysis for the 'Oat1LRCBD' dataset, relating to a
# RCBD experiment

# Loading the packages and data
library(statforbiology)
dataset <- getAgroData("Oat1LRCBD")
dataset$Block <- factor(dataset$Block)
head(dataset)
##   Genotype Block Yield
## 1        A     1  4.50
## 2        A     2  4.65
## 3        A     3  4.59
## 4        B     1  3.70
## 5        B     2  3.38
## 6        B     3  3.58

# Model fitting
mod2 <- lm(Yield ~ Genotype + Block, data = dataset)
```

```
# Residuals and RSS
epsilon <- residuals(mod2)
RSS <- sum(epsilon^2)
RSS
## [1] 0.07878333

# RMSE (sigma)
summary(mod2)$sigma
## [1] 0.1145886
```

Expectedly, the residuals from this model are smaller than those from the previous one, as the block effect contributed to a better description of the dataset. If we remove the block term, the RSS increases from 0.079 to 0.137. Consequently, the sum of squares for the block effect is equal to 0.137 − 0.079 = 0.058. If we re-include the block term and remove the genotype term, we confirm that the increase in RSS with respect to the full model is 2.200 (Code Box 4.9). If we remove both effects and fit the null model, the residual sum of squares increases to 2.338 (total sum of squares, see Code Box 4.5).

Code Box 4.9

```
# Example 4.4 [continuation]
# Variance partitioning

# Removing the blocks
mod3 <- lm(Yield ~ Genotype, data = dataset) # Same model as
        before
deviance(mod3)
## [1] 0.1374
SS_b <- deviance(mod3) - RSS
SS_b
## [1] 0.05861667

# Removing the genotypes
mod4 <- lm(Yield ~ Block, data = dataset)
deviance(mod4)
## [1] 2.27925
SS_g <- deviance(mod4) - RSS
SS_g
## [1] 2.200467
```

The number of degrees of freedom is, respectively, 11 for the total sum of squares SS_{tot}, 3 for the genotypes, and 2 for the blocks; by subtraction, we calculate that the residual sum of squares for the full model has 6 DF. Now, we have all the elements to calculate the mean squares and the two F-ratios; in practice, we can skip all hand calculations and obtain the final ANOVA table by the anova() function, as mentioned earlier (Code Box 4.10).

Code Box 4.10

```
# Example 4.4 [continuation]
# Variance partitioning with R

anova(mod2)
## Analysis of Variance Table
##
## Response: Yield
##           Df  Sum Sq Mean Sq F value    Pr(>F)
## Genotype   3 2.20047 0.73349 55.8612 8.916e-05 ***
## Block      2 0.05862 0.02931  2.2321 0.1885
## Residuals  6 0.07878 0.01313
```

The F-ratios suggest that the causal effect of genotypes is high, while the block effect is very low. The P-value for the genotype effect is lower than 0.05, implying that this effect is statistically significant.

4.7 Interaction Between Experimental Factors

In multifactorial experiments with two (or more) crossed factors, several replicates are usually available for each factor combination, and consequently, the situation is somewhat different from that of the previous example, where only one replicate was available for each genotype in each block. In the presence of those replicates, apart from the causal effects of the two factors under investigation, it is also possible to evaluate their **interaction**, which is a very relevant piece of information and represents the main reason why performing a single factorial experiments is preferred over setting up two separate experiments, one for each experimental factor.

To gain an understanding of the interaction effect, we can examine Fig. 4.2, which displays three possible situations, related to the combinations between factor A with two levels (A1 and A2) and factor B with two levels (B1 and B2). Each symbol represents a combination; for example, in the left panel, we see that the A1B1 combination yielded a response of 10, while the A2B1 combination yielded

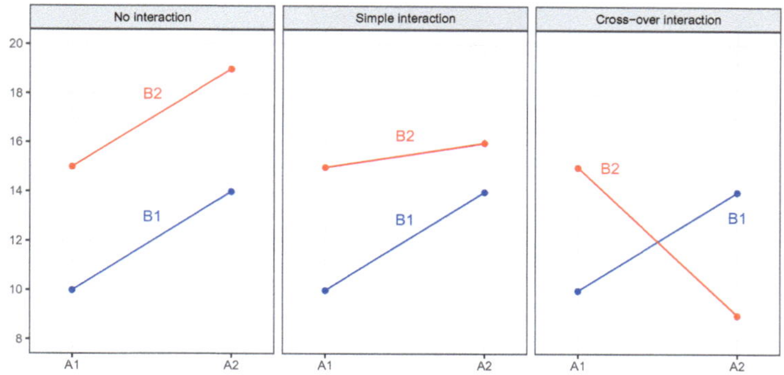

Fig. 4.2 Possible relationships between the two experimental factors A (with the two levels A1 and A2) and B (with the two levels B1 and B2)

a response of 14. Therefore, passing from A1 to A2 (with B1) gave an effect of +4 units. Likewise, we see that the yield of A1B2 was 15, and thus, passing from B1 to B2 had an effect of +5 units. Accordingly, we can predict the yield of A2B2 by summing up the yield of A1B1, the effect of passing from A1 to A2, and the effect of passing from B1 to B2, i.e., $10+4+5 = 19$. In this case A and B do not interact with each other, and their effects are purely additive.

Now, let us look at the central panel. Passing from A1B1 to A2B1 and from A1B1 to A1B2 produced the same effects as in the previous case (respectively, +4 and +5 units). However, we can no longer predict the response of A2B2, as the observed value of 16 differs from the expected value of 19 under additivity. There must be some effect that hinders the response of this specific combination A2B2, and such an effect is known as the **interaction between factors A and B** (or "A $\times$ B" interaction). We can quantify this interaction effect as $16 - 19 = -3$ units; this is an example of a negative interaction, as the observed response is lower than the expected response. Furthermore, this is an example of **simple interaction**, where the expected response is lower, but the ranking of treatments remains unaffected; indeed, A2 is always higher than A1, regardless of B, and B1 is always lower than B2, regardless of A.

If we look at the right panel, we see that the interaction effect is even more dramatic: For A2B2, we observe a value of 9 instead of 19, which means that the interaction effect is -10 units, and it causes a change in ranking: A2 is higher than A1 when B is equal to B1, while the ranking is reversed when B is equal to B2. Whenever the interaction effect modifies the ranking of treatments, we refer to it as a **crossover interaction**.

Why are we so concerned by the interaction? Let us take a further look at the third situation, as seen in the right panel of Fig. 4.2. Table 4.2 shows the means for the four combinations (A1B1, A1B2, A2B1, and A2B2) that are traditionally named **cell means**, together with the means for main factor levels (A1, A2, B1, and B2), usually named **marginal means**, as well as the overall mean.

Table 4.2 Crossover interaction between experimental factors

	B1	B2	Average
A1	10.0	15.0	12.5
A2	14.0	9.0	11.5
Average	12.0	12.0	12.0

If we examine the marginal means, we might get the wrong impression that factor A has only a minor effect while factor B is ineffective. Indeed, both factors have a very wide effect, although the presence of a crossover interaction mitigates it.

That is why we are so concerned about possible interactions between the experimental factors: These effects can be highly misleading when examining the marginal means of A and B.

4.7.1 Example 4.5: A Multi-environment Experiment

Let us consider that the experiment in Example 4.3 was repeated in another location by using a completely randomized design in both locations. The observed data are available as "Oat2L" in the `statforbiology` package.

For such a multisite experiment, the observed yields in the kth replicate of the ith genotype and jth location are subjected to the causal effect of:

1. Genotypes
2. Locations
3. "Genotype by location" interactions

Accordingly, a linear model can be written as

$$Y_{ijk} = \mu + \alpha_i + \beta_j + \alpha\beta_{ij} + \varepsilon_{ijk} \tag{4.17}$$

In this model, μ is the intercept, α_i is the effect of the ith genotype, β_j is the effect of the jth location, and $\alpha\beta_{ij}$ is the interaction effect of the combination between the ith genotype and jth location. The unknown random effects are represented by the residuals ε_{ij}, with a mean equal to 0 and a standard deviation equal to σ.

To estimate model parameters with R, we need to consider that the interaction between two factors (e.g., A and B) is coded by using the ":" operator:

```
Y ~ A + B + A:B
```

We can use the "*" operator as the short form to specify, altogether, the main effects and their interaction (see Code Box 4.11):

```
Y ~ A * B
```

Code Box 4.11

```
# Example 4.5
# A genotype experiment in two locations

# Loading the packages and data
library(statforbiology)
dataset <- getAgroData("Oat2L")
head(dataset)
##   Location Genotype Yield
## 1     LOC1        A  4.50
## 2     LOC1        A  4.65
## 3     LOC1        A  4.59
## 4     LOC1        B  3.70
## 5     LOC1        B  3.38
## 6     LOC1        B  3.58

# Fitting a two-way model with interaction
mod <- lm(Yield ~ Genotype * Location, data = dataset)

# Exploring parameter estimates
coef(mod)
##           (Intercept)             GenotypeB
##           4.580000000          -1.026666667
##             GenotypeC             GenotypeD
##          -0.496666667           0.016666667
##          LocationLOC2 GenotypeB:LocationLOC2
##           0.420000000           2.260000000
## GenotypeC:LocationLOC2 GenotypeD:LocationLOC2
##          -0.003333333           0.583333333

summary(mod)$sigma
## [1] 0.4598958
```

Calculating the sum of squares for all effects is performed by repeatedly fitting the model and omitting effects (as we have done so far). In the presence of interactions, we should obey the marginality restrictions, considering that the interaction is marginal to the main effects that are involved in it. Consequently, it should be omitted first, and it should not be left in the model when one of the involved main effects is removed (Code Box 4.12).

Code Box 4.12

```
# Example 4.5 [continuation]
# Variance partitioning

# Residual sum of squares for the full model
RSS <- deviance(mod)

# removing the interaction
modred <- lm(Yield ~ Genotype + Location, data = dataset)
SSint <- deviance(modred) - RSS
SSint
## [1] 5.147233

# removing the genotype AND the interaction
modred <- lm(Yield ~ Location, data = dataset)
SSloc <- deviance(modred) - RSS - SSint
SSloc
## [1] 2.113233

# removing the location AND the interaction
modred <- lm(Yield ~ Genotype, data = dataset)
SSgen <- deviance(modred) - RSS - SSint
SSgen
## [1] 7.6614
```

As in the previous examples, we have partitioned total data variability into four terms, three of which relate to causal effects, while the fourth relates to all other random effects. In practice, we do not need to perform those hand calculations, and we can use the `anova()` method in R (Code Box 4.13). In the following table, the only element that we have not mentioned before is the number of degrees of freedom for the interaction term, which is **equal to the product of the number of DF for the main effects**.

Code Box 4.13

```
# Example 4.5 [continuation]
# Variance partitioning with R

anova(mod)
## Analysis of Variance Table
```

```
##
## Response: Yield
##                   Df Sum Sq Mean Sq F value    Pr(>F)
## Genotype           3 2.1132  0.7044  3.3305  0.046228 *
## Location           1 7.6614  7.6614 36.2234 1.788e-05 ***
## Genotype:Location  3 5.1472  1.7157  8.1121  0.001646 **
## Residuals         16 3.3841  0.2115
```

4.8 Unbalanced Data

Before concluding this chapter, it is necessary to point out that there are several methods for calculating the sum of squares for model effects, and they do not necessarily yield the same results, particularly when the data are unbalanced, i.e., there are a different number of replicates for each treatment group. The method proposed in this book is based on:

1. Fitting the full model to the observed data
2. Removing the effect under study and fitting the reduced model
3. Subtracting the residual sum of squares of the full model from the residual sum of squares of the reduced model

This approach produces the so-called *marginal sum of squares*, and although we have so far obtained the same results, it is not the same as the approach used with the `anova()` function in R. Indeed, this latter function produces the so-called *sequential sum of squares*, which are the same as marginal sum of squares only with balanced data (the same number of replicates for all treatment groups). With unbalanced data, we strongly recommend using the *marginal sum of squares*, which are produced by the `Anova()` function (note the capital letter) in the `car` package.

4.8.1 *Example 4.6: Fitting an ANOVA Model to Unbalanced Data*

Suppose that we have conducted an experiment to evaluate the selectivity of a postemergence herbicide for weed control in maize, depending on the timing of intervention (2-, 4-, 6-, and 8-leaf stage, plus an untreated, hand-weeded control). The experimental design was randomized in complete blocks, and one value is missing at random from the response variable (weight in grams per plant, at the end of June). The missing value is represented as "NA" (Code Box 4.14).

If a model with two nominal predictors is fitted to this data, the `anova()` method in base R leads to different ANOVA tables, depending on the order in which the two effects (genotype and block) are entered into the model (see Code Box 4.14). Since we have no rationale for deciding which effect should be entered first, the conclusions obtained with the anova() function are purely arbitrary, which is unacceptable.

Code Box 4.14

```
# Example 4.6
# Variance partitioning with unbalanced data

# Loading the packages
library(statforbiology)
library(car)

# Loading the data
dataset <- getAgroData("Timings_77490")
dataset$Block <- factor(dataset$Block)
head(dataset)
##   Plot   Timing Block Height_30 Weight_30 FinalYield
## 1    3 2-Leaves     1    192.50     81.70   96.38328
## 2    7 2-Leaves     2    200.00        NA  135.29526
## 3   15 2-Leaves     3    202.50     89.94  141.77501
## 4   18 2-Leaves     4    213.75     81.81  132.06582
## 5    2 4-Leaves     1    183.75     65.78  129.86594
## 6   10 4-Leaves     2    197.25     72.36  140.52353

# Fitting two models with a different ordering of model terms
mod1 <- lm(Weight_30 ~ Timing + Block, data = dataset)
mod2 <- lm(Weight_30 ~ Block + Timing, data = dataset)

# Variance partitioning
anova(mod1)
## Analysis of Variance Table
##
## Response: Weight_30
##           Df Sum Sq Mean Sq F value   Pr(>F)
## Timing     4 1790.7  447.67  9.3601 0.001511 **
## Block      3  230.5   76.83  1.6065 0.244040
## Residuals 11  526.1   47.83

anova(mod2)
## Analysis of Variance Table
##
## Response: Weight_30
```

```
##            Df  Sum Sq Mean Sq F value    Pr(>F)
## Block      3  169.46   56.49  1.1811 0.361390
## Timing     4 1851.72  462.93  9.6792 0.001318 **
## Residuals 11  526.10   47.83
```

The approach proposed earlier, based on removing the two predictors, one at a time, leads to the sum of squares shown in Code Box 4.15; these sum of squares (for the timing and the block effects) are the same, regardless of the order with which the two effects were included in the full model. To reproduce these results, the `Anova()` function needs the `type = 2` argument (the default). Further information about the types of sum of squares can be found in Langsrud (2003).

Code Box 4.15

```
# Example 4.6 [continuation]

# Removing the predictors one at a time (from 'mod1')
RSS <- deviance(mod1)
mod1.red <- lm(Weight_30 ~ Block, data = dataset)
# Removing the timing
SS_g <- deviance(mod1.red) - RSS
SS_g
## [1] 1851.715
mod1.red2 <- lm(Weight_30 ~ Timing, data = dataset)
# Removing the block
SS_b <- deviance(mod1.red2) - RSS
SS_b
## [1] 230.5048

# Removing the predictors one at a time (from 'mod2')
RSS <- deviance(mod2)
mod2.red <- lm(Weight_30 ~ Block, data = dataset)
# Removing the timing
SS_g <- deviance(mod2.red) - RSS
SS_g
## [1] 1851.715
mod2.red2 <- lm(Weight_30 ~ Timing, data = dataset)
# Removing the block
SS_b <- deviance(mod2.red2) - RSS
SS_b
## [1] 230.5048
```

```
# Using the Anova() method in the 'car' package
Anova(mod1, type = 2)
## Anova Table (Type II tests)
##
## Response: Weight_30
##           Sum Sq Df F value   Pr(>F)
## Timing    1851.7  4  9.6792 0.001318 **
## Block      230.5  3  1.6065 0.244040
## Residuals  526.1 11

Anova(mod2, type = 2)
## Anova Table (Type II tests)
##
## Response: Weight_30
##           Sum Sq Df F value   Pr(>F)
## Block      230.5  3  1.6065 0.244040
## Timing    1851.7  4  9.6792 0.001318 **
## Residuals  526.1 11
```

4.9 Conclusions

In this chapter, we have presented a method for assessing whether a dataset obtained from a controlled experiment can reasonably support the existence of cause-effect relationships between the variables under study.

This method consists of:

1. Fitting a reasonable cause-effect model into the observed data
2. Using the variance partitioning (ANOVA) method to obtain the mean squares (variances) for all causal effects under investigation and the mean square for all the other effects of random nature (residual mean square)
3. Comparing the mean squares for the causal effects with the mean square for random effects by using F-ratios. The higher the F-ratio, the stronger the cause-effect relationship.

For the variance partitioning method with R, there are two available functions, `anova()` in base R and `Anova()` in the `car` package. These two functions give the same results with balanced data, but the second one is highly recommended when the data are not balanced.

4.10 Questions and Exercises

1. What is the difference between joint variation and causation?
2. In numbers, what do we intend by saying "treatment effect?"
3. Describe with a few sentences what the ANOVA is and why it is used.
4. What is the definition of "interaction between two experimental factors"? Explain briefly.
5. Consider the "`rimsulfuron`" data in the `statforbiology` package, relating to a field experiment comparing 14 herbicides and two untreated checks, with four replicates per treatment. The experiment was designed in a randomized complete block design. Considering the yield variable, perform the ANOVA with R, and evaluate the relevance of the herbicide effect.
6. A field experiment was conducted to evaluate the effect of fertilization timing (early, optimal, late) on two genotypes (A and B). The experiment was designed as a randomized complete block design, and the data represent the amount of absorbed nitrogen by the plant. Fit the appropriate linear model, assess whether the timing of fertilization exerted a relevant effect and whether the relative ranking of fertilizers was influenced by the genotype. The dataset is available as "`FertilizationTiming`" in the `statforbiology` package.
7. A chemical process requires one alcohol and one base, and a study is organized to evaluate the factorial combinations of three alcohols (1–3) and two bases (A and B) on the process efficiency, expressed as a percentage. The experiment is completely randomized. Assess the relevance of the two main effects and their interaction. The dataset is available as "`AlcoholBase`" in the `statforbiology` package.
8. An experiment with a completely randomized design and two replicates was conducted to compare two maize genotypes (G1 and G2) under two different fertilization strategies (F1 and F2). Calculate the mean squares and F-ratios for the genotype and fertilization effects and for their interaction. Are the causal effects relevant? The dataset is shown below. Enter the data in R manually, and create a dataframe. Analyze this dataframe to answer the previous questions.

Genotype	Fertilizer	Yield
G1	F1	11.29
G1	F1	12.78
G1	F2	12.58
G1	F2	9.15
G2	F1	14.93
G2	F1	15.01
G2	F2	12.93
G2	F2	12.95

References

Faraway J (2025) Linear Models with R, 3rd edn. CRC Press, Boca Raton

Gavasso-Rita YL, Papalexiou SM, Li Y, Elshorbagy A, Li Z, Schuster–Wallace C (2024) Crop models and their use in assessing crop production and food security: a review. Food Energy Secur 13(1):e503. https://doi.org/10.1002/fes3.503. https://onlinelibrary.wiley.com/doi/10.1002/fes3.503

Gherman IM, Abdallah ZS, Pang W, Gorochowski TE, Grierson CS, Marucci L (2023) Bridging the gap between mechanistic biological models and machine learning surrogates. PLOS Comput Biol 19(4):1–16. https://doi.org/10.1371/journal.pcbi.1010988

Langsrud O (2003) ANOVA for unbalanced data: use type II instead of Type III sums of squares. Stat Comput 13(2):163–167

Pasley H, Brown H, Holzworth D, Whish J, Bell L, Huth N (2023) How to build a crop model. A review. Agron Sustain Develop 43(1):2. https://doi.org/10.1007/s13593-022-00854-9. https://link.springer.com/10.1007/s13593-022-00854-9

Ratkowsky DA (1990) Handbook of Nonlinear Regression Models. Dekker, New York

Shadish W, Cook T, Campbell D (2002) Experimental and Quasi-Experimental Designs for Generalized Causal Inference, 2nd edn. Cengage Learning, Boston

Zaniletti I, Larson DR, Lewallen DG, Berry DJ, Maradit Kremers H (2023) How to distinguish correlation from causation in orthopaedic research. J Arthropl 38(4):634–637. https://doi.org/10.1016/j.arth.2022.11.019. https://linkinghub.elsevier.com/retrieve/pii/S0883540322010403

Chapter 5
Stochastic Models

Models are wrong, but some are useful
—G. Box

Abstract Although a model can predict the expected outcome of an experiment, the residuals have a purely random nature, and consequently, the observable outcome is entirely unpredictable. However, it is usually assumed that, although random, the residuals follow a particular distribution of probability, allowing us to understand which outcomes are more likely to occur. This chapter introduces the Gaussian density function and demonstrates how it can be used to calculate probabilities and simulate future experimental outcomes, through the adoption of Monte Carlo methods.

At this point, an obvious question is can we make use of a fully specified model to make predictions, i.e., to forecast the outcome of a future experiment of the same type? The answer is not so obvious; indeed, we can use the deterministic part of the model to make predictions about the expected outcome (Y_E), which is produced under a cause-effect relationship. Unfortunately, the actual outcome (Y_O) is entirely unpredictable due to the effects of the stochastic elements ε, which change randomly at each sampling effort and confound our observations.

Although we have no way to predict a random outcome, we can make some reasonable guesses. Let us imagine that the expected value, as predicted by the model, is $Y_E = 120$; we should expect that if the model is correct, it is very likely to observe a value of 119 or 121 ($\varepsilon = \pm 1$), less likely to observe 100 or 140 mg/L ($\varepsilon = \pm 20$), very unlikely to observe 80 or 160 mg/L ($\varepsilon = \pm 40$). Consequently, it should be possible to assign a value of probability to each possible ε value (and thus to each possible Y_O outcome) by using some probability function.

A. Onofri, *Field Research Methods in Agriculture*,
https://doi.org/10.1007/978-3-032-08199-5_5

5.1 Probability Functions

In contrast to cause-effect models, probability functions do not predict the outcomes of experiments; instead, they associate each possible outcome with its corresponding probability level. We may be familiar with probability functions for discrete events, which can only take one of a finite list of possible values y. For example, considering that the probability of a discrete event E is the number of outcomes favorable to E divided by the total number of possible outcomes (frequentist definition of probability), we can derive the probability of drawing an ace from a deck of 52 cards. There are four aces in the deck, and thus, the probability of drawing one of those is $4/52 = 0.077$. It is also easy to calculate the probability of getting two heads in two coin tosses: As we have four possible outcomes (head/head, head/tail, tail/head, and tail/tail), that probability is 1/4 = 0.25.

Calculating probabilities for quantitative outcomes, such as yield, is not straightforward, as there is an infinite number of possible outcomes, and the probability of obtaining a precise outcome value (e.g., 12 t/ha and not 12.0000001 or 11.999999) is infinitesimal. However, let us imagine that the population of yields is composed by a very high and finite number of individuals; in that case, we can calculate the probability of measuring a value included within a specific finite interval, e.g., from 11 to 12, by counting the number of individuals with a yield level included in that interval and dividing that number by the total number of individuals. The problem is that the width of the interval is always arbitrary, and, therefore, we could divide the probability in the interval by the width of that interval to obtain the so-called *probability density* (probability per unit width). The top-left graph in Fig. 5.1 displays the density histogram; as mentioned in Chap. 3, the area of each bar represents the probability within that interval.

Now, what happens to the density when the interval becomes smaller and smaller? Figure 5.1 shows that as the interval width approaches 0, the density tends to a finite value resulting in a smooth density curve (see the red shape in Fig. 5.1, bottom-right).

The smooth **Probability Density Function** (PDF) represented in Fig. 5.1 is the Gaussian PDF, which is so common in agriculture and biology that it is usually referred to as the **normal curve**. The equation is

$$\phi(y) = \frac{1}{\sigma\sqrt{2\pi}} \exp\left[-\frac{(y-\mu)^2}{2\sigma^2}\right] \tag{5.1}$$

In this equation, $\phi(y)$ is the density of the point-event y, μ is the mean, and σ is the standard deviation. The Gaussian PDF is bell-shaped, with a shape depending only on the two values μ and σ (see Fig. 5.2 for two examples).

To calculate the Gaussian density with R, we can use the `dnorm()` function; for example, if we want to know the probability density of an individual yield measure

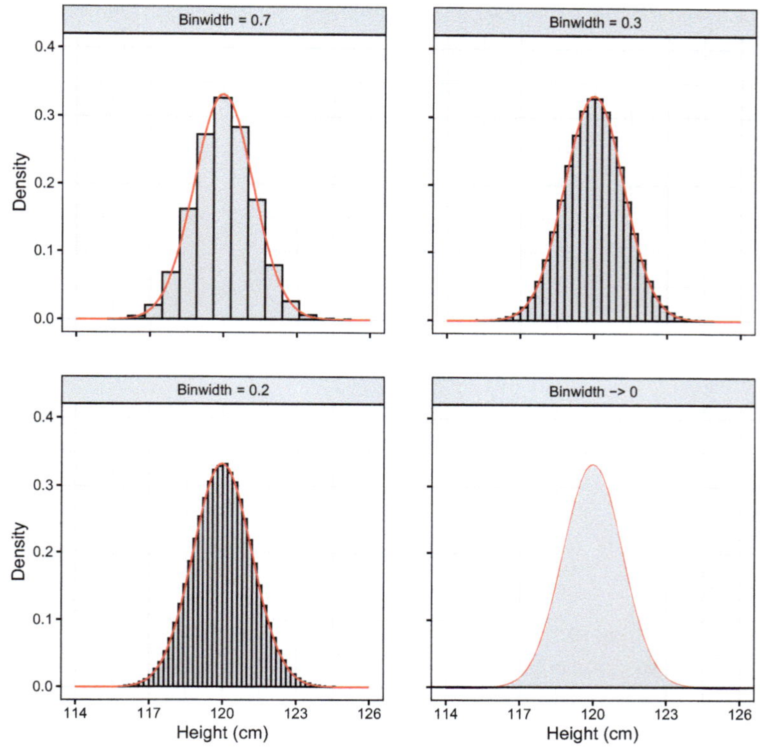

Fig. 5.1 Probability density function for a binned continuous variable, depending on bin width. When the bin width tends to zero, the density function tends to become a smooth curve

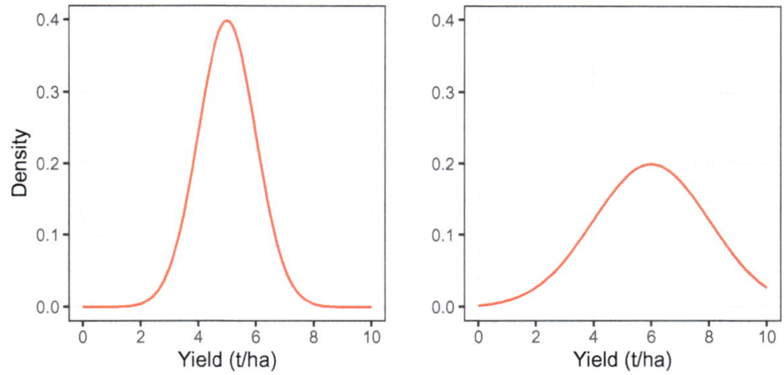

Fig. 5.2 The shape of the Gaussian function depends on the mean and standard deviation (left: mean $= 5$ and SD $= 1$; right: mean $= 6$ and SD $= 3$)

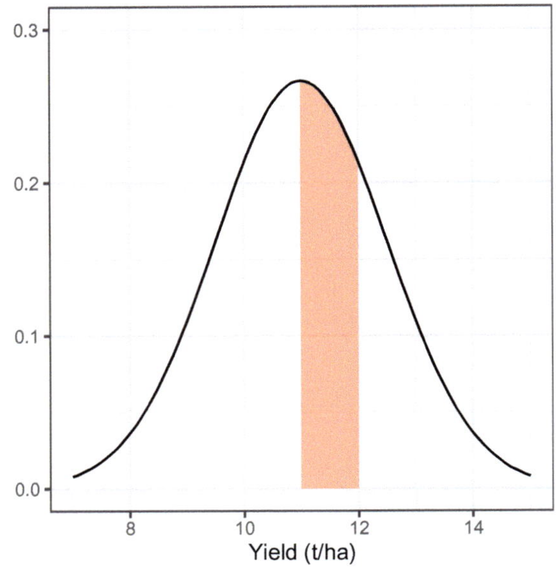

Fig. 5.3 Area-under-the-curve for a Gaussian PDF, depicting the probability of sampling an individual within the interval from 11 to 12 when the mean of the distribution is 11 and the standard deviation is 1.5

equal to, e.g., 12 t/ha, sampled from a population of yields with a mean equal to 11 and a standard deviation equal to 1.5, we can use the code provided in Code Box 5.1.

Code Box 5.1

```
# Gaussian density calculator

dnorm(12, mean = 11, sd = 1.5)
## [1] 0.2129653
```

The density is not a real probability, and it is not interesting in itself (at least, not in absolute terms). However, the PDF has the advantage that it returns the probability of interval events as the area-under-the-curve (AUC). For example, Fig. 5.3 highlights the AUC between 11 and 12, illustrating the probability of sampling an individual within that interval from a population with a mean of 11 and a standard deviation of 1.5.

The AUC and, hence, the probability can be calculated by integrating the Gaussian curve over an interval. For example, the probability within the interval between 11 and 12 in Fig. 5.3 is 0.248 (see Code Box 5.2). More simply, the function `pnorm()` returns the AUC between $-\infty$ and any value y (**Cumulative Distribution**

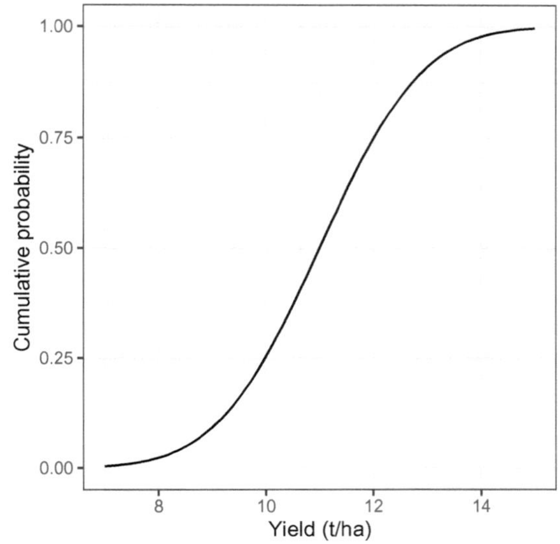

Fig. 5.4 Gaussian cumulative distribution function, with a mean of 11 and a standard deviation of 1.5

Function; see Fig. 5.4), and it can be used to avoid the calculation of an integral (Code Box 5.2).

Code Box 5.2

```
# Integration of the Gaussian density function
AUC <- integrate(function(x) dnorm(x, 11, 1.5), 11, 12)
AUC$value
## [1] 0.2475075

# Use of the cumulative probability function
# (same result as above)
pnorm(12, mean = 11, sd = 1.5)
 - pnorm(11, mean = 11, sd = 1.5)
## [1] 0.2475075
```

The main properties of a Gaussian PDF are:

1. The curve has two asymptotes, and the limits as y approaches $\pm\infty$ are 0. It is implied that every y value is, in theory, observable (its probability is higher than 0), although the probabilities of very small and very high values are negligible.
2. The integral from $-\infty$ to $+\infty$ is 1, as this is the sum of the probability densities for all possible outcomes.

3. The curve is symmetrical around the mode, which is equal to the median and the mean. That is, the probability of obtaining values above the mean is equal to the probability of obtaining values below the mean.
4. For any given μ and σ values, the probability of sampling individuals within the interval from $\mu - \sigma$ to $\mu + \sigma$ is always equal to 0.683, as shown in the example below:

Code box 5.3

```
# Probability of sampling from the interval
# from 'mu - sigma' to 'mu + sigma'

pnorm(120 + 2, 120, 2) - pnorm(120 - 2, 120, 2)
## [1] 0.6826895
```

Now, we come to the most interesting question: What do we do with the Gaussian curve? Dealing with quantitative responses (but, with some prudence, we could also include counts and ratios), we could assume that the stochastic element ε is Gaussian distributed, with a mean equal to 0 and a standard deviation equal to σ:

$$\varepsilon \sim \text{Norm}(0, \sigma) \tag{5.2}$$

Equivalently, we could assume that the outcome of an experiment is Gaussian distributed with a mean equal to Y_E (as predicted by the deterministic part of the model) and a standard deviation equal to σ:

$$Y_O \sim \text{Norm}(Y_E, \sigma) \tag{5.3}$$

The above assumption, whenever reasonable, opens numerous opportunities for researchers. In particular, we can:

1. Calculate probabilities for the observed outcomes.
2. Simulate the results of future experiments.

These can be illustrated with a few examples.

5.2 Calculating Probabilities

In practice, if we assume that a fully specified model can adequately describe a particular phenomenon, we can use that model to predict the expected outcome.

Successively, if we also know the standard deviation of the residual error term, we can use Eq. (5.3) to calculate the probability of any possible observed outcome.

5.2.1 Example 5.1: Calculating the Probability for a Mensurative Experiment

A well is polluted with a xenobiotic substance at a concentration of 120 mg/L. We analyze the concentration by using a measuring instrument with a coefficient of variability of 10%. Answer the following questions:

1. What model can we use to describe such a mensurative experiment?
2. What is the most likely concentration value that could be obtained by chemical analysis (expected value)?
3. What is the probability of finding a water sample with a concentration lower than 100 mg/L?
4. What is the probability of finding a water sample with a concentration higher than 140 mg/L?
5. What is the probability of finding a water sample with a concentration within the interval from 100 to 140 mg/L?
6. What is the 90th percentile, i.e., the concentration value that is very unlikely (10% probability) to be "surpassed"?
7. What are the two values, symmetrical around the mean, which contain the concentrations of 95% of all possible water samples?

For this mensurative experiment, a model of the mean would be appropriate ($Y_E = 120$ mg/L). However, we should consider that such a mechanism is overly simplistic because our chemical instrument is not free from measurement errors; consequently, we should add the stochastic component, as $Y_O = 120 + \varepsilon$, where $\varepsilon \sim \text{Norm}(0, \sigma = 12)$, or $Y_O \sim \text{Norm}(120, 12)$.

The answer to the second question is obvious: The expected value is predicted by the model, i.e., $Y_E = 120$. The solutions to the third question can be obtained by the `pnorm()` function (Code Box 5.4).

For the fourth question, cumulative probabilities are given for the lower curve tail, while we were asked to determine the higher tail. Therefore, either we subtract the lower tail from 1 (the whole area-under-the-curve is 1) or we set the "lower.tail" argument to "FALSE." For the fifth question, the answer is obtained by subtraction (Code Box 5.4).

To calculate the percentiles (Questions 6 and 7; Code Box 5.4), we use the quantile function `qnorm()`.

Code box 5.4

```
# Example 5.1
# Calculating the probability for a mensurative experiment

# Question 3
pnorm(100, mean = 120, sd = 12)
## [1] 0.04779035

# Question 4
1 - pnorm(140, mean = 120, sd = 12)
## [1] 0.04779035
pnorm(140, mean = 120, sd = 12, lower.tail = F)
## [1] 0.04779035

# Question 5
pnorm(140, mean = 120, sd = 12)
- pnorm(100, mean = 120, sd = 12)
## [1] 0.9044193

# Question 6
qnorm(0.8, mean = 120, sd = 12)
## [1] 130.0995

# Question 7
qnorm(0.025, mean = 120, sd = 12)
## [1] 96.48043
qnorm(0.975, mean = 120, sd = 12)
## [1] 143.5196
```

5.2.2 *Example 5.2: Calculating the Probability for a Degradation Experiment*

We know that the concentration C of an herbicide substance in soil at 20 °C drops with time t, according to the nonlinear equation $C = C_0 \times 10^{-0.01\,t}$, where C_0 is the initial herbicide concentration.

Suppose we perform a manipulative experiment and enrich a soil sample with this substance to a concentration $C_0 = 75$ ng g^{-1} and put this sample in an oven at 20 °C. What is the probability that, at 25 days from the start of the experiment, we observe a concentration ≤ 3 ng g^{-1}? As specified in the technical documentation, our measuring instrument is expected to produce a coefficient of variation equal to 10%.

Assuming that the cause-effect relationship is reliable, the expected concentration at 20 days after the treatment should be 4.22 ng g^{-1} (Code Box 5.5). However, the observed result depends on the experimental error, which is a random, unpredictable event; if we assume that the probability function for the observed concentration is Gaussian, with a mean of 4.22 and a standard deviation of 0.422 (i.e., $7.5 \times 10\%$), the probability of obtaining a measure of 3 ng g^{-1} or lower is less than 0.2%, which is a relatively unlikely event.

Code Box 5.5

```
# Example 5.2
# Calculating the probability for a degradation experiment

# Expected concentration
Ct <- 75 * 10^(- 0.05 * 25)
Ct
## [1] 4.21756
# Probability of observing a concentration <= 3
pnorm(3, Ct, Ct * 0.1)
## [1] 0.001945398
```

5.3 Stochastic Simulation

Assuming that random errors are Gaussian, we can also simulate the results of "future" experiments through the so-called Monte Carlo methods based on random number generators. In practice, we can:

1. Simulate the expected results by using the selected cause-effect model for each experimental unit.
2. Attach random variability to the expected outcomes by sampling from a Gaussian PDF.

In R, the Gaussian random number generator is implemented in the `rnorm()` function, which requires three arguments: the number of random values we intend to extract, the mean of the distribution, and its standard deviation.

5.3.1 Example 5.3: Simulating a Mensurative Experiment

Considering the polluted well in Example 5.1, simulate the results of a mensurative experiment where we analyze three replicated water samples, using an instrument with 10% coefficient of variability. In this condition, we can assume that the expected values are generated under the model of the mean $Y_E = 120$, while the errors are Gaussian, with a mean of 0 and a standard deviation of 12 (Code Box 5.6).

At the very beginning of Code Box 5.6, we set the seed to the value of "1234." Indeed, drawing random numbers, by definition, produces different values at each draw unless we set a specific "seed" and force the drawing process to start from the same value. By setting the same seed when working through this book, you can reproduce the same random numbers as I obtained when writing this book.

Code Box 5.6

```
# Example 5.3
# Simulating a mensurative experiment

set.seed(1234)
Y_E <- 120
epsilon <- rnorm(3, 0, 12)
Y_O <- Y_E + epsilon
Y_O
## [1] 105.5152 123.3292 133.0133
```

5.3.2 Example 5.4: Simulating a Fertilization Experiment

Simulate the results of an experiment to compare the yield of wheat treated with four different nitrogen rates (0, 60, 120, and 180 kg/ha); the experimental design is completely randomized with four replicates (16 data in all), and the cause-effect model is

$$Y_O = 25 + 0.15\,X + \varepsilon \tag{5.4}$$

In this model, Y_O is the observed yield, X is the N rate, and $\varepsilon \sim N(0, \sigma = 2.5)$. The solution is shown in Code Box 5.7.

Code Box 5.7

```
# Example 5.4
# Simulating a fertilization experiment

set.seed(1234)

# Creating the vector to host the experimental design
Dose <- rep(c(0, 60, 120, 180), each=4)

# Predicting the expected yield
Yield_E <- 25 + 0.15 * Dose

# Predicting the residuals
epsilon <- rnorm(16, 0, 2.5)

# Predicting the observations
Yield <- Yield_E + epsilon
dataset <- data.frame(Dose, Yield)
dataset
##    Dose    Yield
## 1     0 21.98234
## 2     0 25.69357
## 3     0 27.71110
## 4     0 19.13576
## 5    60 35.07281
## 6    60 35.26514
## 7    60 32.56315
## 8    60 32.63342
## 9   120 41.58887
## 10  120 40.77491
## 11  120 41.80702
## 12  120 40.50403
## 13  180 50.05937
## 14  180 52.16115
## 15  180 54.39874
## 16  180 51.72429
```

5.3.3 Example 5.5: Simulating a Genotype Experiment

Simulate the results of a genotype experiment with five genotypes in four blocks (20 observations in all). The cause-effect relationship is the following:

$$Y_{O(ij)} = \mu + \alpha_i + \gamma_j + \varepsilon_{ij} \tag{5.5}$$

In the previous equation, Y_O is the observed yield for one plot, μ is the average yield of the first genotype in the first block, α is the effect of the genotype in that plot, and γ is the effect of the block to which that plot belongs. Consider that μ is 48 q/ha, α values are, respectively, 0, 1, 3, −2, and −3 for the five genotypes, while the γ values are, respectively, 0, −2, 3, and 1 for the four blocks. The stochastic elements ε are Gaussian distributed with a mean of 0 and $\sigma = 5$.

The process is exactly as outlined above, and the solution is shown in Code Box 5.8.

Code Box 5.8

```
# Example 5.5
# Simulating a genotype experiment

set.seed(1234)

# Prepare the vectors for the experimental design
Genotype <- rep(LETTERS[1:5], each=4)
Block <- rep(1:4, times = 5)

# Input the value of parameters
mu <- 48
alpha <- rep(c(0, 1, 3, -2, -3), each = 4)
gamma <- rep(c(0, -2, 3, 1), times = 5)
sigma <- 5

# Predict the expected yields
Yield_E <- mu + alpha + gamma

# Simulate the residuals and the observed values
epsilon <- rnorm(20, 0, sigma)
Yield <- Yield_E + epsilon
dataset <- data.frame(Genotype, Block, Yield)
dataset
##    Genotype Block    Yield
## 1         A     1 41.96467
```

```
## 2          A      2 47.38715
## 3          A      3 56.42221
## 4          A      4 37.27151
## 5          B      1 51.14562
## 6          B      2 49.53028
## 7          B      3 49.12630
## 8          B      4 47.26684
## 9          C      1 48.17774
## 10         C      2 44.54981
## 11         C      3 51.61404
## 12         C      4 47.00807
## 13         D      1 42.11873
## 14         D      2 44.32229
## 15         D      3 53.79747
## 16         D      4 46.44857
## 17         E      1 42.44495
## 18         E      2 38.44402
## 19         E      3 43.81414
## 20         E      4 58.07918
```

5.4 Conclusions

As a conclusion to this part, the following statements can be made:

1. Models can provide a very handy description of cause-effect relationships, and they can be used to describe the experimental outcomes in a given situation, although they can only predict the expected value.
2. Due to the presence of random effects, the exact outcome of each single individual is unpredictable; however, we can calculate the probability of obtaining one of several possible outcomes by using stochastic models in the form of Probability Density Functions (PDFs).
3. The Gaussian PDF is the most commonly used PDF for continuous variables, but, with due precautions (see later), it can also be used with counts and ratios.

Although this chapter only covered one stochastic model (the Gaussian PDF), several other probability density functions could be used to describe random variability. For example, in the rest of this book, we will encounter the Student's t-distribution and the Fisher-Snedecor F-distribution. Those interested in this topic can find plenty of information in Bolker (2008). Another useful reference for statistical models in agriculture is Schabenberger and Pierce (2002).

5.5 Questions and Exercises

1. Consider a population that is Gaussian distributed with a mean of 155 and a standard deviation of 15. Calculate the probability of drawing individual values from this population that are (i) higher than 170, (ii) lower than 140, and (iii) within the range from 140 and 170.
2. A xenobiotic substance degrades in soil following a first-order kinetic, which is described by the following equation: $Y_E = 100\, e^{-0.07\, t}$, where Y_E is the expected concentration at time t. After spraying this substance in soil, what is the probability that 50 days later, we observe a concentration below the toxicity threshold for mammalians (2 ng/g)? Please consider that all unknown sources of experimental error can be regarded as Gaussian, with a coefficient of variation of 20%.
3. Crop yield is a function of crop density, according to the function $Y_E = 0.8 + 0.8\, X - 0.07\, X^2$, where Y_E is the expected yield and X is the density. Draw the graph, and find the required density to obtain the highest yield (use a simple graphical method). If we make a mensurative experiment at the optimal density level, what is the probability of obtaining a yield between 2.5 and 3 t/ha? Consider that random variability is 12%.
4. The toxicity of a compound changes with the dose, according to the following expression: $Y_E = 1/\left\{1 + \exp\left[-2\, (\log(X) - \log(15))\right]\right\}$, where Y_E is the expected proportion of dead animals, and X is the dose. If we treat 150 animals with a dose of 35 g, what is the probability of finding more than 120 dead animals? Random variability can be approximated by using a Gaussian distribution, with a standard deviation equal to 0.067.
5. Consider the relationship between crop yield and density, as shown in Exercise 2 ($Y_E = 0.8 + 0.8\, X - 0.07\, X^2$). Reproduce the results of a completely randomized (four replicates) sowing density experiment with five densities (2, 4, 6, 8, and 10 plants per square meter), considering that the random variability can be described by a Gaussian distribution, with a mean equal to 0 and a standard deviation equal to 0.25 (common value for all densities).
6. Simulate the possible results of a genotype experiment with five maize genotypes (A, B, C, D, and E) and expected values of, respectively, 12, 13, 12.5, 14, and 11 tons per hectare. Assume that the experimental (random) variability can be described by a Gaussian distribution, with a mean equal to 0 and a standard deviation equal to 1.25 (common value for all genotypes). The experiment is designed as a completely randomized study, with four replicates.

References

Bolker BM (2008) Ecological Models and Data in R. Princeton University Press, Princeton

Schabenberger O, Pierce FJ (2002) Contemporary Statistical Models for the Plant and Soil Sciences. Taylor & Francis/CRC Press, Milton Park/Boca Raton

Chapter 6
A Brief Intro to Statistical Inference

Death is a fact. All else is inference
—W. Farr

Abstract Statistics calculated on a sample do not fully match the corresponding statistics for the population being studied, but they are generally different. When we perform an experiment, we examine a sample of individuals, but our primary interest is to draw general conclusions about the entire population from which our sample was obtained. In other words, the main research question is "*what can we possibly say about the population, after having seen the sample*?" The process by which we look at the results of an experiment to draw more general conclusions is named **statistical inference**, and it is traditionally based on the so-called **frequentist confidence interval**, which is an interval of values that can "capture" the real underlying population value for the statistic under study, with high confidence and small probability of error. In this chapter, simple methods for obtaining confidence intervals are provided, and the limitations of the frequentist confidence intervals are discussed.

In Chaps. 3 and 4, we have examined several methods to describe the dataset at hand and to explore the cause-effect relationships between the observed variables. However, the dataset at hand is seldom interesting in itself, as we typically seek general conclusions that also apply to the entire population of individuals from which our sample was obtained. For example, we have sampled a set of representative field plots to determine the yield of a crop in a specific environment. We can use the mean to express the average yield of the observed sample, but the question is "what is the average yield in the entire environment"?

Even though the sample was selected to be fully representative of the entire population, it is clear that every descriptive statistic calculated for the sample (e.g., mean, standard deviation, correlation coefficient, F-ratio, or model parameters)

A. Onofri, *Field Research Methods in Agriculture*,
https://doi.org/10.1007/978-3-032-08199-5_6

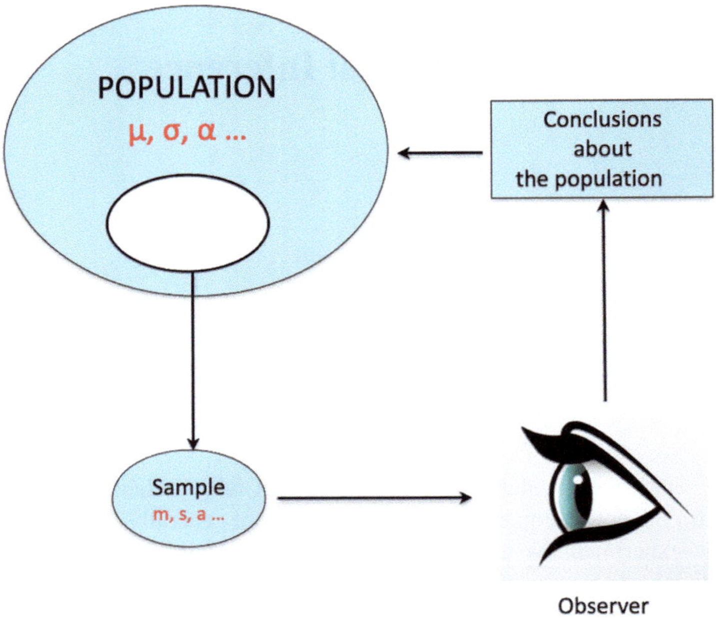

Fig. 6.1 The process of statistical inference, by which we look at a sample to derive the characteristics of the whole population

differs to some extent from the corresponding statistic for the entire population. So "*what can we possibly say about the population after having seen the sample*?"

The process by which we analyze the results of an experiment to draw more general conclusions about the population is known as **statistical inference**, and it is summarized in Fig. 6.1.

Let us reconsider Example 5.3, which concerns a polluted well containing xenobiotic substance at a concentration of $\mu = 120$ mg/L. A mensurative experiment might consist of collecting three water samples and measuring the concentration of that xenobiotic substance with an instrument that has, e.g., a 10% coefficient of variation. This experiment should return a result that is amenable to be described by the "model of the mean" (see Chap. 4), where the expectation is $Y_E = 120$ mg/L, while the observation is $Y_O = Y_E + \varepsilon$; the random element is assumed as Gaussian, with a mean of 0 and a standard deviation of $\sigma = 12$. In Example 5.3, we used Monte Carlo simulation to reproduce the results of such a mensurative experiment, and we obtained the three values 105.5, 123.3, and 133.01 mg/L. If we fit the "model of the mean" to this dataset (Code Box 6.1), the estimate of μ is $m = 120.62$, which differs from the real underlying value $\mu = 120$.

Code Box 6.1

```
# reconsidering the example 5.2

set.seed(1234)
Y_E <- 120
epsilon <- rnorm(3, 0, 12)
Y_O <- Y_E + epsilon

# Fitting the 'model of the mean' to the observed results
mod <- lm(Y_O ~ 1)
coef(mod)
## (Intercept)
##    120.6192
```

In a real research situation, the average concentration μ would be unknown. Based on the observed sample and assuming it is representative (this should not be questioned, as long as we believe that the experiment is valid), a preliminary estimate for the concentration in the whole well might be $\mu = m = 120.62$. The process by which we assign to the population the same value as we observed in the sample is known as **point estimation**, and it is not only legitimate but also insufficient, as we see that μ cannot be precisely equal to the estimate m.

The traditional approach to inference consists of expressing our uncertainty about the population statistic by using an interval of values, which can "capture" the real underlying value with high confidence and a small probability of error (**interval estimation**). Such an interval is called **Confidence Interval** (CI), and it is based on the theories of Karl Pearson (1857–1936), his son Egon Pearson (1895–1980), and Jerzy Neyman (1894–1981), as well as on the work of Ronald Fisher. The CI is one of the foundations of the so-called **frequentist inference**, which is not the only available type of inference, and it is not free from some conceptual inconsistencies (see Morey et al. 2016). However, it is very common and extensively used in most scientific papers.

The term "frequentist" originates from the fact that the CI is constructed by considering how sample estimates change across repeated sampling and the frequency with which different estimates are obtained.

6.1 Repeating Experiments

The Monte Carlo experiment in Example 5.3 and Code Box 6.1 can be repeated a large number of times at no cost to understand how the estimates m change across sampling efforts. The simulation process consists of:

1. Sampling three individuals from a Gaussian distribution with a mean of 120 and a standard deviation of 12
2. Fitting the model of the mean to obtain an estimate m
3. Repeating the simulation 100,000 times to obtain 100,000 estimates
4. Describing this population of estimates

In Code Box 6.2, the above tasks are performed by using an iterative procedure based on the `for()` statement. In practice, all instructions between curly brackets are repeated, while the counter i is updated at each cycle, from 1 to 100,000. In the end, the dataframe "result" contains 100,000 estimates obtained from just as many experiments; this population of sample estimates is called the **sampling distribution**, and it shows how the sample estimates change across repeated sampling when the "real truth" ($\mu = 120$ and $\sigma = 12$) is kept constant.

Exploring this population of sample estimates shows that the sampling distribution (Code Box 6.2):

1. Also includes very low and very high values (from 90.1 to 149.0 mg/L), although such "discrepant" values are relatively infrequent
2. Does not contain any value that is exactly equal to 120 mg/L
3. Has a mean equal to 120 mg/L (approximately)
4. Has a standard deviation equal to 6.94, which is the so-called **standard error** (SE)

Code Box 6.2

```
# Monte Carlo simulation #1
nrep <- 3
mean <- 120
sigma <- 12
set.seed(1234)
result <- rep(0, 100000)
for (i in 1:100000){
  sample <- rnorm(nrep, mean, sigma)
  mod <- lm(sample ~ 1)
  result[i] <- coef(mod)
}

# Characterising the population of estimates
min(result)
## [1] 90.14123

max(result)
## [1] 149.0346
```

```
result[result == 120]
## numeric(0)

mean(result)
## [1] 120.0341

sd(result)
## [1] 6.939063
```

The standard error is an essential "ingredient" in research, as it represents a measure of precision for all estimates: **When the standard error is high, the sampling distribution is flat, and our estimates are somewhat uncertain and highly variable across repeated experiments. Otherwise, when the standard error is low, our estimates are very precise and change very little across repeated experiments.**

6.2 A Theoretical Sampling Distribution

Building an empirical sampling distribution by Monte Carlo simulation is always possible, but it may often be impractical; it is much more convenient to describe the population of sample estimates using a theoretical density function. To gain more information, we can bin the sample means into a series of intervals (from 80 to 160 mg/L with a 2.5 step) and calculate the proportion of means in each interval.

The sampling distribution in Fig. 6.2 is similar to a Gaussian PDF, with a mean of 120 and a standard deviation of approximately 6.94. Such an empirical finding has a theoretical support: The **central limit theorem** states that, regardless of the shape of the original population (whether Gaussian or not), the sampling distribution of several statistics obtained from random and independent samples is **approximately** Gaussian, with a mean equal to the corresponding population statistic.[1]

From this Gaussian sampling distribution, we can take a multiple of the standard error ($k \times$ SE) to form an interval from $\mu - k \times$ SE to $\mu + k \times$ SE, containing 95% of the possible sample estimates m (Fig. 6.3). If the sampling distribution were truly Gaussian, k would equal the 97.5th percentile from a standardized Gaussian distribution (i.e., a Gaussian distribution with a mean of 0 and a standard deviation of 1), which is close to 2 (with R: `qnorm(0.975) = 1.960`). Unfortunately, in most cases the sampling distribution is only approximately Gaussian, so that k must be determined differently (see later).

---

[1] The central limit theorem holds for very large samples. With small samples, the approximation is accurate only when there are more than 20–25 individuals.

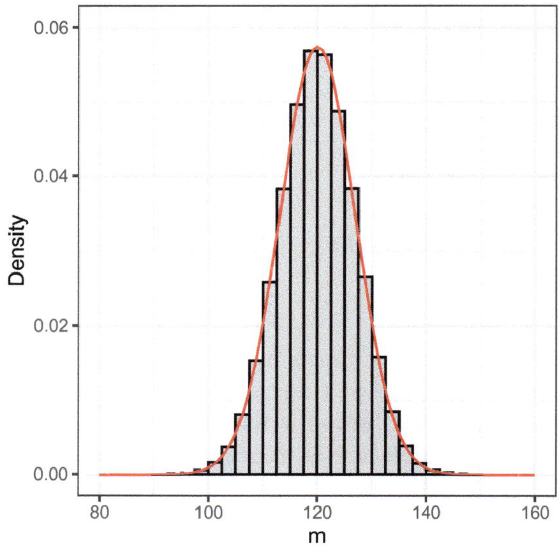

Fig. 6.2 Empirical distribution of 100,000 sample estimates ($n = 3$), drawn from a Gaussian population with mean $= 120$ and SD $= 12$. The solid line shows the theoretical Gaussian PDF, with mean $=$ 120 and SD $= 6.94$

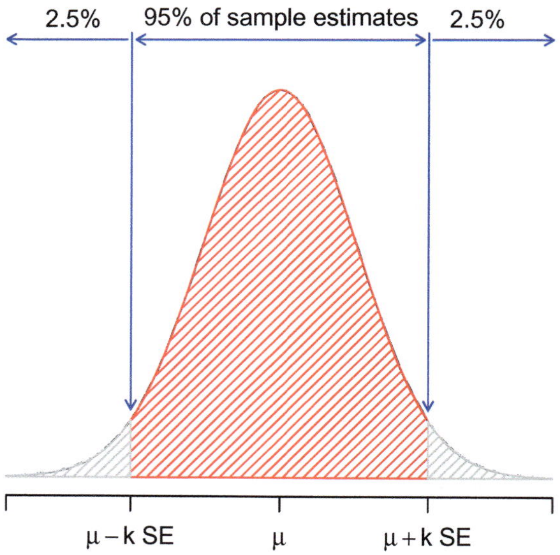

Fig. 6.3 A Gaussian sampling distribution with a mean of 120 and a standard deviation equal to 6.94 the red interval contains 95% of sample means, and it is obtained by adding/subtracting to/from 120, a value equal to k times the standard error. See the text for the determination of the multiplier "k"

6.3 The Frequentist Confidence Interval

The previous finding can be expressed as

$$P\left[\mu - k \times SE \leq m \leq \mu + k \times SE\right] = 0.95 \tag{6.1}$$

From there, with simple math (subtract μ and m from all terms, multiply by -1, and rearrange the terms), we can derive the following expression:

$$P\left[m - k \times SE \leq \mu \leq m + k \times SE\right] = 0.95 \tag{6.2}$$

This latter expression is of extreme importance, as it states that **when we conduct an experiment and obtain an estimate m, by an appropriate selection of k, we can construct an interval around m that is equal to k times the standard error and contains the population value μ with 95% probability**. This interval is known as **frequentist confidence interval** (CI), and, owing to the central limit theorem, it can be extended to all other sample statistics of interest.

Consequently, whenever we have a sample statistic and we want to infer the corresponding population statistic, we need to:

1. Calculate the standard error
2. Calculate a confidence interval by using a multiple of the standard error

By doing so, we can conclude that the population statistic is included in that interval and be confident that this conclusion is wrong in no more than 5% of the cases.

6.4 How Do We Calculate a Standard Error?

In some cases, the standard error can be obtained from simple rules (see Cochran and Cox 1950). For example, in the case of the sample mean, the standard error can be obtained according to the law of propagation of errors (see Sect. 3.3) as

$$SEM = \frac{\sigma}{\sqrt{n}} \tag{6.3}$$

Indeed, considering the previous simulation, the standard error with Eq. (6.3) would be $12/\sqrt{3} = 6.928$, which is very close to the standard deviation of the empirical sampling distribution.

Likewise, it is possible to demonstrate that the standard error for the differences between two independent sample means with the same variance and a number of replicates equal to n_1 and n_2, respectively, is

$$SED = \sqrt{\frac{\sigma^2}{n_1} + \frac{\sigma^2}{n_2}} \tag{6.4}$$

In other cases, calculating the standard error by hand can be more difficult; however, in practice, standard errors are most often produced by the statistical software. In particular, for models fitted with the `lm()` function or with several other fitting functions in R, standard errors for parameter estimates can be obtained by using the summary() function, passing the model object as an argument.

For example, let us reconsider the data in Example 4.3, which relates to a field experiment comparing the yield of four oat genotypes (named A, B, C, and D) on a completely randomized design with three replicates. If we fit a simple one-way ANOVA model to this dataset ($Y_i = \mu + \alpha_j + \varepsilon_i$), the estimates of model parameters with their standard errors can be obtained as shown in Code Box 6.3.

Code Box 6.3

```
# Standard errors for parameter estimates

# Input the data and fit the model (as in Code box 4.3)
library(statforbiology)
dataset <- getAgroData("Oat1L")
mod6.1 <- lm(Yield ~ Genotype, data = dataset)

# Derive estimates and standard errors
summary(mod6.1)
## Coefficients:
##              Estimate Std. Error t value Pr(>|t|)
## (Intercept)  4.58000    0.07566  60.531 6.17e-12 ***
## GenotypeB   -1.02667    0.10700  -9.595 1.16e-05 ***
## GenotypeC   -0.49667    0.10700  -4.642  0.00166 **
## GenotypeD    0.01667    0.10700   0.156  0.88008
##
## Residual standard error: 0.1311 on 8 degrees of freedom
## Multiple R-squared:  0.9412, Adjusted R-squared:  0.9192
## F-statistic: 42.71 on 3 and 8 DF,  p-value: 2.866e-05
```

6.5 How Do We Select a Multiplier?

To select a multiplier k, it is necessary to consider the *coverage* of the confidence interval, i.e., how often the CI "captures" the true-population value. Generally, the higher the k value, the wider the interval and the greater the coverage. Common sense suggests that we should aim at a coverage of 95%, corresponding to a probability of error of 5%; consequently, we should ask ourselves what k value permits to achieve such a coverage.

The coverage can be calculated by using Monte Carlo; in Code Box 6.4, this method is applied to the polluted well data by repeatedly accomplishing the following tasks:

1. Three individuals are sampled from a Gaussian population, with a mean equal to 120 and a standard deviation equal to 12.
2. The model of the mean is fitted to those individuals to derive an estimate of μ, together with its standard error.
3. A CI is built, using a multiplier $k = 2$. If such a CI contains the real value of 120 mg/L, it is successful, and the vector "result" is assigned a value of 1.
4. The steps from 1 to 3 are repeated 100,000 times, and the number of successes is counted.

Code Box 6.4

```
# Monte Carlo simulation - 2
# Coverage of a confidence interval
# depending on the multiplier k

# Sampling 3 reps from a Gaussian with mean=120 and sd=12
mean <- 120
sigma <- 12
nrep <- 3
k <- 2
set.seed(1234)
result <- rep(0, 100000)
for (i in 1:100000){
  sample.i <- rnorm(nrep, mean, sigma)
  mod <- lm(sample.i ~ 1)
  m <- coef(mod)
  se <- summary(mod)$coef[1,2]
  limInf <- m - k * se
  limSup <- m + k * se
  # did we capture the mean?
  result[i] <- ifelse(limInf < 120 & limSup > 120, 1, 0)
}
sum(result)/100000
## [1] 0.81708
```

It is shown that setting $k = 2$ produces low coverage (less than 82%), corresponding to an unacceptable error probability of almost 19%. Indeed, the sample size is very small, and thus, the sampling distribution of m is not reliably approximated by a Gaussian PDF. Indeed, if the same simulation is run with 20 replicates instead of 3, the coverage increases to 94% (not shown). In practice, setting $k = 2$ is regarded as acceptable to obtain "naive" confidence intervals when the sample size is higher than, e.g., 20–25.

For small sample sizes (and in general), an exact 95% coverage can be achieved by using the 97.5th percentile of a Student's t-distribution, which is calculated by using the `qt()` function in R. This function requires, at minimum, two arguments: The first one is the desired percentile, while the second one represents the number of degrees of freedom for the standard error. Concerning the previous simulation with three replicates, the number of DF is $3 - 1 = 2$, and the 97.5th percentile from a Student's t-distribution is `qt(0.975, 2) = 4.303`, which is much higher than 2. This multiplier decreases as the number of degrees of freedom increases, approaching a limit of 1.96, as the number of DF approaches ∞.

A further Monte Carlo simulation may confirm that using $k = 4.303$ results in exact 95% coverage (not shown).

We can also construct a 99% confidence interval, which reduces our risk of error, by using the 99.5th percentile from a Student's t-distribution. In general, if α is the desired confidence level, the corresponding percentile is $q_\alpha = 1 - (1 - \alpha/2)$ (e.g., $q_{0.05} = 1 - (1 - 0.95)/2 = 0.975$ or $q_{0.99} = 1 - (1 - 0.99)/2 = 0.995$).

6.6 What Are the Limitations?

The frequentist confidence interval is widely used in scientific literature, while point estimation is most often regarded as unacceptable. For example, the guidance for the authors of Weed Research, a high ranking international journal on the topic of plant science, says *"all estimated values (e.g., model parameters, means, differences, etc.) should be presented together with an appropriate measure of variability in text, tables, and graphs."*[2] Intervals are very often presented in the simplest form "estimate $\pm$ SE," although the coverage of such an interval is pretty low.

Nonetheless, it is necessary to be aware of the limitations of a frequentist confidence interval (Hastie et al. 2009) that needs to be interpreted with reference to a sampling distribution, i.e., to the hypothetical repetitions of the same experiment with different samples, as shown in Code Box 6.4. On the contrary, it is not possible to interpret the CI with reference to each sampling effort, i.e., we cannot say that the specific CI that was determined for a single experiment contains the true-population parameter with 95% probability because this is untrue (please note that the CI changes at each sampling effort; see Code Box 6.4 and see also Morey et al. 2016).

[2] Taken from the guidance for authors of Weed Research, see https://onlinelibrary.wiley.com/page/journal/13653180/homepage/forauthors.html (accessed on April 24, 2025).

6.7 Confidence Intervals in Practice

6.7.1 Example 6.1: CI for a Sample Mean

A mensurative experiment was conducted to determine the average yield of sunflowers in a macro-environment of central Italy. A sample of 20 random fields was selected from that environment to determine the yield values (Code Box 6.5); based on the results of such an experiment, what is the expected yield in the whole macro-environment?

For this example, the sample mean is $m = 58.68$, which is a reliable point estimate of the average yield across the entire macro-environment. To calculate a CI, we need:

1. The SE, which can be easily calculated by using the simple equation (6.3); σ is unknown, but we can plug in the standard deviation of the sample, which is 3.47
2. A multiplier k, which is obtained as the 97.5th quantile from a Student's t-distribution (i.e., 2.09)

Accordingly, the two limits of the CI are, respectively, $58.68 - 2.09 \times 0.775 = 57.1$ and $58.68 + 2.09 \times 0.775 = 60.3$. The conclusion is that, with 95% confidence, the yield in the macro-environment falls within the interval between 57.1 and 60.3.

Code Box 6.5

```
# Example 6.1
# Confidence interval for a sample mean

# Input the sample and calculate the mean
Y <- c(54.08, 66.31, 56.17, 56.32, 52.01, 58.91, 58.74, 57.49,
       59.57, 61.71, 56.89, 54.82, 56.88, 60.05, 59.39, 57.19,
       64.76, 61.36, 62.03, 58.83)
m <- mean(Y)
m
## [1] 58.6755

# Calculate the standard error
s <- sd(Y)
SEM <- s/sqrt(length(Y))
SEM
## [1] 0.7754783

# Determine the multiplier
k <- qt(0.975, length(Y) - 1)
k
```

```
## [1] 2.093024

# Calculate the limits of the CI
# Lower limit
mean(Y) -  k * SEM
## [1] 57.05241

# Higher limit
mean(Y) +  k * SEM
## [1] 60.29859
```

We can also achieve the same result more easily within a model fitting strategy by using the `confint()` function (Code Box 6.6).

Code box 6.6

```
# Example 6.1 [continuation]

# Retrieving confidence intervals from model fit

mod <- lm(Y ~ 1)
confint(mod)
##                 2.5 %   97.5 %
## (Intercept) 57.05241 60.29859
```

6.7.2 *Example 6.2: CIs for Model Parameters*

The same approach as in Code Box 6.6 can be used with all linear models and with most models in R. For example, let us reconsider the "Oat1L" data (Example 4.3) and fit a one-way ANOVA model as in Code Box 4.3. The confidence intervals for parameter estimates can be obtained using the `confint()` function in R (Code Box 6.7).

Code Box 6.7

```
# Example 6.2
# CIs for model parameters for the 'Oat1l' data
```

```
# Load libraries and data
library(statforbiology)
dataset <- getAgroData("Oat1L")

# Fit the model
mod6.1 <- lm(Yield ~ Genotype, data = dataset)

# CIs for model parameters
confint(mod6.1)
##                  2.5 %     97.5 %
## (Intercept)  4.4055191  4.7544809
## GenotypeB   -1.2734199 -0.7799134
## GenotypeC   -0.7434199 -0.2499134
## GenotypeD   -0.2300866  0.2634199
```

6.8 Other Approaches

The approach proposed in this chapter relies on the prerequisites that (i) the sampling distribution is Gaussian (at least, approximately; large sample approximation) and (ii) a standard error is available through the statistical software or it can be easily calculated by some simple rules.

For cases where these two prerequisites are not fulfilled, alternative methods to calculate confidence intervals exist, such as the Monte Carlo method (as used in Code Box 6.2) and the "bootstrap" method (Chernick 2011). Furthermore, it is worth mentioning the "Credible Interval," which is the counterpart of the frequentist confidence interval in Bayesian statistics (Kruschke 2011).

These computer-intensive methods of obtaining confidence intervals may be helpful in some circumstances, although they will not be explored in detail because they are beyond the scope of this introductory book.

6.9 Questions and Exercises

1. Explain briefly the difference between the standard error (SE) and the standard deviation (SD).
2. Consider the following statement: "The confidence interval goes from 13 to 18." What does this mean? Discuss briefly.
3. A chemical analysis was repeated three times, with the following results: 125, 169, and 142 ng/g. Calculate the mean, variance, standard deviation, standard error, and confidence intervals ($P = 0.95$ and $P = 0.99$).

4. An experiment was conducted to compare the yield of four wheat genotypes (in tons per hectare), and the results are reported below. For each genotype, calculate the mean, deviance, variance, standard deviation, standard error, and confidence interval (P = 0.95). [Hint: Do the calculation without fitting a model].

Genotype	Rep 1	Rep 2	Rep 3	Rep 4
A	4.39	6.06	6.10	5.46
B	6.02	6.00	5.78	6.07
C	4.50	4.59	4.93	5.28
D	6.63	6.39	6.15	6.20

5. We have measured the lengths of 30 maize seedlings treated with a water solution enriched with selenium (the observed lengths are reported below). Calculate the mean, variance, standard deviation, standard error, and confidence interval (P = 0.95 and P = 0.99).

```
LENGTH <- c(2.07, 2.23, 2.04, 2.16, 2.12, 2.33, 2.21, 2.22,
            2.29, 2.28, 2.44, 2.04, 2.02, 1.49, 2.12, 2.38,
            2.51, 2.27, 2.55, 2.44, 2.28, 2.20, 2.03, 2.35,
            2.34, 2.34, 1.99, 2.44, 2.44, 1.91)
```

6. Consider Examples 4.2 and 4.3, and calculate the standard errors and confidence intervals for the estimates of model parameters.

References

Chernick MR (2011) An Introduction to Bootstrap Methods with Applications to R. Wiley, Hoboken

Cochran WG, Cox GM (1950) Experimental Design. Wiley, Hoboken

Hastie T, Tibshirani R, Friedman J (2009) The Elements of Statistical Learning. Springer Series in Statistics. Springer Science + Business Media, Cham, CA

Kruschke JK (2011) Doing Bayesian Data Analyses. A Tutorial with R and BUGS. Academic, Burlington, MA

Morey RD, Hoekstra R, Rouder JN, Lee MD, Wagenmakers EJ (2016) The fallacy of placing confidence in confidence intervals. Psychon Bull Rev 23(1):103–123. https://doi.org/10.3758/s13423-015-0947-8. http://link.springer.com/10.3758/s13423-015-0947-8

Chapter 7
Making Decisions Under Uncertainty

> *The null hypothesis is never proved or established, but it is possibly disproved, in the course of experimentation. Every experiment may be said to exist only to give the facts a chance of disproving the null hypothesis.*
>
> —R.A. Fisher

Abstract In this chapter, Formal Hypothesis Testing (FHT) is briefly presented as a method for taking decisions in the presence of random experimental errors. The null and alternative hypotheses are defined, and FHT is introduced using Monte Carlo methods, to illustrate how decisions are made by considering the sampling distribution of test statistics under the null hypothesis. Examples are provided for Wald t-tests, traditional t-tests, and F-tests in ANOVA.

In the previous chapter, we saw that experimental errors and, above all, sampling errors produce uncertainty in the estimation process, which we must account for by determining and displaying standard errors or confidence intervals along with all point estimates. Similarly, we need to be able to make decisions in the presence of uncertainty; is the effect of a treatment statistically significant? Is the effect of a treatment higher/lower than the effect of another treatment?

Making such decisions is called **Formal Hypothesis Testing** (FHT), and it is primarily based on the so-called **P-value**. Let us introduce this technique with a few examples commonly encountered in research work.

7.1 Example 7.1: A Comparison Between Two Genotypes

Let us imagine we have conducted a small plot experiment to compare the yield of genotype A with that of genotype P on a completely randomized design with five replicates. The ten plots should be regarded as a sample from a broader population

A. Onofri, *Field Research Methods in Agriculture*,
https://doi.org/10.1007/978-3-032-08199-5_7

of plots, and we aim to draw conclusions of general validity. Is the yield level of the two genotypes significantly different?

The results of such an experiment (in quintals per hectare) are shown in Code Box 7.1, together with all the main descriptive statistics of interest.

Code Box 7.1

```
# Example 7.1
# A comparison between two genotypes

# Load the data
A <- c(65, 68, 69, 71, 78)
P <- c(80, 81, 84, 88, 94)

# Descriptive statistics for A
m1 <- mean(A)
s1 <- sd(A)
n1 <- length(A)
m1; s1; n1
## [1] 70.2
## [1] 4.868265
## [1] 5

# Descriptive statistics for P
m2 <- mean(P)
s2 <- sd(P)
n2 <- length(P)
m2; s2; n2
## [1] 85.4
## [1] 5.727128
## [1] 5
```

To elucidate the causal effect of the genotype factor, we can fit a simple one-way ANOVA model, as shown in Chap. 4:

$$Y_i = \mu + \delta_j + \varepsilon_i \tag{7.1}$$

In this model, Y_i is the yield of the ith plot (i goes from 1 to 10), μ is the expected yield for genotype A ($\mu_A = \mu$), while δ_j is the genotype effect (with j going from 1 to 2) that is constrained to be 0 for genotype A ($\delta_1 = 0$), and, for the second genotype, it is equal to the yield difference between the two genotypes ($\delta_2 = \mu_P - \mu_A$). Consequently, the expected yield for P is $\mu_P = \mu + \delta_2$, and the residuals

ε_i represent all the other unknown sources of variability that are independent and specific to each plot. The residuals are assumed as Gaussian, with a mean of 0 and a standard deviation equal to σ. The choice of using $\delta_1 = 0$ is purely arbitrary: We could have just also set $\delta_2 = 0$ so that δ_1 would have been equal to the opposite of δ_2, as obtained with the previous parameterization.

The estimation of model parameters can be performed by using the `lm()` function in R, as shown in Chap. 4 (Code Box 7.2).

Code Box 7.2

```
# Example 7.1 [continuation]

# Fitting a model with one nominal predictor
# to the data at Code box 7.1

yield <- c(A, P)
genotype <- rep(c("A", "P"), each = 5)
mod <- lm(yield ~ genotype)
summary(mod)
## Coefficients:
##             Estimate Std. Error t value Pr(>|t|)
## (Intercept)   70.200      2.377  29.533 1.87e-09 ***
## genotypeP     15.200      3.362   4.522  0.00195 **
##
## Residual standard error: 5.315 on 8 degrees of freedom
## Multiple R-squared:  0.7188, Adjusted R-squared:  0.6836
## F-statistic: 20.45 on 1 and 8 DF,  p-value: 0.001945

confint(mod)
##                 2.5 %   97.5 %
## (Intercept) 64.718691 75.68131
## genotypeP    7.448258 22.95174
```

It is important to note that the residual standard deviation (σ), with confusing terminology, is indicated in the R output as the "residual standard error" ($\sigma = 5.315$). It is also important to note that, under the specification of our model, the standard deviation of residuals is unique and common to all observations; thus, the model assumes that the genotype effect influences the yield level but not its variability across replicates. Such an assumption is known as **homoscedasticity**, and it should be carefully checked, as will be explained later in this book.

The estimate of δ_2, which we can refer to as d_2, is 15.2. However, this is just a sample statistic and is insufficient for our purposes, as we aim to draw general conclusions from it. The CI for the genotype effect is $7.45 - 22.95$, and it does not contain 0, which is indirect evidence that such an effect is significant, although a more formal test is needed to confirm this significance.

7.1.1 The "Null" Hypothesis

According to the Popperian falsification principle, experiments should be planned to test and potentially falsify hypotheses. Therefore, we select the hypothesis that there is no difference between the two genotypes (**null hypothesis**: H_0) and, consequently, $H_0 : \delta_2 = 0$. Accordingly, the point estimate d_2 is different from 0 only due to random fluctuations. Based on the observed data, is it possible to falsify such a hypothesis?

7.1.2 The t-Test

We are trying to demonstrate that one model parameter equals 0, when, in reality, our point estimate is further away from 0. It is intuitively clear that a certain degree of discrepancy between reality and observation may be an inherent characteristic of the sampling process. However, it is also clear that the higher the discrepancy, the lower the probability that the "null" hypothesis is true. In particular, our intuition is that a parameter is significantly different from 0 when its value is much bigger than the uncertainty with which we have estimated it.

We can formalize such an intuition by defining the T statistic:

$$T = \frac{d_2}{SE_{d_2}} = \frac{15.2}{3.362} = 4.521727 \tag{7.2}$$

If the null hypothesis were true, we would expect to observe $T = 0$, whereas we have observed $T = 4.522$. Can we reject the null? We do not know; it depends on how likely it is to obtain such a discrepant value when the null is true. Therefore, we need to ask ourselves **what is the sampling distribution for T under the null hypothesis?**

7.1.3 Monte Carlo Simulation

The empirical sampling distribution for T can be constructed by using Monte Carlo simulation, assuming that if the null hypothesis is true, the ten observations belong to a single group with a mean of 77.8 and a standard deviation of 9.45 (Code Box 7.3).

Code Box 7.3

```
# Example 7.1 [ continuation]

# We assume a single group, with no genotype distinction
# and calculate the descriptive statistics

mu <- mean(yield)
devStAP <- sd(c(A, P))
mu; devStAP
## [1] 77.8
## [1] 9.44928
```

The `for()` statement is used in Code Box 7.4 to repeat the experiment 100,000 times. In each experiment, the null is regarded as true, and the constraint $\delta_2 = 0$ is imposed so that the observed result is simulated by attaching to the overall observed mean (77.8) a set of subject-specific random values, drawn from a Gaussian distribution with mean equal to 0 and standard deviation equal to 9.44928 (Code Box 7.4; it is to be noted that this simulation is based on three fundamental constraints: The errors are independent, Gaussian, and homoscedastic, which correspond to the assumptions made by this test). For each experiment, a simple one-way ANOVA model is fitted, and an estimate δ_2 is obtained. This estimate is used to calculate a T-value, which is stored in the "result" vector. In the end, this vector represents the sampling distribution for T, assuming that the null is true; clearly, any value of T that differs from 0 is only due to random "noise."

Code Box 7.4

```
# Example 7.1 [ continuation]

# Building a sampling distribution for T
# assuming that the null hypothesis is true

set.seed(34)
result <- rep(NA, 100000)
for (i in 1:100000){
  epsilon <- rnorm(10, 0, devStAP)
  Yo <- mu + epsilon
```

```
    mod <- lm(Yo ~ genotype)
    d2 <- coef(mod)[2]
    SE <- summary(mod)$coefficients[[2,2]]
    Ti <- d2 / SE
    result[i] <- Ti
}
mean(result)
## 0.001230418

min(result)
## -9.988315

max(result)
## 9.993187
```

What values did we obtain for T? As expected, the values are close to 0, but there are also several relatively high or low values (close to 10 and -10), which prove that random sampling fluctuations can also bring very "odd" results. For our real experiment, we obtained $T = 4.522$; however, the positive sign is an artifact related to how we formulated our model: We could have also obtained $T = -4.522$ if we had reversed the ordering of the two genotypes, setting the constraint $\delta_2 = 0$, instead of $\delta_1 = 0$.

Ronald Fisher proposed that we should reject the null hypothesis based on the probability of obtaining values as extreme or more extreme than those we observed when the null hypothesis is true. Examining the vector "result," we see that the proportion of values lower than -4.521727 and higher than 4.521727 is $0.00095 + 0.00082 = 0.00177$. This proportion represents the probability that we need to use when making statistical decisions, and it is referred to as the **P-value** or **P-level** (Code Box 7.5).

Code Box 7.5

```
# Example 7.1 [ continuation]

# P-value with Monte Carlo simulation

T_obs <- 4.521727
upperTail <- length(result[result > T_obs]) / 100000
lowerTail <- length(result[result < - T_obs]) /100000
upperTail + lowerTail
## [1] 0.00177
```

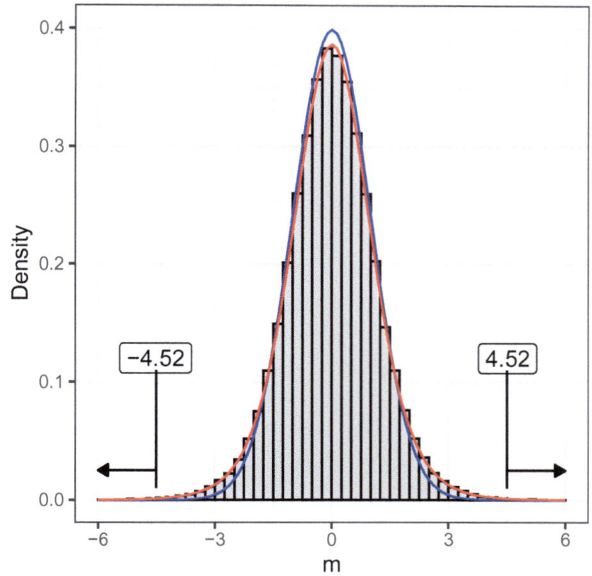

Fig. 7.1 Empirical sampling distribution for the T statistic, compared to a standardized Gaussian (blue line) and a Student's t-distribution with 8 degrees of freedom (red line). The observed T-values have been highlighted, and the total probability (area-under-the-curve) of sampling outside the interval from −4.522 to 4.522 represents the P-value

Let us summarize. We have seen that when the null is true, the sampling distribution for T contains a very low proportion of values outside the interval from −4.522 to 4.522. Therefore, our observation fell within an improbable range, corresponding to a probability of 0.00177 (the so-called P-value). As **the usual yardstick for decision is 0.05**, we reject the null hypothesis because if this were true, we would have obtained a very unlikely result.

7.1.4 A Formal Solution

A new question: Is there any formal Probability Density Function (PDF) that we can use in place of our empirical, Monte Carlo-based sampling distribution for T? Let us take a closer look at the "result" vector. In particular, we can bin this continuous variable and plot the empirical distribution of frequencies (see Fig. 7.1).

The empirical sampling distribution is not approximated by a standardized Gaussian distribution, but it can be approximated by using the Student's t-distribution. In more detail, this distribution was devised by the "Student," i.e., William Sealy Gosset (1876–1937), who used such a pseudonym in his scientific papers while working at the Guinness Brewery in Dublin; it is similar to a standardized Gaussian distribution but with heavier tails, and the weight in the tails is inversely proportional to the parameter ν (the number of DF), so that this distribution approaches a Gaussian when ν approaches ∞.

For our problem, we can use the Student's t-distribution with 8 DF to calculate the P-value rather than performing a time-consuming Monte Carlo simulation (Code Box 7.6). The results obtained with the two methods are very similar, and the P-values are already available for all estimated parameters in the output of the `summary()` method applied to the linear model object (Code Box 7.2).

Code Box 7.6

```
# Example 7.1 [continuation}

# P-value from the Student's t distribution

pt(T_obs, df=8, lower.tail = FALSE)
 # probability that T > 4.522
## [1] 0.0009727353
pt(-T_obs, df=8) # probability that T < -4.522
## [1] 0.0009727353
2 * pt(abs(T_obs), df=8, lower.tail = F) # P-value
## [1] 0.001945471
```

In conclusion to this part, it is necessary to reinforce the idea that the P-level obtained from a t-test makes **three basic assumptions**: Residuals are independently sampled from a normal distribution (independence and normality), the standard deviation is unique, and it is not affected by the treatment level (homoscedasticity).

If the observed data do not meet these assumptions, the sampling distribution for T does not correspond to a Student's t-distribution, and consequently, the P-level is invalid. Methods to check the validity of these assumptions will be presented in Chap. 8.

7.1.5 The Traditional Student's t-Test

The t-test we have just shown is primarily intended to support model fitting procedures, and it allows us to test the hypothesis that one of the parameters is not significantly different from 0. The traditional Student's t-test is relatively old technique (dating back to 1908) used for comparing two sample means without fitting any model to the observed data. Although it is now regarded as somewhat outdated, we would like to show how the `t.test()` function in R can be used to obtain the same results as before regarding the δ parameter (Code Box 7.7).

Code Box 7.7

```
# Example 7.1 [continuation]

# Traditional Student's t-test with R

t.test(A, P, var.equal = T)
##
##  Two Sample t-test
##
## data:  A and P
## t = -4.5217, df = 8, p-value = 0.001945
## alternative hypothesis: true difference in means
    is not equal to 0
## 95 percent confidence interval:
##  -22.951742  -7.448258
## sample estimates:
## mean of x mean of y
##      70.2      85.4
```

The argument `var.equal = T` specifies a homoscedastic Student's t-test, which assumes that the variances of the two samples are homogeneous. One advantage of this traditional t-test is that it can be easily extended to situations where the two samples have different variances, a problem known as heteroscedasticity (heteroscedastic t-test, also referred to as the Welch test). The main difference between the two tests (Student's and Welch's) lies in the number of degrees of freedom, which for the Welch test is approximated by using the Satterthwaite method (Satterthwaite 1946). Due to its higher level of robustness, the Welch test is routinely preferred to the Student's t-test, and it is, thus, the default option in R.

Code Box 7.8

```
# Example 7.1 [continuation]

# Heteroscedastic t-test (Welch test) with R

t.test(A, P, var.equal = F)
##
##  Welch Two Sample t-test
##
## data:  A and P
```

```
## t = -4.5217, df = 7.7977, p-value = 0.002076
## alternative hypothesis: true difference in means is not
   equal to 0
## 95 percent confidence interval:
##  -22.986884  -7.413116
## sample estimates:
## mean of x mean of y
##      70.2      85.4
```

In some cases, two measures are taken on the same subject, e.g., at different times or in several positions ("paired sample"), and we are interested in knowing whether there is a significant difference between the first and second measures. Under these conditions, we need to perform a paired t-test, as shown in the following example.

7.2 Example 7.2: Paired Measurements During a Dietary Program

Let us imagine that we have examined a sample of 20 mice, taking weight measurements at the beginning and the end of a particular dietary program; at the end of this experiment, we have two paired measurements for each individual, totaling 40 values. A traditional t-test assumes that the measurements in the two groups are independent, while this is not true for this example, as we have 40 measures but only 20 independent mice. We can perform a paired t-test using the same function as in Code Box 7.7, setting the "paired" argument to TRUE, as shown in Code Box 7.9. Please note that the number of degrees of freedom is 19 (20 independent subjects minus 1).

Code Box 7.9

```
# Example 7.2
# Paired measurements during a dietary program

before <- c(171.8, 228.3, 181.5, 182.2, 162.3, 194.1, 193.3,
            187.6, 197.2, 207.1, 184.8, 175.3, 184.8, 199.4,
            196.3, 186.2, 221.1, 205.5, 208.5, 193.7)
after <- c(400.2, 452.7, 423.4, 384.8, 363.5, 385.8, 387.8,
           397.5, 397.9, 404.3, 413.5, 454.6, 377.7, 362.2,
           382.7, 379.4, 401.7, 379.6, 417.1, 364.1)
t.test(before, after, paired = T, var.equal = F)
##
```

```
##  Paired t-test
##
## data:  before and after
## t = -33.637, df = 19, p-value < 2.2e-16
## alternative hypothesis: true mean difference is not equal
   to 0
## 95 percent confidence interval:
##  -216.1358 -190.8142
## sample estimates:
## mean difference
##        -203.475
```

7.3 Example 7.3: Testing Differences Between Model Parameters

The Welch test can be generalized to test the difference between two independent estimates. For example, let us imagine that we have fitted a model to measure the growth rate of sugar beet with two different agronomic practices and obtained the estimates $\rho_1 = 0.22$ with a standard error of 0.013 and $\rho_2 = 0.31$ with a standard error of 0.029. A T ratio can be obtained as

$$T = \frac{0.31 - 0.22}{\sqrt{0.031^2 + 0.029^2}} = -2.12 \tag{7.3}$$

If we cannot determine the number of degrees of freedom for T (which is not always easy) and if the sample size is the same for the two samples, and is sufficiently large, we can use a Gaussian approximation to derive the P-level, as shown in Code Box 7.10.

It may be useful to mention that, to compare model parameters across nonlinear regression fits, it is possible to use the `compParm()` function in the `drm` package, or the `compCoefs()` function in the `statforbiology` package.

Code Box 7.10

```
# Example 7.3
# testing differences between model parameters

T_obs <- (0.22 - 0.31)/sqrt(0.031^2 + 0.029^2)
2 * pnorm(abs(T_obs), lower.tail = F)
## [1] 0.033994
```

7.4 Example 7.4: The F-Test in ANOVA

The F-ratio is a measure of the strength of a causal relationship between a set of nominal/quantitative predictors and a quantitative response (see Chap. 4). Whenever the observed data represent a sample from a broader population, the observed F value is just an instance of an infinite number of possible F values, which define a sampling distribution. What does such sampling distribution look like?

For example, let us reconsider the genotype experiment presented earlier (Example 4.3) in Chap. 4, with four oat genotypes ("oat1L" data); the F-ratio in ANOVA (Code Box 4.7) for the genotype effect is 42.71, with 3 degrees of freedom at the numerator and 8 degrees of freedom at the denominator.

For this experiment, the null hypothesis would correspond to a situation where, at the population level, it is

$$H_0 : \mu_1 = \mu_2 = \mu_3 = \mu_4$$

which amounts to saying that all treatment effects are equal to 0:

$$H_0 : \alpha_1 = \alpha_2 = \alpha_3 = \alpha_4 = 0$$

The observed F-ratio contradicts the null hypothesis; however, we must consider the range of values the F-ratio could assume when the null hypothesis is true. We need to ask ourselves what is the sampling distribution for the F-ratio when the null is true?

Such a sampling distribution could be constructed by Monte Carlo simulation; however, employing a theoretical CDF is a more straightforward approach. The American mathematician George Snedecor demonstrated that when the null is true and the residuals are independent, Gaussian distributed, and homoscedastic, the sampling distribution for the F-ratio can be described by the F-distribution (Fisher-Snedecor distribution), which is only defined for positive values and has an asymmetric shape (right-skewed), depending on the number of degrees of freedom. An example is shown in Fig. 7.2.

The exact P-value can be calculated using the cumulative distribution function in R, as follows: `pf(42.707, 3, 8, lower.tail = F)` $= 2.87 \times 10^{-5}$. This value is lower than 0.05, and thus, we reject the null.

7.5 Conclusions

The inherent uncertainty in all experimental data prevents us from drawing conclusions and making decisions without risk of error. As we aim to reject hypotheses, we must protect ourselves as much as possible against the possibility of incorrect rejection. To do so, we need to:

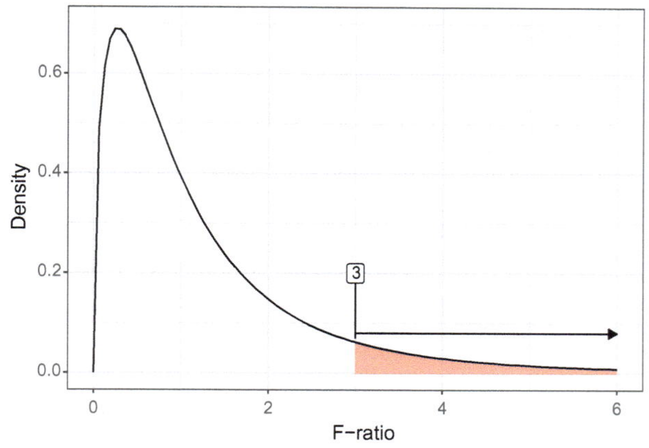

Fig. 7.2 Fisher-Snedecor density function with 3 and 8 degrees of freedom. Considering a hypothetical F-ratio of 3, the total probability (area-under-the-curve) above this value represents the P-value, that is, 0.095

1. Calculate a useful statistic to summarize the results of an experiment (as the T-value or the F-ratio).
2. Identify a sampling distribution for that statistic under the null hypothesis. That sampling distribution could be a theoretical cumulative probability function or, in case the former is not found, an empirical distribution from Monte Carlo simulation.
3. Use the selected sampling distribution to derive the probability of events as extreme or more extreme than the one we just observed.

Before concluding, we would like to point out four main issues that we should always bear in mind:

1. The P-value is regarded as the probability of wrongly rejecting the null (so-called type I error rate: false positive). However, we should interpret such a probability with reference to the sampling distribution rather than a single experiment. It follows that we can conclude "*if the null hypothesis is true and we repeat the experiment an infinite number of times, we have less than a 5% probability of obtaining such a high T or F-ratio.*" However, we cannot legitimately conclude "*there is less than a 5% probability that we have reached wrong conclusions.*" Indeed, we do not (and will never) know whether we have reached correct conclusions in our specific experiment, while our "false-positive" probability is only valid in the long run.
2. The P-value is valid if the basic assumptions of independent, normally distributed, and homoscedastic residuals are met.
3. As mentioned in Chap. 1, Neyman and Pearson proposed adopting an alternative hypothesis that is held to be true when the null hypothesis is rejected. For example (see Sect. 7.1), if the null is $H_0 : \delta_2 = 0$, the alternative is $H_0 : \delta_2 \neq 0$.

		REALITY	
		The two genotypes A and B have the same yield performances	The two genotypes A and B have different yield performances
NULL HYPOTHESIS There is no difference between the two genotypes	NULL is accepted	RIGHT DECISION	TYPE II ERROR (false negative)
	NULL is rejected	TYPE I ERROR (false positive)	RIGHT DECISION

Fig. 7.3 The two types of statistical errors

More complex alternative hypotheses are also possible, such as $H_1 : \delta_2 > 0$ or $H_1 : \delta_2 < 0$, although these complex alternative hypotheses can only be adopted when there is some prior knowledge that justifies them. In all cases, we should avoid the common misconception that rejecting the null implies that either the alternative is demonstrated or the alternative is true with a probability $P_{alt} = 1 -$ P-value (Gigerenzer 2018).

4. "Statistical" decisions do imply not only the risk of committing a false-positive error (type I error) but also the risk of committing a false-negative error (type II error) whenever a false null hypothesis is not rejected (Fig. 7.3). These two error types are interrelated, and the higher the protection against the false-positive error, the higher the risk of committing a false-negative error. In general, we should always be careful to decide which of the two errors might be more dangerous for our specific aim.

7.6 Questions and Exercises

1. The observed T-value for the null is 2.79, and the number of DF is 12. We want to test the hypothesis that the T-value is not significantly different from 0; what is the probability of type I error?
2. Our best estimate of a model parameter is $g = -7.2$, with a standard error equal to 2.8, with 16 degrees of freedom. Is it possible that the population-based parameter is $\gamma = 0$? What is the P-value for the null? Do we have to accept it, or should we reject it?
3. Our best estimate for δ is $d = 13.5$, with a standard error of 8.4; however, we have no idea about the degrees of freedom for the SE. Test the hypothesis that $\delta = 0$, under the assumption that the sample size is large enough to adopt a Gaussian approximation.

4. We have compared two herbicides for weed control in maize. With the first herbicide (A), we observed the following weed coverings: 9.3, 10.2, and 9.7%, while, with the second, we observed 12.6, 12.3, and 12.5%. Are the means for the two herbicides significantly different ($\alpha = 0.05$)?
5. The observed F-ratio in ANOVA is 3.57, with 3 DF and 8 DF. The null hypothesis is that the experimental treatments are not significantly different; what is the P-level? Do we reject the null?
6. A plant pathologist studied the crop performances with (A) and without (NT) a fungicide treatment. The yield results in 100 kg per hectare were A = [65, 71, 68) and NT = [54, 51, 59]. Considering these results, decide whether the treatment effect is significant ($\alpha = 0.05$).
7. A laboratory experiment has shown that the degradation rate of a xenobiotic substance is $k_1 = -0.071 \pm 0.012$, whereas a similar substance has shown a degradation rate of $k_2 = -0.153 \pm 0.024$. Test the hypothesis that the degradation rates of the two substances are not significantly different, assuming that the sample size was sufficiently high to adopt a Gaussian approximation.
8. The observed F value is 4.58, with 6 and 9 DF, respectively, at the numerator and denominator. Do we reject the null? What is the P-level?
9. Serum cholesterol levels were measured for eight dairy cows before and after a 3-month dietary program. Considering the observed values (see later), decide whether the therapy was significant or not.

```
Before <- c(167.3,186.7,105.0,214.5,148.5,171.5,
      161.5,243.6)
After <- c(126.7,154.2,107.9,209.3,138.5,121.3,
     112.4,190.5)
```

10. A plant breeder conducted an experiment to compare three wheat genotypes, i.e., GUERCINO, ARNOVA, and BOLOGNA, using a completely randomized design with ten replicates. Considering the results below, by way of an F-test, decide whether the three genotypes show at least one significant difference.

Guercino	Arnova	Bologna
53.2	53.1	43.5
59.1	51.0	41.0
62.3	51.9	41.2
48.6	55.3	44.8
59.7	58.8	40.2
60.0	54.6	37.2
55.7	53.0	45.3
55.8	51.4	38.9
55.7	51.7	42.9
54.4	64.7	39.3

References

Gigerenzer G (2018) Statistical Rituals: the replication delusion and how we got there. Adv Methods Pract Psychol Sci 1(2):198–218. https://doi.org/10.1177/2515245918771329. https://journals.sagepub.com/doi/10.1177/2515245918771329

Satterthwaite FE (1946) An approximate distribution of estimates of variance components. Biom Bull 2(6):110. https://doi.org/10.2307/3002019. http://www.jstor.org/stable/10.2307/3002019?origin=crossref

Chapter 8
Checking Fitted Models

> *An approximate answer to the right problem is worth a good deal more than an exact answer to an approximate problem*
> —J. Tukey

Abstract Fitted models must be thoroughly checked to ensure that they provide a good description of the experimental data and, conversely, that the data adhere to the basic assumptions that the models make. Without this check, we cannot be sure that the fitted models can provide a reliable answer to the research questions we intend to ask. In this chapter, a checking routine is proposed for model residuals based on several types of graphs that are easily accessible in R, together with a few simple formal statistical tests for normality and homoscedasticity. Variance stabilizing transformations are introduced as a swift remedy for model violations, and guidance is provided on how to select the most suitable type of transformation, based on the widely used Box-Cox method.

In the previous chapters, models were introduced as "tools" to describe cause-effect relationships among the experimental variables and to make inferences and test relevant hypotheses. However, we have also seen that **statistical models make assumptions**, which must be reasonably respected for the models to be used reliably to achieve their intended aims.

In particular, the basic assumptions are:

1. The model provides a good description of the experimental data (**goodness of fit**).
2. The residuals are independent of one another (**independency**).
3. The residuals have a Gaussian distribution of probability (**normality**).
4. All the residuals have the same variance (**homoscedasticity**).

Apart from the above assumptions, the observed data must also respect another essential requirement: the absence of "gross" **outliers**, which are observations that differ remarkably from all the other observations in the same treatment group. These

A. Onofri, *Field Research Methods in Agriculture*,
https://doi.org/10.1007/978-3-032-08199-5_8

outliers produce huge negative or positive residuals, which can be highly influential, both for the previous assumptions and for the reliability of the estimation process.

Unfortunately, problems relating to the above issues are anything but infrequent.

8.1 Deviations from Basic Assumptions

Lack-of-fit may occur when model predictions appear to systematically deviate from the observed data, such as, when a straight line is fitted to a curvilinear response. In case of lack-of-fit, we should conclude that the data and the model do not support each other and, thus, that the model "does not enable the researcher to answer the scientific questions at hand" (Kass et al. 2016).

Lack of independence arises when the residuals contain not only random errors but also a systematic component. For example, if a block effect exists but is not accounted for in the model, the residuals will reflect this systematic block effect. As a result, residuals from the same block will tend to be more similar to each other than to residuals from different blocks. Consequently, those residuals cannot be considered genuinely independent (see also Chap. 12).

Such a deviation may occur because of (i) systematic intrusions, (ii) grouping factors that have not been accounted for in the model, (iii) systematic lack-of-fit due to the wrong selection of the model function, or (iv) lack of proper randomization (see also Sect. 4.6 and Chap. 12). Lack of independence is considered one of the most dangerous assumptions to violate, leading to an inflated risk of type I error (Frey et al. 2024), i.e., an increased risk of wrongly rejecting a true null hypothesis (false positive).

Normality is violated when model residuals do not "reflect" the typical shape of a Gaussian distribution, i.e., when they are asymmetric (skewed distribution: the mean is not equal to the median) or when the tails are too heavy (platykurtic distribution: too many extreme values) or too light (leptokurtic distribution: the values are too "concentrated" around the mean) (Fig. 8.1; see also Chap. 5). In the absence of "gross" outliers (see later), non-normality is considered less detrimental than other deviations (Knief and Forstmeier 2021), as it does not provoke strong bias in parameter estimation or an inflated risk of type I error. Nonetheless, a cautious attitude is always recommended, as deviations from normality may be associated with other types of more dangerous deviations, such as heteroscedasticity.

Deviations from normality may also occur due to the presence of "gross" outliers related to random errors of an exceptional entity (e.g., faulty procedures, poor control, or intrusions of any kind). These outliers pull away means and standard deviations, potentially provoking misinterpretations of the experimental results (Cochran 1947).

Heteroscedasticity may occur, for example, when experimental treatments produce effects on both the mean and the standard deviations (e.g., multiplicative effects) so that these two statistics become proportional to each other. Other common causes of heteroscedasticity include pest attacks and other intrusions, as

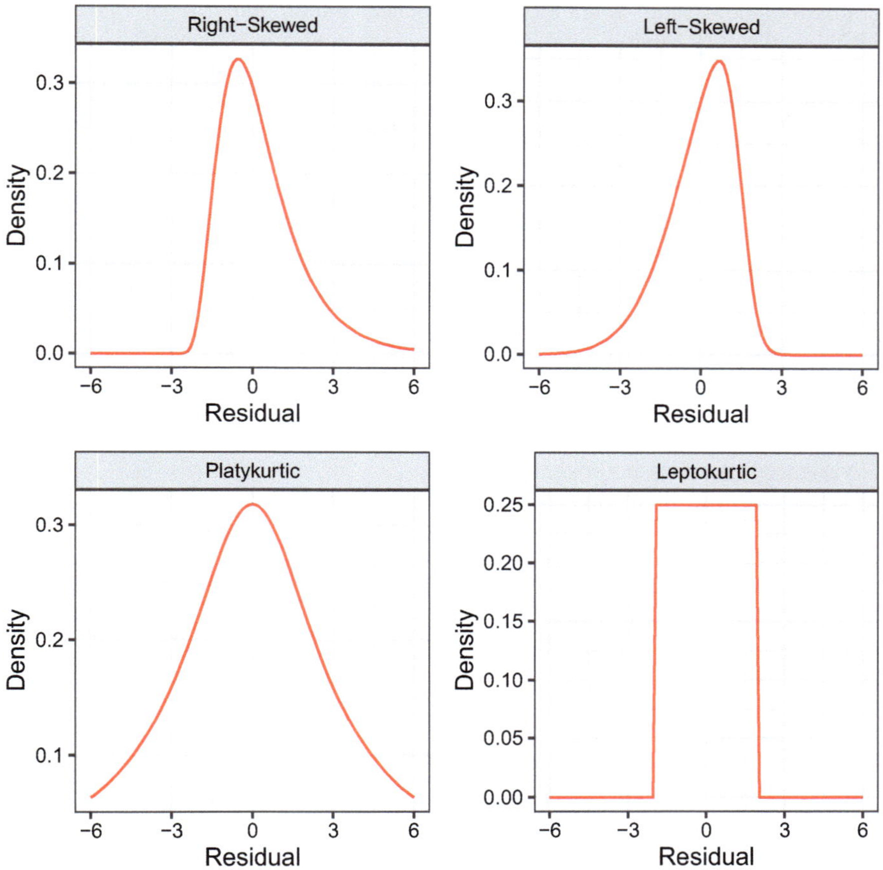

Fig. 8.1 Different non-normal shapes for model residuals: right-skewed: the median is lower than the mean, left-skewed: the median is higher than the mean; platykurtic: tails are too heavy, with too many extreme values; leptokurtic: tails are too light and values are too "concentrated" near to the mean

well as a lower degree of control in certain parts of the field experiment. It has been shown that heteroscedasticity results in a biased estimate of the residual standard deviation and invalid P-values, so that the actual error rate can be very different from the nominal one (Glass et al. 1972).

8.2 Detecting Violations

For the reasons mentioned in the previous paragraphs, it is fundamental to detect problems with the basic assumptions of linear models, using the most suitable diagnostic methods.

Possible departures from the independence assumption can be detected by verifying that the experimental design is correct and that the model is adequate for the design. In particular, it is important to ensure that all grouping factors and other constraints to complete randomization are included in the model (e.g., the blocks and the main-plots) and are not omitted, even if their effect is not found to be statistically significant (Frey et al. 2024).

Apart from independence, possible problems with the other assumptions (systematic lack-of-fit, non-normality, or heteroscedasticity) are detected by a careful check of model residuals, which needs to be particularly accurate in three conditions:

1. When the response is made of counts or ratios, which are very rarely normal and homoscedastic
2. When the response is quantitative, and the differences between group means are very high (e.g., higher than one order of magnitude) because, for this data, variances are rarely homogeneous
3. When we have fitted a regression model, which might systematically deviate from the observed responses

Inspection methods can be divided into two groups: graphical and numerical (Anscombe and Tukey 1963). Both will be considered in the following sections.

8.2.1 Graphical Inspection Methods

Graphical methods are very simple yet powerful enough to reveal substantial deviations, while slight deviations can usually be tolerated. For their clarity and simplicity, it is recommended that a graphical inspection of residuals is routinely performed after every model fitting process.

Among the possible graphs of residuals, the following sections will cover the three main types of simple plots that can easily be produced with R or other plotting software.

8.2.1.1 Plot of Predicted and Observed Values

For all types of regression models, the most important tool for checking the goodness of fit is a scatterplot of the observed response against the predictor, augmented with predictions from the model fit. In this graph, predictions should closely follow the observed data (Fig. 8.2A) without showing any sign of systematic deviations, as illustrated in Fig. 8.2B, C, and D.

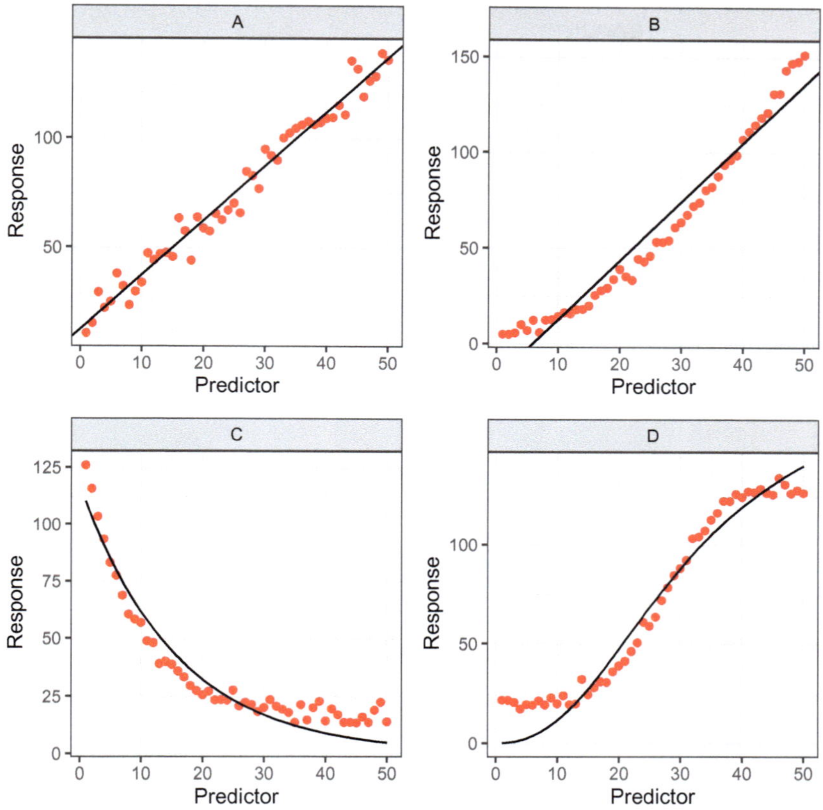

Fig. 8.2 Scatterplots of the observed responses (symbols) against a quantitative predictor, augmented with model predictions (solid black lines). Panel A displays a well-fitting linear regression model, while Panel B shows a linear regression model that systematically deviates from a curvilinear response. Panels C and D show two curvilinear regression models that are not suitable to describe two curvilinear asymptotic responses

8.2.1.2 Plot of Residuals Against Expected Values

Residuals from the model fit can be plotted against the expected values. Suppose there are no systematic errors, and variances are homogeneous across treatments. In this case, the points in this graph should be randomly scattered, with no visible systematic patterns (Fig. 8.3, top-left).

Every possible deviation from such a random pattern should be carefully inspected; for example, the presence of outliers is indicated by a few "isolated points," as shown in Fig. 8.3 (top-right). Otherwise, when the cloud of points takes the form of a "funnel" (Fig. 8.3, bottom-left), the variances are proportional to the expected values, and therefore, they are not homogeneous across treatments (heteroscedasticity). Last but not least, lack-of-fit may be indicated by, for example,

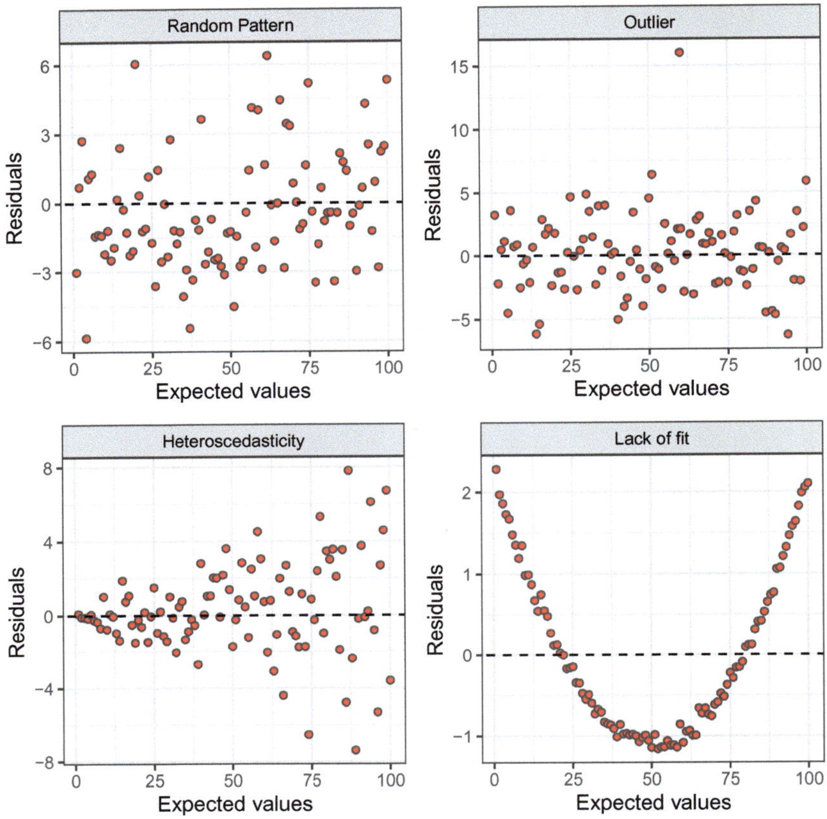

Fig. 8.3 A plot of residuals against expected values: Randomly scattered symbols support the respect of the basic assumptions (top, left). An outlying observation is visible as an isolated point with a very high residual (top, right). Heteroscedasticity is shown by residuals that tend to increase on one side of the graph (bottom, left). Lack-of-fit is revealed by, e.g., clusters of residuals of the same sign (bottom, right)

residuals that tend to be systematically negative in a part of their range and systematically positive elsewhere (Fig. 8.3, bottom-right). This pattern corresponds, for example, to the situation depicted in Fig. 8.2B, and it is more common with regression models than with models with nominal predictors.

8.2.1.3 QQ-Plot

The so-called QQ-plot (quantile-quantile plot) is used to detect possible problems with the basic assumption of normality. It is a scatterplot of the standardized residuals (on the y-axis) against the corresponding percentiles of a normal distribution (on the x-axis). For the sake of simplicity, details on how to draw a QQ-plot are not

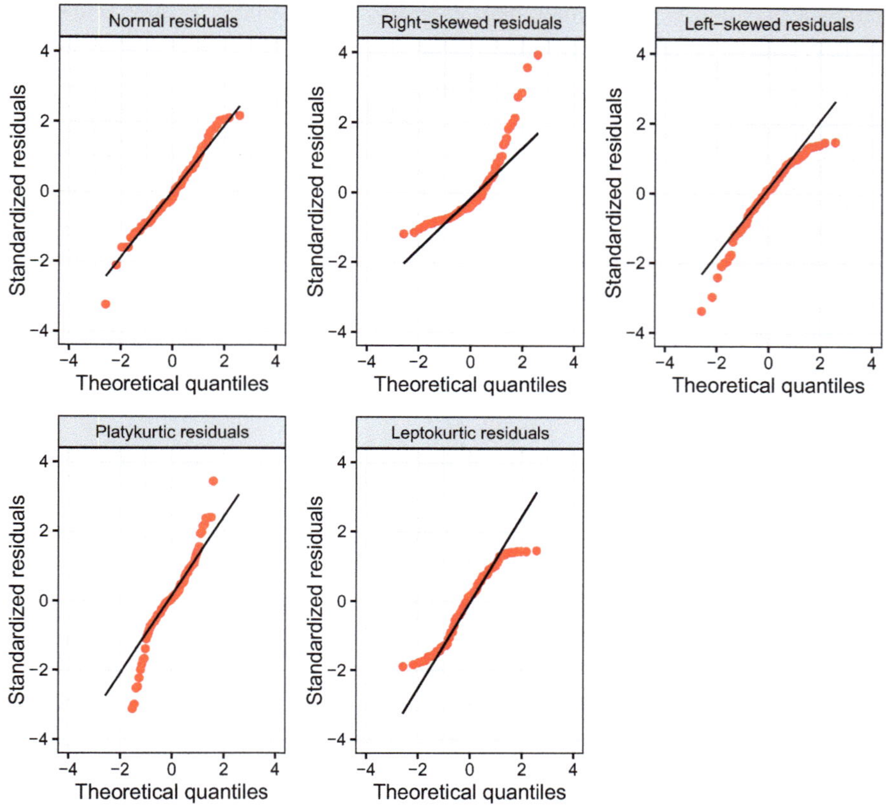

Fig. 8.4 QQ-plot for normal residuals (top-left) and for residuals that show several types of deviations from normality (see also Fig. 8.1)

given here; they can be found in the companion blog.[1] In terms of interpretation, Gaussian residuals should approximately lie along the diagonal (e.g., see Fig. 8.4, top-left). Any systematic deviations from the diagonal suggest that the normality assumption may not hold (see Fig. 8.4, all panels except top-left).

8.2.2 *Formal Statistics and Hypothesis Testing*

Apart from graphical inspection methods, several formal statistical testing procedures are available to test the hypotheses of homoscedasticity and normality formally. In theory, the most significant advantage of these procedures over

[1] Go to https://www.statforbiology.com/2020/stat_general_percentiles/.

graphical techniques is that they permit decisions based on a P-value. However, all that glitters is not gold, and these tests may create more problems than they solve. For example, they typically require large sample sizes and make stringent assumptions so that, in the end, the reliability of their results is often questionable (Kozak and Piepho 2018). For these reasons, their use is not recommended, and it should be reserved for complex situations where graphical methods do not provide clear answers.

The procedures presented in this chapter were selected because they are widely used and readily available in R.

8.2.2.1 Levene's Test for Homoscedasticity

According to the simulation study of Conover et al. (1981), Levene's test is one of the most reliable procedures for testing the hypothesis of homoscedasticity in models with nominal predictors. The F statistic is obtained by fitting the original model to a pseudo-response variable, which is obtained by replacing each original response value with the absolute value of its difference with the center of its group (centered data).

The rationale of this test is that the group means of group-centered data are zero for all treatment groups. However, if we remove the signs, these means become positive and tend to increase when the group variances are higher. In the original Levene work, the center of each treatment group was defined as the mean of that group. However, in later work, Brown and Forsythe (1974) suggested that the mean be replaced with the median to obtain a more robust test for non-normal residuals. Both the tests are available in the `leveneTest()` function in the R package `car`, but the second one is regarded as the default.

An example of this test is provided in Code Box 8.3, which compares two maize genotypes in a completely randomized design with 11 replicates. The second genotype (B) has a higher variance, and Levene's test turns out to be significant (the P-value is lower than 0.05, and the null hypothesis of homoscedasticity is rejected). The two tests (centering with the means or centering with the medians) yield similar results, which may suggest that the original data do not deviate significantly from normality.

Code Box 8.1

```
# Testing hypotheses about model residuals
# Levene's test for homoscedasticity
library(car)

# Entering the data
dataset <- data.frame(Genotype = c("A", "A", "A", "A", "A",
                                   "A", "A", "A", "A", "A",
                                   "A", "B", "B", "B", "B",
```

```
                                        "B", "B", "B", "B", "B",
                                        "B", "B"),
                          Yield = c(10.0, 10.7, 11.9, 10.3,
                                   10.0, 7.8, 10.4, 9.7,
                                   10.0, 9.2, 9.7, 15.0,
                                   11.2, 13.7, 11.9, 9.4,
                                   10.6, 12.6, 10.1, 9.9,
                                   15.3, 12.2))
head(dataset)
##   Genotype Yield
## 1        A  10.0
## 2        A  10.7
## 3        A  11.9
## 4        A  10.3
## 5        A  10.0
## 6        A   7.8

# Fitting the model
mod <- lm(Yield ~ Genotype, data = dataset)

# Centering the data by subtracting, for each genotype
# the group mean (Levene's test)
GroupMeans <- tapply(dataset$Yield, dataset$Genotype,
     mean)
YieldC <- dataset$Yield - rep(GroupMeans, each = 11)

# Re-fitting the same model to the absolute values of
# centered data and run an ANOVA
modlevene <- lm(abs(YieldC) ~ dataset$Genotype)
anova(modlevene)
## Analysis of Variance Table
##
## Response: abs(YieldC)
##                  Df  Sum Sq Mean Sq F value  Pr(>F)
## dataset$Genotype  1  5.2129  5.2129  5.8944 0.02475 *
## Residuals        20 17.6878  0.8844

# Centering the data by subtracting, for each genotype
# the group median (Brown-Forsythe's test)
GroupMedians <- tapply(dataset$Yield, dataset$Genotype, median)
YieldC <- dataset$Yield - rep(GroupMedians, each = 11)

# Re-fitting the same model to the absolute values of
# centered data and run an ANOVA
modlevene <- lm(abs(YieldC) ~ dataset$Genotype)
anova(modlevene)
## Analysis of Variance Table
```

```
##
## Response: abs(YieldC)
##                  Df  Sum Sq Mean Sq F value  Pr(>F)
## dataset$Genotype  1  5.2041  5.2041  5.7245 0.02666 *
## Residuals        20 18.1818  0.9091

# Non-robust Levene's test with R (centering with means)
leveneTest(mod, center = "mean")
## Levene's Test for Homogeneity of Variance
   (center = "mean")
##       Df F value  Pr(>F)
## group  1  5.8944 0.02475 *
##       20

# Levene's test with R (centering with medians; default)
leveneTest(mod)
## Levene's Test for Homogeneity of Variance
    (center = median)
##       Df F value  Pr(>F)
## group  1  5.7245 0.02666 *
##       20
#
```

8.2.2.2 Shapiro-Wilk's Test for Normality

The Shapiro-Wilks test for normality provides the W statistic and a P-value for the null hypothesis that the residuals are normally distributed. The testing procedure is not as straightforward as the procedure for Levene's test and hand calculations are not as easy to perform. However, we can make use of the `shapiro.test()` function in R, passing the model residuals as an argument.

8.2.2.3 Other Tests

It is worth mentioning some numerical techniques for detecting outliers, such as the methods proposed by Anscombe and Tukey (1963) and Grubbs (1969).

8.2.3 Example 8.1: Checking the Residuals for the "Mixture" Data

A pot experiment was performed to compare the weed control efficacy of two herbicides used alone and in a mixture. A control was also added as a reference, and thus, the four treatments were:

1. Metribuzin
2. Rimsulfuron
3. Metribuzin + rimsulfuron
4. Untreated control

Sixteen uniform pots were prepared and sown with *Solanum nigrum*. When the plants reached the 4-true-leaf stage, the pots were treated with the above herbicides or left untreated, according to a completely randomized design with four replicates. Three weeks after the treatments, the plants in each pot were harvested and weighed; the lower the weight, the higher the efficacy of the herbicides (Onofri et al. 1995).

For this experiment, a linear model with one nominal predictor (the herbicide treatment) can be fitted (see Eq. (4.6) in Chap. 4), as shown in Code Box 8.2.

Code Box 8.2

```
# Example 8.1
# Checking the residuals for the 'mixture' data

# Loading the packages
library(statforbiology)
library(car)

# Loading and transforming the data
mixture <- getAgroData("mixture")
mixture$Treat <- factor(mixture$Treat)
head(mixture)
##                Treat Weight
## 1 Metribuzin__348  15.20
## 2 Metribuzin__348   4.38
## 3 Metribuzin__348  10.32
## 4 Metribuzin__348   6.80
## 5     Mixture_378   6.14
## 6     Mixture_378   1.95

# Model fitting
mod1 <- lm(Weight ~ Treat, data = mixture)
```

After fitting, swift graphical analyses of model residuals can be obtained by using the `plot()` function, passing the model object as the first argument, while the `which` argument can be set to 1 or 2: The former produces a plot of residuals

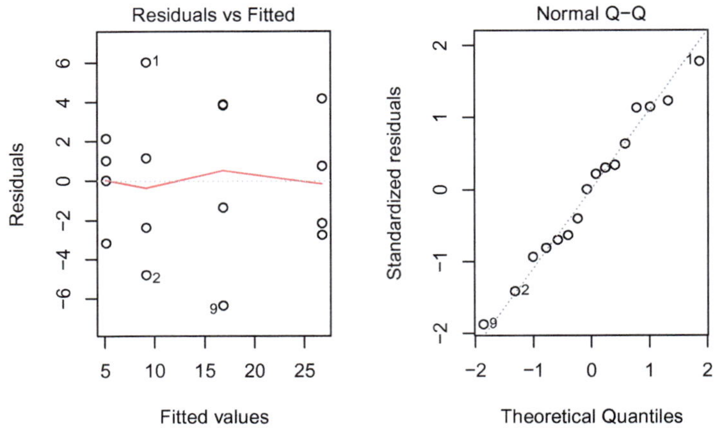

Fig. 8.5 Graphical analyses of residuals for the "mixture" data

against expected values, while the latter makes a QQ-plot (Code Box 8.2), which are displayed in Fig. 8.5.

Code Box 8.3

```
# Example 8.1 [continuation]

# Graphical analyses of residuals in R
plot(mod1, which = 1)
plot(mod1, which = 2)
```

Neither of the two graphs suggests deviations from the basic assumptions. Considering that we have a quantitative variable with small differences (less than one order of magnitude) between group means, we conclude that there are no problems with the basic assumptions. Although this would not be necessary, we can confirm our conclusion by running the Levene's and Shapiro-Wilk's tests (Code Box 8.4). Please note that the model object is passed as an argument to the `leveneTest()` function, while the residuals need to be passed to the `shapiro.test()` function.

Code Box 8.4

```
# Example 8.1 [continuation]

# Levene's test and Shapiro-Wilk's test

leveneTest(mod1)
## Levene's Test for Homogeneity of Variance
   (center = median)
##       Df F value Pr(>F)
## group  3  1.0698 0.3984
##       12

shapiro.test(residuals(mod1))
##
##  Shapiro-Wilk normality test
##
## data:  residuals(mod1)
## W = 0.97615, p-value = 0.9257
```

8.2.4 *Example 8.2: Checking the Residuals for the "Insects" Data*

Plants of tobacco were treated with three different insecticides according to a completely randomized design with five replicates (15 plants in total), and the number of insects over the surface of leaves in each plant was counted 3 weeks after the treatments. To elucidate the causal effect of the insecticides, a model with the "Insecticide" variable as a nominal predictor was fitted to the observed data (Code Box 8.5).

In this case, checking for deviations from the basic assumptions requires great care, as the response variable is a count, and the descriptive statistics indicate that the standard deviations are somewhat proportional to the means (not shown). The graphical analyses of residuals in Fig. 8.6 show clear signs of heteroscedasticity (left plot) and right-skewed residuals (right plot). These deviations are confirmed by Levene's test (P-value $= 0.043$) and Shapiro-Wilks' test (P-value $= 0.048$).

Code Box 8.5

```
# Example 8.2
# checking the residuals for the 'insects' data

# Loading the packages
library(statforbiology)
library(car)

# Loading and transforming the data
insects <- getAgroData("insects")
insects$Insecticide <- factor(insects$Insecticide)
head(insects)
##   Insecticide Rep Count
## 1          T1   1   448
## 2          T1   2   906
## 3          T1   3   484
## 4          T1   4   477
## 5          T1   5   634
## 6          T2   1   211

# Fitting a model
mod2 <- lm(Count ~ Insecticide, data = insects)

# Graphical analyses of residuals (Fig. 8.7)
plot(mod2, which = 1)
plot(mod2, which = 2)

# Levene's test
leveneTest(mod2)
## Levene's Test for Homogeneity of Variance
  (center = median)
##       Df F value Pr(>F)
## group  2  1.0263 0.3878
##       12

# Shapiro-Wilks' test
shapiro.test(residuals(mod2))
##
##  Shapiro-Wilk normality test
##
## data:  residuals(mod2)
## W = 0.87689, p-value = 0.04265
```

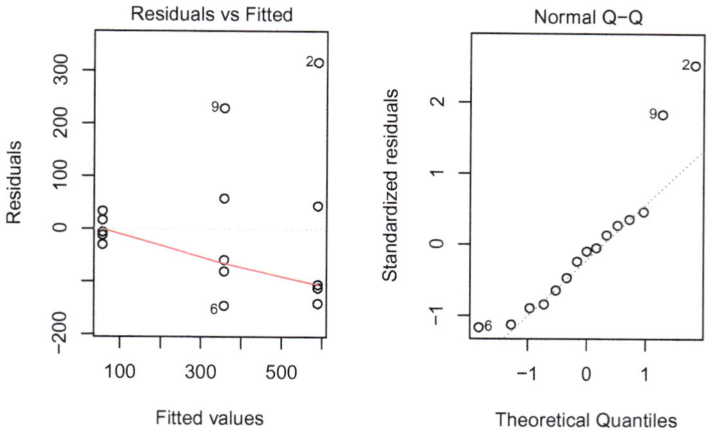

Fig. 8.6 Graphical analyses of residuals for the "insects" dataset

8.3 Correcting Measures

Whenever the basic assumptions are not met, appropriate correcting measures must be taken, to prevent misinterpretations and flawed conclusions.

In the presence of "gross" outliers, it is necessary to decide whether they should either be neglected, given a lower weight during the analysis stage, or even removed from the dataset. This latter solution is not recommended and should only be considered after careful thought to avoid losing important information and/or artificially decreasing the variability of the data while unduly increasing the power of statistical testing. In particular, it is always necessary to make sure that any outlying observation (i) is not a part of the population under study, (ii) is only caused by the effect of random errors or intrusions, and (iii) has no relationship with the effects of the experimental treatments under study. Furthermore, the removal of outliers should concern only a very low number of observations; otherwise, it might be wise to discard the entire experiment and conduct a new one.

Regarding the other basic assumptions, the most traditional method for dealing with non-normality and heteroscedasticity is through the so-called **variance stabilizing transformations**, which involve changing the metric of the observations to make them more consistent with the basic assumptions for linear models.

Traditional textbooks (e.g., Snedecor and Cochran 1991) recommend selecting the transformation based on the type of data available; for example, the square root transformation is usually recommended for counts, the arcsin-square root transformation (angular transformation; Ahrens et al. 1990) is suggested for proportions, and the logarithmic transformation is recommended for log-normal data, when variances increase with means.

More recently, the availability of high computing power permits the empirical selection of the best transformation method based on a direct comparison of several possible alternatives; for example, it is possible to consider the Box-Cox family of transformations (Box and Cox 1964), which is

$$W = \begin{cases} \frac{Y^{\lambda}-1}{\lambda} & \text{if } \lambda \neq 0 \\ \log(Y) & \text{if } \lambda = 0 \end{cases} \tag{8.1}$$

In this equation, W is the transformed variable, Y is the original variable, and λ is the transformation parameter, which can be changed to fit the transformation needs of the dataset at hand.[2] It is easy to note that if λ equals 1, the transformation only consists of subtracting a constant value, which does not alter the metric of the original data. Instead, if λ is between 0 and 1, the upper end of observations is pulled in, while the lower end is stretched out, which permits the correction of right-skewed residuals and breaks the proportionality between variances and means. On the other hand, if λ is higher than 1, it will have an opposite effect and will correct left-skewed residuals with variances that are inversely proportional to the means.

Box and Cox (1964) suggested a maximum likelihood method to select the optimal λ value for the dataset at hand, which is implemented in the `boxcox()` function in the `MASS` package.

8.3.1 *Example 8.1 (Continued)*

Although the previous analyses showed that the "mixture" data did not significantly deviate from the basic assumptions for linear models, we can also run the `boxcox()` function in the MASS package, passing the model object as an argument (Code Box 8.6). This function returns a graph of the likelihoods associated with different λ values (Fig. 8.7).

Code Box 8.6

```
# Example 8.1 [continuation]

# Selecting the optimal transformation by the Box-Cox method
library(MASS)
boxcox(mod1)
```

[2] Note that the limit of $(Y^{\lambda} - 1)/\lambda$ for $\lambda \to 0$ is $\log(y)$.

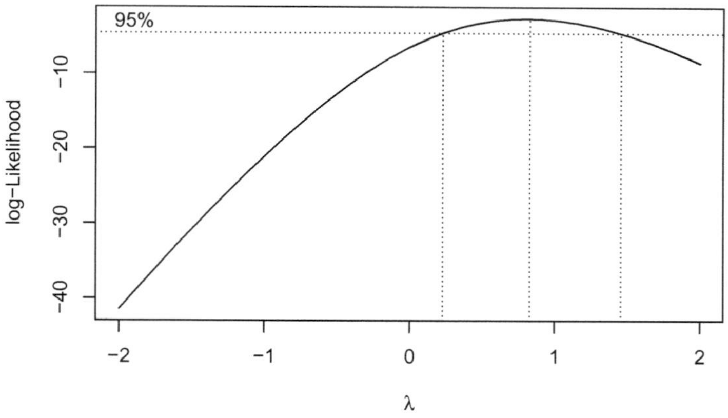

Fig. 8.7 Selecting the maximum likelihood "lambda" value (Box and Cox 1964) for the "mixture" data. The central vertical dotted line identifies the optimal "lambda" value, while the two lateral vertical dotted lines identify the 95% confidence limits

From that graph, it is possible to see that the maximum likelihood λ value is slightly lower than 1. However, the 95% confidence interval (included between the two lateral vertical dotted lines) goes from slightly above 0 to approximately 1.5. Consequently, $\lambda = 1$ can be regarded as an acceptable value for the transformation, which supports the idea that a transformation is not needed.

8.3.2 Example 8.2 (Continued)

The Box-Cox method for the "insects" data returns the graph in Fig. 8.8; the maximum likelihood value is $\lambda = 0.14$, and the 95% confidence interval goes from slightly below zero to roughly 0.5. Thus, for the sake of simplicity, we select $\lambda = 0$, which corresponds to a logarithmic transformation.

The process of data analysis proceeds by transforming the data into their logarithms, refitting the model and reanalyzing the new residuals (Code Box 8.7). Please note that the transformation is performed inside the model fitting command, which is helpful for reasons that will be discussed in the next chapter. A graphical inspection of model residuals for the transformed data (not shown) confirms that there are no apparent deviations from the basic assumptions. The ANOVA table suggests that there are significant differences among the insecticides ($P = 1.49 \times 10^{-6}$; Code Box 8.7).

It may be interesting to compare the ANOVA on transformed data with the ANOVA on untransformed data (Code Box 8.7); apart from the fact that this latter analysis is wrong because the basic assumptions of linear models are not respected,

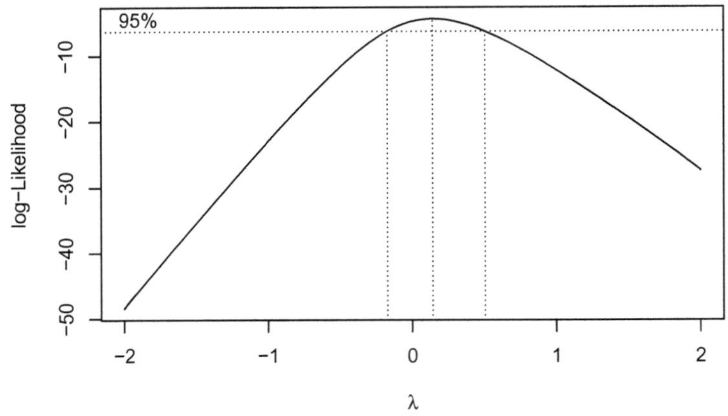

Fig. 8.8 Selecting the maximum likelihood "lambda" value (Box and Cox 1964) for the "insects" data

it is possible to see that the analysis on transformed data is more powerful (lower P-value). However, this conclusion is not general, but it is specific to this dataset.

Code Box 8.7

```
# Adopting a stabilizing transformation

mod2t <- lm(log(Count) ~ Insecticide,
 data = insects)
anova(mod2t)
## Analysis of Variance Table
##
## Response: log(Count)
##             Df  Sum Sq Mean Sq F value    Pr(>F)
## Insecticide  2 15.8200  7.9100  50.122 1.493e-06 ***
## Residuals   12  1.8938  0.1578

# Comparing with ANOVA on the untransformed data
anova(mod2)
## Analysis of Variance Table
##
## Response: Count
##             Df Sum Sq Mean Sq F value    Pr(>F)
## Insecticide  2 714654  357327  18.161 0.0002345 ***
## Residuals   12 236105   19675
```

It may be helpful to give some reasonable suggestions for the cases where the optimal λ value is neither 1 nor 0. For those cases, the transformation $W = (Y^\lambda - 1)/\lambda$ can be simplified to $W = Y^\lambda$, with no change in terms of distributional assumptions. Consequently, $\lambda = 0.5$ would correspond to a square root transformation, while $\lambda = -1$ would be analogous to a reciprocal transformation, with a remarkable increase in terms of simplicity and clarity. An example of such an equivalence is provided in Code Box 8.8, where the two transformations $W = (Y^{0.5} - 1)/0.5$ and $W = Y^{0.5}$ produce the same F and P-values.

Code Box 8.8

```
# Equivalence of the ANOVA with two different transformations

mod.1 <- lm(sqrt(Count) ~ Insecticide, data = insects)
mod.2 <- lm((Count^0.5 - 1)/0.5 ~ Insecticide, data = insects)
anova(mod.1)
## Analysis of Variance Table
##
## Response: sqrt(Count)
##             Df Sum Sq Mean Sq F value    Pr(>F)
## Insecticide  2 724.22  362.11  35.022 9.791e-06 ***
## Residuals   12 124.08   10.34

anova(mod.2)
## Analysis of Variance Table
##
## Response: (Count^0.5 - 1)/0.5
##             Df Sum Sq Mean Sq F value    Pr(>F)
## Insecticide  2 2896.9 1448.44  35.022 9.791e-06 ***
## Residuals   12  496.3   41.36
```

Another critical remark is that the Box-Cox family of transformations does not work when the data are negative or equal to zero. In these cases, it is possible to select a constant value, k, to be added to the original observations so that they become strictly positive. For example, if the lowest negative observation is -0.9, we can use the transformation $W = \log(y + 1)$.

8.3.3 Other Possible Approaches

Stabilizing transformations were very much in fashion in the previous century and were mainly used with counts, proportions, and quantitative heteroscedastic data.

Even today, due to their high simplicity, they remain a very handy tool that should not be neglected.

For several decades, an alternative approach to addressing problems with basic assumptions has been to utilize the so-called nonparametric methods of data analysis, which make little or no assumptions about the distribution of residuals (Siegel and Castellan 1988). However, they are slightly less efficient than the traditional parametric methods discussed in this book.

Nowadays, the availability of high computing power enables the use of alternative methods of data analysis that relax the usual assumptions of normality and homoscedasticity, such as Generalized Linear Models (GLMs) and Generalized Least Squares (GLS) models (Venables and Ripley 2002). These methods are innovative, because they permit the modeling of both the distribution of errors and the relationship between means and standard deviations, as well as the comparison of alternative formulations. However, these methods are too advanced, and they are beyond the scope of this introductory book.

8.4 Questions and Exercises

1. Consider the exercises from 5 to 7 in Chap. 4. For all these exercises, verify that the basic assumptions for linear models are met, by using graphical methods and formal hypothesis testing.

References

Ahrens WH, Cox DJ, Budwar G (1990) Use of the arcsin and square root trasformation for subjectively determined percentage data. Weed Sci 38(38):452–458

Anscombe FJ, Tukey JW (1963) The examination and analysis of residuals. Technometrics 5(2):141–160

Box GEP, Cox DR (1964) An analysis of transformations. J R Stat Soc B 26:211–252

Brown MB, Forsythe AB (1974) Robust tests for the equality of variances. J Am Stat Assoc 69(346):364–367

Cochran WG (1947) Some consequences when the assumptions for the analysis of variance are not satisfied. Biometrics 3(1):22. https://doi.org/10.2307/3001535. https://www.jstor.org/stable/3001535?origin=crossref

Conover WJ, Johnson ME, Johnson MM (1981) A comparative study of tests for homogeneity of variances, with applications to the outer continental shelf bidding data. Technometrics 23(4):351–361

Frey J, Hartung J, Ogutu J, Piepho H (2024) Analyze as randomized—why dropping block effects in designed experiments is a bad idea. Agron J 116(3):1371–1381. https://doi.org/10.1002/agj2.21570. https://acsess.onlinelibrary.wiley.com/doi/10.1002/agj2.21570

Glass G, Peckham P, Sanders J (1972) Consequences of failure to meet assumptions underlying the fixed effects analyses of variance and covariance. Rev Educ Res 42(3):237–288

Grubbs FE (1969) Procedures for detecting outlying observations in samples. Technometrics 11(1):1–21

Kass RE, Caffo BS, Davidian M, Meng XL, Yu B, Reid N (2016) Ten simple rules for effective statistical practice. PLOS Comput Biol 12(6):e1004961. https://doi.org/10.1371/journal.pcbi.1004961. https://dx.plos.org/10.1371/journal.pcbi.1004961

Knief U, Forstmeier W (2021) Violating the normality assumption may be the lesser of two evils. Behav Res Methods 53(6):2576–2590. https://doi.org/10.3758/s13428-021-01587-5. https://link.springer.com/10.3758/s13428-021-01587-5

Kozak M, Piepho H (2018) What's normal anyway? Residual plots are more telling than significance tests when checking ANOVA assumptions. J Agron Crop Sci 204(1):86–98. https://doi.org/10.1111/jac.12220. https://onlinelibrary.wiley.com/doi/10.1111/jac.12220

Onofri A, Covarelli L, Tei F (1995) Efficacy of rimsulfuron and metribuzin against Solanum nigrum L. at different growth stages in tomato. In: International Meeting on Weed Control. Proceedings 16th COLUMA Conference, Reims, ANPP, Reprints, pp 993–1000

Siegel S, Castellan NJ (1988) Nonparametric Statistics for the Behavioral Sciences. McGraw-Hill, Columbus

Snedecor GW, Cochran WG (1991) Statistical Methods, 8th edn. IOWA State University Press, Ames

Venables WN, Ripley BD (2002) Modern Applied Statistics with S. Statistics and Computing, 4th edn. Springer, New York

Chapter 9
Linear/Nonlinear Combinations of Model Parameters

The aim of science is to seek the simplest explanation of complex facts. Seek simplicity and distrust it
—A.N. Whitehead

Abstract Once a model has proven to provide a good description of the experimental data, it is possible to test several relevant hypotheses that can be "translated" into linear or nonlinear combinations of model parameters. This chapter presents examples of the relevance of such combinations and how they can be implemented in R, using several functions of interest, such as the `glht()` function in the `multcomp` package, the `gnlht()` function in the `statforbiology` package, and the `emmeans()` and `contrast()` functions in the `emmeans` package. Particular attention is given to least squares means, orthogonal contrasts, pairwise comparisons, back-transformations, predictions, and inverse predictions, which can all be defined in terms of linear or nonlinear combinations of the estimated model parameters.

Once a model has proven to provide a good description of the experimental data, it is possible to test several relevant hypotheses that can be "translated" into linear or nonlinear combinations of model parameters. These combinations are functions involving the parameters and a set of coefficients; to understand this concept and its importance, let us start with an example.

9.1 Example 9.1: Determining the Average Effect of Herbicides

Let us reconsider the pot experiment of Example 8.1 with the "mixture" data; four herbicide treatments (metribuzin, rimsulfuron, their mixture, and the untreated control) were compared, based on their activity against a common weed species in tomato (*Solanum nigrum*). In Chap. 8, a simple model with one nominal predictor

A. Onofri, *Field Research Methods in Agriculture*,
https://doi.org/10.1007/978-3-032-08199-5_9

was fitted to this dataset, and both graphical and numerical methods were used to demonstrate that the basic assumptions for linear models were met. After these checks and based on the results of an ANOVA, the null hypothesis $H_0 : \mu_1 = \mu_2 = \mu_3 = \mu_4$ can be rejected (P < 0.0001; Code Box 9.1).

Code Box 9.1

```
# Example 9.1
# Determining the average effect of herbicides in the
  'mixture' data

# Loading the packages
library(statforbiology)
library(multcomp)

# Loading the data
dataset <- getAgroData("mixture")

# Fitting a one-way ANOVA model
model <- lm(Weight ~ Treat, data=dataset)
summary(model)
## Coefficients:
##                       Estimate Std. Error t value Pr(>|t|)
## (Intercept)              9.175      1.959   4.684 0.000529 ***
## TreatMixture_378        -4.047      2.770  -1.461 0.169679
## TreatRimsulfuron_30      7.685      2.770   2.774 0.016832 *
## TreatUnweeded           17.598      2.770   6.352 3.65e-05 ***

# Variance partitioning
anova(model)
## Analysis of Variance Table
##
## Response: Weight
##           Df  Sum Sq Mean Sq F value    Pr(>F)
## Treat      3 1089.53  363.18  23.663 2.509e-05 ***
## Residuals 12  184.18   15.35
```

A relevant question is "Is weed control (on average) an effective practice?" This question can be answered by building a linear combination of model parameters, as follows.

The estimated parameters are $\mu = 9.175$, $\alpha_2 = -4.0475$, $\alpha_3 = 7.685$, and $\alpha_4 = 17.5975$, where μ is the mean for the first herbicide (in alphabetical order), α_2, α_3, and α_4 are, respectively, the differences between the means of the second, third, and fourth treatment and the mean of the first one (see Chap. 4). With these estimates, we can calculate the mean of untreated pots as $\mu_u = \mu + \alpha_4$ and the mean of treated pots as $\mu_t = [\mu + (\mu + \alpha_2) + (\mu + \alpha_3)]/3$, that is, $\mu_t = \mu + 1/3\,\alpha_2 + 1/3\,\alpha_3$. Consequently, the difference between treated and untreated pots is equal to the following linear combination: $\delta_{tu} = \mu_t - \mu_{ut} = 1/3\,\alpha_2 + 1/3\,\alpha_3 - \alpha_4$. The result of this combination (δ_{tu}) answers the previous question: If we menage to reject the hypothesis that $\delta_{tu} = 0$, we can conclude that the herbicide treatment is, on average, effective in reducing the biomass of *Solanum nigrum*.

To code and test a linear combination of model parameters with R (and with other software), it is helpful to use the sum of the products of a set of parameters by a set of coefficients:

$$C = 0 \cdot \mu + \frac{1}{3} \cdot \alpha_2 + \frac{1}{3} \cdot \alpha_3 - 1 \cdot \alpha_4 \tag{9.1}$$

The matrix of coefficients is

$$K = [0 \;\; 1/3 \;\; 1/3 \;\; -1] \tag{9.2}$$

From there, we obtain $C = \delta_{tu} = -16.385$, which is a sample estimate. A standard error for this quantity can be obtained by using the law of propagation of errors, considering the variances and covariances of model parameters. For the sake of simplicity, the detail about the propagation of errors is not given, but it can be found in the companion blog.[1]

To fit this linear combination in R, we need a model object and a matrix of coefficients that can be passed to the `glht()` function in the `multcomp` package, as shown in Code Box 9.2. A 95% confidence interval for the EMMs can also be obtained by using the `confint()` function.

Code Box 9.2

```
# Example 9.1 [continuation]

# Fitting linear combinations with the 'glht()' function in R
library(multcomp)

# Setting the matrix of coefficients
K <- matrix(c(0, 1/3, 1/3, -1),
            nrow = 1, ncol = 4, byrow = T)
row.names(K) <- c("delta_tu")
K
##          [,1]      [,2]      [,3] [,4]
```

[1] https://www.statforbiology.com/2024/stat_general_errorpropagation/

```
## delta_tu     0 0.3333333 0.3333333   -1

# Fitting the contrast
con <- glht(model, linfct = K)
summary(con)
##   Simultaneous Tests for General Linear Hypotheses
##
## Fit: lm(formula = Weight ~ Treat, data = dataset)
##
## Linear Hypotheses:
##                 Estimate Std. Error t value Pr(>|t|)
## delta_tu == 0  -16.385      2.262  -7.244 1.02e-05 ***

# Confidence intervals
## confint(con)
##   Simultaneous Confidence Intervals
##
## Fit: lm(formula = Weight ~ Treat, data = dataset)
##
## Quantile = 2.1788
## 95% family-wise confidence level
##
##
## Linear Hypotheses:
##                 Estimate lwr      upr
## delta_tu == 0 -16.3850 -21.3132 -11.4568
```

It is important to note that the estimate δ_{tu} can be divided by its standard error to deliver a t-test for the null hypothesis that the observed estimate is not significantly different from zero (see Sect. 7.1). The corresponding P-value is very low, allowing for the rejection of the null hypothesis. Thus, we conclude that the average herbicide effect is statistically significant.

9.2 Example 9.2: Determining the Average Efficacy of Herbicides

The previous concepts can be extended to every other function of model parameters that cannot be reduced to the sum of the products of coefficients by parameters as in Eq. (9.1) but involves nonlinear expressions. The only difference is that, with nonlinear functions, standard errors can only be approximated by using the so-called **delta method** (Weisberg 2005).[2]

In R, a flexible approach for fitting nonlinear combinations of model parameters is to use the `gnlht()` function in the `statforbiology` package, which generalizes the approach of the `glht()` function. This function can also be used to fit linear combinations, although, in this case, it is less computationally efficient than `glht()`.

As an example of nonlinear combinations, let us reconsider the data from the "mixture" experiment and use the model parameters to calculate the percentage reduction of weed growth with respect to the untreated control (herbicide efficacy (HE)). For the first herbicide, it is

$$\text{HE} = \frac{\mu_4 - \mu_1}{\mu_4} \times 100 = \frac{\mu_1 + \alpha_4 - \mu_1}{\mu_1 + \alpha_4} \times 100 = \frac{\alpha_4}{\mu_1 + \alpha_4} \times 100 \tag{9.3}$$

In this expression, the parameters μ_1 and α_4 are in the denominator, and therefore, this combination is nonlinear. The nonlinear expressions for obtaining the HEs for all other herbicides can be derived using simple mathematics (Code Box 9.3).

These nonlinear combinations are coded as a list and passed as the argument `func` to the `gnlht()` function (Code Box 9.3). The name of parameters used in those combinations and the position of parameter estimates in the model object (as given in the `coef` function) are matched by using the `parameterNames` argument. The three herbicide efficacies are, respectively, 65%, 80%, and 37%, and they are all significantly different from 0 (Code Box 9.3)

Code Box 9.3

```
# Example 9.2
# Determining the average efficacy of herbicides in the 'mixture
  data

# Loading the packages and data
library(statforbiology)
dataset <- getAgroData("mixture")

# Fitting a one-way ANOVA model
model <- lm(Weight ~ Treat, data=dataset)

# Fitting nonlinear combinations with 'gnlht()'

library(statforbiology)
funList <- list(~ a4/(mu1 + a4) * 100,
                ~ (a4 - a2)/(mu1 + a4) * 100,
```

[2] Those who are interested can find information about the delta method in the companion blog, at https://www.statforbiology.com/2024/stat_general_thedeltamethod_edit/.

```
                    ~ (a4 - a3)/(mu1 + a4) * 100)
gnlht(model, funList, parameterNames = c("mu1", "a2", "a3", "a4"))
#                              Form Estim.    SE  t-val   p-value
# 1          a4/(mu1 + a4) * 100 65.730 7.734  8.498 2.014e-06
# 2 (a4 - a2)/(mu1 + a4) * 100 80.848 7.450 10.853 1.470e-07
# 3 (a4 - a3)/(mu1 + a4) * 100 37.025 8.647  4.282 1.065e-03
```

9.3 Some Combinations of General Interest

Coding linear and nonlinear functions of model parameters can be very useful to answer specific research questions, as shown in the previous examples. In particular, for linear combinations, the `glht()` function exhibits a high level of flexibility, provided that we can code the appropriate matrix of coefficients, which can be a highly tedious task. Luckily, the R software provides a set of facilities that help us code some linear or nonlinear combinations of general interest, such as:

1. Least squares means
2. Orthogonal contrasts
3. Pairwise comparisons
4. Back-transformations
5. Predictions and inverse predictions

9.4 Example 9.3: Least Squares Means for the "Mixture" Data

For every model with nominal predictor(s), it is usually relevant to estimate the population means for each treatment level (e.g., μ_1, μ_2, μ_3, ..., μ_n, where n is the number of treatment levels). Although the arithmetic means can be used as estimators (see the `tapply()` function in Chap. 3), we must be aware that these estimators are biased in certain circumstances, such as when the data are unbalanced (different number of replicates for each treatment group). **Least Squares Means** (also named **Expected Marginal Means**, i.e., EMMs) represent an important alternative: They are equal to the arithmetic means when the data are balanced, while they provide better estimators of population means when the data are unbalanced. EMMs can be easily obtained as linear combinations of model parameters, as shown in the following example.

If we go back to the "mixture" data, in Example 9.1, we see that the estimated parameters are $\mu = 9.175$, $\alpha_2 = -4.0475$, $\alpha_3 = 7.685$, and $\alpha_4 = 17.5975$. Considering the biological meaning of these estimates (see Example 9.1), the four EMMs can be obtained by the following linear combinations:

$$\begin{cases} C_1 = \mu_1 = 1 \cdot \mu + 0 \cdot \alpha_2 + 0 \cdot \alpha_3 + 0 \cdot \alpha_4 = 9.18 \\ C_2 = \mu_2 = 1 \cdot \mu + 1 \cdot \alpha_2 + 0 \cdot \alpha_3 + 0 \cdot \alpha_4 = 5.13 \\ C_3 = \mu_3 = 1 \cdot \mu + 0 \cdot \alpha_2 + 1 \cdot \alpha_3 + 0 \cdot \alpha_4 = 16.86 \\ C_4 = \mu_4 = 1 \cdot \mu + 0 \cdot \alpha_2 + 0 \cdot \alpha_3 + 1 \cdot \alpha_4 = 26.77 \end{cases} \tag{9.4}$$

The matrix of coefficients is

$$K = \begin{bmatrix} 1\,0\,0\,0 \\ 1\,1\,0\,0 \\ 1\,0\,1\,0 \\ 1\,0\,0\,1 \end{bmatrix} \tag{9.5}$$

In principle, this set of linear combinations can be fitted using the general `glht()` function in the `multcomp` package, as shown in Code Box 9.4.

Code Box 9.4

```
# Example 9.3
# Least squares means for the 'mixture' data

# Loading the packages
library(statforbiology)
library(multcomp)

# Loading the data
dataset <- getAgroData("mixture")

# Fitting a one-way ANOVA model
model <- lm(Weight ~ Treat, data=dataset)

# Estimating EMMs with the 'glht()' function

# Setting the matrix of coefficients
K <- matrix(c(1,0,0,0,1,1,0,0,1,0,1,0,1,0,0,1),
            nrow = 4, ncol = 4, byrow = T)
row.names(K) <- c("mu1", "mu2", "mu3", "mu4")
K
##      [,1] [,2] [,3] [,4]
## mu1     1    0    0    0
## mu2     1    1    0    0
## mu3     1    0    1    0
## mu4     1    0    0    1
```

```
# Fitting the linear combination
con <- glht(model, linfct = K)
summary(con)
##
##   Simultaneous Tests for General Linear Hypotheses
##
## Fit: lm(formula = Weight ~ Treat, data = dataset)
##
## Linear Hypotheses:
##          Estimate Std. Error t value Pr(>|t|)
## mu1 == 0    9.175      1.959   4.684  0.00199 **
## mu2 == 0    5.127      1.959   2.618  0.08143 .
## mu3 == 0   16.860      1.959   8.607  < 0.001 ***
## mu4 == 0   26.773      1.959  13.668  < 0.001 ***
## ---
## Signif. codes:
## 0 '***' 0.001 '**' 0.01 '*' 0.05 '.' 0.1 ' ' 1
## (Adjusted p values reported -- single-step method)

# Confidence intervals
confint(con)
##
##   Simultaneous Confidence Intervals
##
## Fit: lm(formula = Weight ~ Treat, data = dataset)
##
## Quantile = 2.8936
## 95% family-wise confidence level
##
##
## Linear Hypotheses:
##          Estimate lwr     upr
## mu1 == 0  9.1750   3.5069 14.8431
## mu2 == 0  5.1275  -0.5406 10.7956
## mu3 == 0 16.8600  11.1919 22.5281
## mu4 == 0 26.7725  21.1044 32.4406
```

However, especially when the number of means is very high, coding the matrix of coefficients from scratch can be a daunting task; thus, for the calculation of EMMs, the `emmeans()` function in the `emmeans` package is preferred (Lenth 2016) because it is much simpler to use. It needs two basic arguments: the model object and the predictor for which we want to calculate the EMMs (Code Box 9.5).

Code Box 9.5

```
# Example 9.3 [continuation]

# EMMs with the 'emmeans()' function

library(emmeans) # Load the package
muj <- emmeans(model, ~Treat)
muj
##  Treat            emmean   SE df lower.CL upper.CL
##  Metribuzin__348    9.18 1.96 12     4.91     13.4
##  Mixture_378        5.13 1.96 12     0.86      9.4
##  Rimsulfuron_30    16.86 1.96 12    12.59     21.1
##  Unweeded         26.77 1.96 12    22.50     31.0
##
## Confidence level used: 0.95
```

Apart from being reliable estimates of population means, the EMMs can also serve as the starting point to build further linear or nonlinear combinations, which will be examined in the following sections.

9.5 Example 9.4: Contrasts of Means for the "Mixture" Data

In Example 9.1, we have seen that a linear combination of model parameters can be used to answer a relevant question based on the difference between the mean of the untreated pots and the mean of treated pots. Comparing means or groups of means is the most common task for models based on nominal predictors; for example, for "mixture" data, three such comparisons are relevant:

1. Treated (on average) vs. untreated
2. Single treatment (on average) vs. mixture
3. Metribuzin vs. rimsulfuron

Instead of combining model parameters to code the three previously listed differences, as we did in Example 9.1 for the first difference, it is much more straightforward to combine the means. If we consider the ordering with which the four means appear in the dataframe "muj" in Code Box 9.5, the three linear combinations can be written as

$$\begin{cases} C_1 = \frac{1}{3}\,\mu_1 + \frac{1}{3}\,\mu_2 + \frac{1}{3}\,\mu_3 - \mu_4 \\ C_2 = \frac{1}{2}\,\mu_1 - \mu_2 + \frac{1}{2}\,\mu_3 - 0 \cdot \mu_4 \\ C_3 = \mu_1 - 0 \cdot \mu_2 - \mu_3 - 0 \cdot \mu_4 \end{cases} \tag{9.6}$$

Each of the linear combinations C_1, C_2, and C_3 has the typical property that its coefficients sum to zero. Consequently, the result must be zero when the differences between the involved means, or groups of means are equal to zero, and a *t-test* can be used to assess this null hypothesis. Linear combinations of this type are typically referred to as **contrasts**.

The three contrasts above have the further characteristic that their coefficients are mutually uncorrelated; thus these contrasts are named **orthogonal contrasts**. Orthogonality used to be regarded as a desirable property because the sum of squares of all orthogonal contrasts for the levels of a treatment factor can be summed to return the sum of squares for the treatment effect (see Code box 9.7). Thus, the application of orthogonal contrasts used to be regarded as an elegant and efficient method for exploiting the entire information contained in the data without conducting too many simultaneous tests of hypothesis (Chew 1976). Nowadays, the emphasis on orthogonality is lower, but it may be helpful to provide example of how orthogonal contrasts can be fitted in R, using the `contrast()` function in the `emmeans` package.

Going again back to the "mixture" data, we need to:

1. Prepare a list with the coefficients, assigning a name to each contrast (please note that this is a difference with respect to the `glht()` function in Code Box 9.2, which requires a matrix)
2. Use the `contrast()` function in the `emmeans` package, passing the following arguments: (i) the object resulting from the call to the `emmeans()` function (see above), (ii) the list of contrasts K, as the `method` argument, and (iii) the type of adjustment (we will talk about this later; so far, please use the command as shown in Code Box 9.6)

Code Box 9.6

```
# Example 9.4
# Orthogonal contrasts with the 'emmeans()' function

# Loading the packages
library(statforbiology)
library(multcomp)
```

```
# Loading the data
dataset <- getAgroData("mixture")

# Fitting a one-way ANOVA model
model <- lm(Weight ~ Treat, data=dataset)

# Creating a vector of coefficients for each contrast
C1 <- c(1/3, 1/3, 1/3, -1)
C2 <- c(1/2, -1, 1/2, 0)
C3 <- c(1, 0, -1, 0)

# Creating a list of contrasts (NOT a matrix)
K <- list("U vs T" = C1,
          "mix vs single" = C2,
          "met vs rim" = C3)

# Fitting the contrasts, using the 'muj' object
muj <- emmeans(model, ~Treat)
con <- contrast(muj, method = K, adjust="none")
con
##  contrast      estimate   SE df t.ratio p.value
##  U vs T          -16.39 2.26 12  -7.244  <.0001
##  mix vs single     7.89 2.40 12   3.289  0.0065
##  met vs rim       -7.68 2.77 12  -2.774  0.0168

# Confidence intervals
confint(con)
##  contrast      estimate   SE df lower.CL upper.CL
##  U vs T          -16.39 2.26 12   -21.31   -11.46
##  mix vs single     7.89 2.40 12     2.66    13.12
##  met vs rim       -7.68 2.77 12   -13.72    -1.65
##
## Confidence level used: 0.95
```

Orthogonal contrasts can also be fitted by using the `aov()` function in R. In this case, the list of contrasts needs to be transformed into a matrix and associated with the experimental factor by way of the `C()` function (note the capital letter; see Code Box 9.7). By using this coding, it is possible to see that the sum of squares for the treatment effect is fully partitioned into three parts, one for each contrast, yielding identical P-values as shown in Code Box 9.6.

Code Box 9.7

```
# Example 9.4 [continuation]

# Fitting orthogonal contrasts and partitioning
# the sum of squares for the treatment effect

# Creating a vector of coefficients for each contrast (as in
  Code box 9.6)
C1 <- c(1/3, 1/3, 1/3, -1)
C2 <- c(1/2, -1, 1/2, 0)
C3 <- c(1, 0, -1, 0)

# Creating a list of contrasts (as in Code box 9.6)
K <- list("U vs T" = C1,
          "mix vs single" = C2,
          "met vs rim" = C3)

# Transform the list of contrasts into a matrix
Kmat <- do.call(rbind, K)

# Associate the matrix of coefficients to the treatment
factor dataset$Treat2 <- C(factor(dataset$Treat), t(Kmat))

# Fit the model with the 'aov()' function
mod <- aov(Weight ~ Treat2, dataset)
summary(mod, split = list(Treat2 = list(1,2,3)))
##               Df Sum Sq Mean Sq F value   Pr(>F)
## Treat2         3 1089.5   363.2  23.663 2.51e-05 ***
##   Treat2: C1   1  805.4   805.4  52.476 1.02e-05 ***
##   Treat2: C2   1  166.0   166.0  10.816  0.00647 **
##   Treat2: C3   1  118.1   118.1   7.696  0.01683 *
## Residuals     12  184.2    15.3
```

9.6 Example 9.5: Pairwise Comparisons for the "mixture" Data

Orthogonal contrasts may not be able to provide answers to all relevant research questions. For example, for the "mixture" data, we cannot compare the mixture against either the herbicides used alone because these two contrasts would not be orthogonal. Consequently, it may be relevant to test all possible **pairwise comparisons** between the means, i.e., to consider any pair of herbicide means μ_i and μ_j (with $j > i$) and determine whether the observed difference is statistically significant. This technique is named **Multiple Comparison Testing** (MCT) or **Multiple Comparison Procedure** (MCP). There are two main approaches: the "all-pairwise-comparisons" approach (usually named Tukey's method in the R literature) and the "all-against-one" approach, where each mean is compared only with the best/worst treatment level or with the control level (usually named Dunnett's method) (Hsu 1996).

With Tukey's method, the number of contrasts is very high, and it is equal to $n \times (n-1)/2$, where n is the number of means to be compared. The number of contrasts is reduced to $k = n - 1$ with Dunnett's method, and such a reduction might be important for reasons that will be described later on.

The adoption of pairwise comparisons is not particularly elegant because it implies a lot of unplanned tests without clear focus (a sort of "spray and pray"; Cousens 1988). Furthermore, according to the English scientist John Tukey, "*all we know about the world teaches us that the effects of A and B are always different in some decimal place for any A and B. Thus asking "are the effects different?" is foolish.*" Nonetheless, pairwise comparisons may be very handy; they have been in fashion for almost a century, and thus, it is worthwhile to become acquainted with them.

For the "mixture" example, there are four means to compare and, thus, a total of six pairwise comparisons that can be defined as follows:

$$\begin{cases} C_1 = \mu_1 - \mu_2 = 1 \cdot \mu_1 - 1 \cdot \mu_2 + 0 \cdot \mu_3 + 0 \cdot \mu_4 \\ C_2 = \mu_1 - \mu_3 = 1 \cdot \mu_1 - 0 \cdot \mu_2 - 1 \cdot \mu_3 + 0 \cdot \mu_4 \\ C_3 = \mu_1 - \mu_4 = 1 \cdot \mu_1 - 0 \cdot \mu_2 + 0 \cdot \mu_3 - 1 \cdot \mu_4 \\ C_4 = \mu_2 - \mu_3 = 0 \cdot \mu_1 + 1 \cdot \mu_2 - 1 \cdot \mu_3 + 0 \cdot \mu_4 \\ C_5 = \mu_2 - \mu_4 = 0 \cdot \mu_1 + 1 \cdot \mu_2 + 0 \cdot \mu_3 - 1 \cdot \mu_4 \\ C_6 = \mu_3 - \mu_4 = 0 \cdot \mu_1 + 0 \cdot \mu_2 + 1 \cdot \mu_3 - 1 \cdot \mu_4 \end{cases} \tag{9.7}$$

The matrix of coefficients is

$$K = \begin{bmatrix} 1 & -1 & 0 & 0 \\ 1 & 0 & -1 & 0 \\ 1 & 0 & 0 & -1 \\ 0 & 1 & -1 & 0 \\ 0 & 1 & 0 & -1 \\ 0 & 0 & 1 & -1 \end{bmatrix} \tag{9.8}$$

Luckily, there is no need to code the matrix K from scratch; with `emmeans()`, it is only necessary to specify the type of approach (Tukey or Dunnett) by assigning the corresponding value to the "method" argument. The Dunnett method, by default, compares all means against the first in alphabetical order, which may not be what is desired. However, it is possible to change the reference level by setting the `ref` argument.

For the "mixture" example, the primary interest is in comparing all herbicides with the mixture (the second in alphabetical order), so the `ref` argument is set to 2. Confidence intervals can be obtained by assigning the result of the `contrast()` function to a variable and exploring this variable with the `confint()` function.

Code Box 9.8

```
# Example 9.5
# Pairwise comparisons for the 'mixture' data

# Loading the packages
library(statforbiology)
library(multcomp)

# Loading the data
dataset <- getAgroData("mixture")

# Fitting a one-way ANOVA model
model <- lm(Weight ~ Treat, data=dataset)

# Determining the least square means
muj <- emmeans(model, ~Treat)

# All-pairwise comparisons (Tukey's method)
# Follows from Code box 9.5

contrast(muj, adjust="none", method="tukey")
#
## contrast                     estimate   SE df t.ratio p.value
## Metribuzin - Mixture             4.05 2.77 12   1.461  0.1697
## Metribuzin - Rimsulfuron        -7.68 2.77 12  -2.774  0.0168
## Metribuzin - Unweeded          -17.60 2.77 12  -6.352  <.0001
## Mixture - Rimsulfuron          -11.73 2.77 12  -4.235  0.0012
## Mixture - Unweeded             -21.64 2.77 12  -7.813  <.0001
## Rimsulfuron - Unweeded          -9.91 2.77 12  -3.578  0.0038

## Comparisons all-against-one (Dunnett's method)
con <- contrast(muj, adjust="none", method="dunnett", ref = 2)
con
#
## contrast               estimate   SE df t.ratio p.value
## Metribuzin - Mixture       4.05 2.77 12   1.461  0.1697
## Rimsulfuron - Mixture     11.73 2.77 12   4.235  0.0012
## Unweeded - Mixture        21.64 2.77 12   7.813  <.0001

## Confidence intervals
confint(con)
#
## contrast              estimate   SE df lower.CL upper.CL
```

```
## Metribuzin - Mixture      4.05 2.77 12    -1.99     10.1
## Rimsulfuron - Mixture    11.73 2.77 12     5.70     17.8
## Unweeded - Mixture       21.64 2.77 12    15.61     27.7
```

9.6.1 Letter Display for MCPs

When the number of means is high, reporting all pairwise comparisons may be impractical. Therefore, the so-called **letter display** can be helpful; it consists of augmenting the table of means with significance letters so that *means followed by different letters are significantly different from each other* at a certain predefined protection level, which is usually $\alpha = 0.05$.

A letter display can be easily added by hand according to the following procedure:

1. Sort the means in increasing/decreasing order.
2. Start from the uppermost mean, and add the A letter to this mean and all the following ones, as long as the difference with the first one is not significant.
3. Go on to the second mean, and add the B letter to this mean and to all the following ones, as long as the difference with the second one is not significant.
4. Continue like this until all means have received their letters.

The above procedure works well with balanced experiments, but we prefer using the "insert-and-absorb" algorithm (Piepho 2004), as implemented in the `cld()` function of the `multcomp` package. In this case, it is necessary to provide the selected method of adjustment (see the next section) and a third argument (`Letters = 'LETTERS'`; pay attention to small and capital letters) to invoke the most widespread capital letters display, instead of the default numbering display.

Code Box 9.9

```
# Example 9.5 [continuation]

# Compact letter display
library(multcomp)
cld(muj, adjust="none", Letters=LETTERS)
##  Treat              emmean   SE df lower.CL upper.CL .group
##  Mixture_378          5.13 1.96 12     0.86      9.4  A
##  Metribuzin__348      9.18 1.96 12     4.91     13.4  A
##  Rimsulfuron_30      16.86 1.96 12    12.59     21.1   B
##  Unweeded            26.77 1.96 12    22.50     31.0    C
```

The letter display is handy, but it can only answer questions about the significance of differences, providing no hints about the direction and magnitude of those differences. For this reason, using the letter display is sometimes regarded as an inelegant practice in presenting the experimental results.

9.6.2 Multiplicity Correction

When we perform a set of MCPs, we simultaneously test a very high number of hypotheses. Let us consider one of those hypotheses and imagine that the null is rejected with a P-value of 0.04, which would be the **comparisonwise error rate** (P_c), i.e., the probability of a wrong rejection. If the null were rejected with a P-value of 0.04 for all the n simultaneous contrasts, we would define the probability of wrong rejection for at least one of those hypotheses, i.e., the so-called **familywise error rate** (P_f). We can get a sense that the familywise error rate is higher than the comparisonwise error rate, especially when n is high; in particular, the relationship between P_c and P_f is

$$P_f = 1 - (1 - P_c)^n \tag{9.9}$$

and it is obtained by considering that the probability of one correct rejection is $1 - P_c$, while, for n hypotheses, the probability of all correct rejections is $(1 - P_c)^n$ (joint probability of independent events). Consequently, the probability of having at least one wrong rejection is the complement of such an event.

In practice, if we have $n = 10$ contrasts and each one is rejected at $P_c = 0.04$, the probability that we make at least one wrong decision is `1 - (1 - 0.04)^10` = 0.3351674, which is incredibly high. This issue is generally known as the **multiplicity problem**: Whenever we make a large number of simultaneous inferences, the probability that we make at least one mistake (i.e., a wrong rejection) is much higher than the error rate for each test. **Generally, ignoring the problem of multiplicity, as I did in Code Boxes 9.8 and 9.9, is not considered an acceptable practice.**

Since long ago, there has been a broad consensus in the literature that we should address the multiplicity problem by making decisions based on the familywise[3] error rate instead of the comparisonwise error rate (see, e.g., Chew 1976). In other words, the null is rejected when $P_f < 0.05$ and not when $P_c < 0.05$. In particular, a familywise error rate protection is preferred when (Onofri et al. 2010):

[3] With the term familywise error rate, I refer to the overall type I error rate for a specified collection of hypothesis tests, which does not necessarily coincide with all the possible tests of hypothesis for an entire experiment. Instead, the term experimentwise error rate should be used to refer to the familywise error rate for the entire experiment. In practice, the two terms are often used interchangeably.

- We have a relatively high number of simultaneous tests, especially when the overall conclusion tends to be wrong when at least one single test is wrong.
- We need to compare genotypes or agricultural techniques, and we want to avoid wrongly excluding a genotype or technique from the group of the best ones. Indeed, when the number of treatments is high, the probability that at least one treatment is wrongly excluded from the lot of the best ones may be very high.
- We want to avoid false positives (i.e., wrong rejections), which might be numerous if we do not address the multiplicity problem.
- We want to draw conclusions that refer to the entire set of simultaneous contrasts. For example, we have used a letter display and wish to state that "treatments followed by different letters are significantly different ($P < 0.05$)." In this case, the conclusion applies to the entire set of comparisons, and the comparisonwise error rate is invalid.

On the contrary, we might like to stick to a comparisonwise error rate protection when:

- Only a few comparisons or contrasts are to be tested, each having a strong biological relevance (single-contrast problems).
- We need to compare genotypes or agricultural techniques, and we want to avoid wrongly including a genotype or technique in the group of the best ones.
- We want to avoid false negatives (i.e., wrong acceptances), which might be numerous, if we do not address the multiplicity problem.

If we decide to use the familywise error rate, we must adjust the observed P-value based on the number of simultaneous inferences being made. The most natural method is to utilize the relationship between P_c and P_f, which is known as Sidak's correction. In Code Box 9.10, we apply this correction through hand calculations, considering that the number of simultaneous contrasts is 6. We also use R by manipulating the "`adjust`" argument in the `contrast()` function.

Code Box 9.10

```
# Example 9.5 [continuation]

# Correcting for multiplicity: Sidak's method

# Correction by hand (six simultaneous contrasts)
con <- contrast(muj, method = "pairwise", adjust = "none")
Pc <- as.data.frame(con)[,6]
Pf <- 1 - (1 - Pc)^6
Pf
#
## [1] 6.722991e-01 9.683462e-02 2.190543e-04
## [4] 6.923077e-03 2.869757e-05 2.255183e-02
```

```
# With R
contrast(muj, method = "pairwise", adjust = "sidak")
#
## contrast                    estimate   SE df t.ratio p.value
## Metribuzin - Mixture            4.05 2.77 12   1.461  0.6723
## Metribuzin - Rimsulfuron       -7.68 2.77 12  -2.774  0.0968
## Metribuzin - Unweeded         -17.60 2.77 12  -6.352  0.0002
## Mixture - Rimsulfuron         -11.73 2.77 12  -4.235  0.0069
## Mixture - Unweeded            -21.64 2.77 12  -7.813  <.0001
## Rimsulfuron - Unweeded         -9.91 2.77 12  -3.578  0.0226
```

We observe that applying this type of multiplicity correction renders the second contrast no longer significant. An alternative, more straightforward, and much more widespread procedure is the so-called Bonferroni's correction, which is based on the following heuristic:

$$\alpha_E = \alpha_C \cdot k \tag{9.10}$$

Code Box 9.11

```
# Example 9.5 [continuation]

# Correcting for multiplicity: Bonferroni's method

Pc * 6
## [1] 1.018071e+00 1.009900e-01 2.190743e-04
## [4] 6.943132e-03 2.869792e-05 2.276671e-02

contrast(muj, method = "pairwise", adjust = "bonferroni")
## contrast                    estimate   SE df t.ratio p.value
## Metribuzin - Mixture            4.05 2.77 12   1.461  1.0000
## Metribuzin - Rimsulfuron       -7.68 2.77 12  -2.774  0.1010
## Metribuzin - Unweeded         -17.60 2.77 12  -6.352  0.0002
## Mixture - Rimsulfuron         -11.73 2.77 12  -4.235  0.0069
## Mixture - Unweeded            -21.64 2.77 12  -7.813  <.0001
## Rimsulfuron - Unweeded         -9.91 2.77 12  -3.578  0.0228
```

Both Sidak's and Bonferroni's methods are rather conservative in the sense that they provide overestimated P_f values since they do not account for the correlation between contrasts. Other correction procedures exist (e.g., Holm, Hochberg, Hommel; Hsu 1996), but all of them are more or less conservative.

In recent times, a group of American scientists has developed a method for accounting for the correlation between contrasts. This method is based on the multivariate Student's t-distribution (Bretz et al. 2011) and yields approximately correct familywise error rates. It is applied by default in the `contrast()` function, without the need for any specification (Code Box 9.12).

Code Box 9.12

```
# Example 9.5 [continuation]

# Correcting for multiplicity: default method
# based on the multivariate t distribution

contrast(muj, method="pairwise")
## contrast                  estimate   SE df t.ratio p.value
## Metribuzin - Mixture          4.05 2.77 12   1.461  0.4885
## Metribuzin - Rimsulfuron     -7.68 2.77 12  -2.774  0.0698
## Metribuzin - Unweeded       -17.60 2.77 12  -6.352  0.0002
## Mixture - Rimsulfuron       -11.73 2.77 12  -4.235  0.0055
## Mixture - Unweeded          -21.64 2.77 12  -7.813  <.0001
## Rimsulfuron - Unweeded       -9.91 2.77 12  -3.578  0.0173
##
## P value adjustment: tukey method for comparing a family of
    4 estimates

contrast(muj, method="dunnett", ref = 2)
## contrast               estimate   SE df t.ratio p.value
## Metribuzin - Mixture       4.05 2.77 12   1.461  0.3711
## Rimsulfuron - Mixture     11.73 2.77 12   4.235  0.0032
## Unweeded - Mixture        21.64 2.77 12   7.813  <.0001
##
## P value adjustment: dunnettx method for 3 tests
```

Before concluding this part, we need to point out that the multiplicity problem does not only relate to MCPs but may be a concern for all experiments, whenever a high number of hypotheses are simultaneously tested.

9.6.3 Traditional Multiple Comparison Procedures

In this book, pairwise comparisons are placed within the framework of linear contrasts, as done, e.g., in Hsu (1996). In earlier times, MCPs were not regarded as contrasts, and they were based on the determination of a critical difference: Whenever the observed difference was higher than the critical difference, it was deemed significant. The following multiple comparison procedures are still very much widespread in scientific literature:

1. Fisher's Least Significant Difference (LSD)
2. Tukey's Honest Significant Difference (HSD)
3. Dunnett's test
4. Duncan's test
5. Newman-Keuls' test
6. Tukey's MCP

The connection with the pairwise contrast methods we have described in the previous section is that for balanced experiments, Fisher's LSD corresponds to pairwise contrasts with no multiplicity correction (comparisonwise error rate protection), while Tukey's HSD and Dunnett's test, for balanced data, produce the same results as the default multiplicity correction in R. The traditional Tukey HSD for balanced data can be calculated in R by using the `aov()` function to fit the model and the `TukeyHSD()` function to produce a multiple comparison test with familywise error rate protection (Code Box 9.13).

Code Box 9.13

```
# Example 9.5 [continuation]

# Tukey HSD for a linear model fitted with the 'aov()' function
mod2 <- aov(Weight ~ Treat, data = dataset)

TukeyHSD(mod2)
##   Tukey multiple comparisons of means
##     95% family-wise confidence level
##
## Fit: aov(formula = Weight ~ Treat, data = dataset)
##
## $Treat
##                                 diff        lwr       upr     p adj
## Mixture_378-Metribuzin__348   -4.0475 -12.271978  4.176978 0.4884620
## Rimsulfuron_30-Metribuzin__348  7.6850  -0.539478 15.909478 0.0698118
## Unweeded-Metribuzin__348      17.5975   9.373022 25.821978 0.0001854
## Rimsulfuron_30-Mixture_378    11.7325   3.508022 19.956978 0.0055015
## Unweeded-Mixture_378          21.6450  13.420522 29.869478 0.0000247
## Unweeded-Rimsulfuron_30        9.9125   1.688022 18.136978 0.0172572
```

All the other tests employ a mechanism that increases the critical difference to account for a certain degree of multiplicity. However, they do not control either the comparisonwise or the familywise error rate but remain in between. For this reason, their use should be discouraged (see Hsu 1996).

As a final comment on multiple comparison procedures, it is necessary to consider that these methods have often been abused in previous years, and debates with editors and reviewers are still common today. In particular, the use of pairwise comparisons is strongly discouraged when the experimental treatment is represented by a quantitative series of rates, doses, times, or other quantitative variables. Indeed, even though a small number of "doses" were selected to be included in the experiment, the primary interest lies in the determination of the pattern of responses across the whole range of possible "doses," and fitting a regression model instead of making pairwise comparisons is much more meaningful and respectful of the original aims and data.

We should also avoid making all pairwise comparisons for the combined levels of the experimental factors in a multifactorial experiment. In this case, the number of multiple comparisons is very high, and consequently, the adjustment for multiplicity needs to be very stringent, resulting in decreased power and increased risks of type II errors. In this situation, we should prefer comparing the means of one factor within (and not across) the levels of the other factor(s) (see Example 10.3 in Chap. 10).

9.7 Example 9.6: Back-Transformations for the "Insects" Data

Whenever a stabilizing transformation has been made, to respect the basic assumptions for linear models, the EMMs will also be in the transformed scale, and they might not be meaningful for the presentation and interpretation of results. Therefore, it might be convenient to back-transform them by using the inverse transformation; for example, if the data were square root transformed, the EMMs can be squared to go back to the original measurement unit.

Back-transformations can be viewed as nonlinear combinations of model parameters, and thus, they can be performed with the `gnlht()` function. More efficiently, back-transformations can be seen as nonlinear combinations of means, and hence, they can be fitted using the `emmeans()` function, by setting the `type = "response"` argument.

As an example, let us continue the analyses of the "insect" data (Example 8.2); the number of insects in tobacco leaves of plants treated with one of three insecticides was counted and used to parameterize a simple linear model with one nominal predictor (Code Box 8.5). The graphical and statistical analyses of residuals showed that a logarithmic transformation was necessary to meet the basic assumptions of linear models (Code Box 8.5 and Figs. 8.6 and 8.7), and, therefore, model fitting and variance partitioning were performed on log-transformed data, so that the EMMs are, as well, on a logarithmic scale (Code Box 9.13).

The inverse transformation (the anti-logarithmic transformation) for, e.g., the first mean would be EMM $= e^{6.34} = 568.6$. In Code Box 9.14, this combination is fitted with the `emmeans()` function by setting the `type = "response"` argument.

Code Box 9.14

```
# Example 9.6
# Back-transformations for the 'insects' data

# Loading the packages
library(statforbiology)
library(emmeans)

# Loading the data
dataset <- getAgroData('insects')


# Model fitting on transformed data
modt <- lm(log(Count) ~ Insecticide, data = dataset)

# Calculate the EMMs
treatMeans <- emmeans(modt, ~Insecticide)
treatMeans
##  Insecticide emmean    SE df lower.CL upper.CL
##  T1            6.34 0.178 12     5.96     6.73
##  T2            5.81 0.178 12     5.43     6.20
##  T3            3.95 0.178 12     3.56     4.34
##
## Results are given on the log (not the response) scale.
## Confidence level used: 0.95

# Back-transformation
retroMeans <- emmeans(modt, ~Insecticide,
                      type = "response")
retroMeans
##  Insecticide response     SE df lower.CL upper.CL
##  T1             568.6 101.01 12    386.1    837.3
##  T2             335.1  59.54 12    227.6    493.5
##  T3              51.9   9.22 12     35.2     76.4
##
## Confidence level used: 0.95
## Intervals are back-transformed from the log scale
```

```
# Comparison with EMMs on the original data
emmeans(lm(Count ~ Insecticide, data = dataset),
        ~Insecticide)
##  Insecticide emmean   SE df lower.CL upper.CL
##  T1           589.8 62.7 12    453.1      726
##  T2           357.4 62.7 12    220.7      494
##  T3            56.6 62.7 12    -80.1      193
##
## Confidence level used: 0.95
```

Back-transformed means are different from EMMs in the original (untransformed) scale (see Code Box 9.14), and they should be regarded as estimators of the medians on the original scale rather than the means,[4] which is an advantage. In fact, as the data in the original scale were skewed (which is why a transformation was needed), the medians represent better descriptors of central tendency than the means.

Before concluding this section, it is necessary to mention that the technique shown in Code Box 9.14 is feasible whenever the transformation has been performed inside the model fitting function (please note the code line: `modt <- lm(log(Count) ~ Insecticide, data = dataset)`), and it is one of the transformations that are auto-detected by the `emmeans()` function. Otherwise, when the transformation is not auto-detectable or it has not been performed inside the `lm()` function, we need to:

1. Make the transformation before fitting the model
2. Fit the model to the transformed variable
3. Update the “reference grid” for the model and specify what type of transformation has been made (e.g., `tran = "inverse"`)
4. Pass the updated grid to the `emmeans()` function (Code Box 9.15)

Code Box 9.15

```
# Example 9.6 [continuation]

# The transformation to the reciprocal is not auto-detected
modt2 <- lm(1/Count ~ Insecticide, data = dataset)
emmeans(modt2, ~Insecticide, type = "response")
##  Insecticide  emmean      SE df lower.CL upper.CL
##  T1          0.00182 0.00279 12 -0.00426  0.00789
```

[4] If the data are Gaussian in the transformed scale, the mean and the median coincide in that scale. When we back-transform with a monotonic function, we alter the mean, but the ordering of observations remains the same, and thus, the central value (the median) does not change.

```
## T2            0.00317 0.00279 12 -0.00291  0.00924
## T3            0.02120 0.00279 12  0.01513  0.02727
##
## Confidence level used: 0.95

# Updating the emmeans grid
dataset$invCount <- 1/dataset$Count
modt3 <- lm(invCount ~ Insecticide, data = dataset)
updGrid <- update(ref_grid(modt3), tran = "inverse")
emmeans(updGrid, ~Insecticide, type = "response")
## Insecticide response    SE df lower.CL upper.CL
## T1             550.9 845.9 12    126.8      Inf
## T2             315.8 278.0 12    108.2      Inf
## T3              47.2   6.2 12     36.7       66
##
## Confidence level used: 0.95
## Intervals are back-transformed from the inverse scale
```

The method shown in Code Box 9.15 can be used with several types of transformations, such as "identity," "1/mu^2," "inverse," "reciprocal," "log10," "log2," and "asin.sqrt" (angular transformation). For other transformations, such as the Box-Cox transformation in its simplified version ($W = Y^{\lambda}$, wherever $\lambda \neq 0$ or $\lambda \neq 0.5$), the back-transformation is possible by the `make.tran()` function, as shown in Code Box 9.16.

Code Box 9.16

```
# Example 9.6 [continuation]

# Another possibility for back-transformation
dataset$lCount <- dataset$Count^0.25
mod4 <- lm(lCount ~ Insecticide, data = dataset)
updGrid <- update(ref_grid(mod4),
                  tran = make.tran("power", 0.25))
emmeans(updGrid, ~Insecticide, type = "response")
## Insecticide response   SE df lower.CL upper.CL
## T1             573.5 78.7 12    420.3    765.3
## T2             340.5 53.2 12    238.5    472.1
## T3              53.1 13.2 12     29.6     88.3
##
## Confidence level used: 0.95
## Intervals are back-transformed from the mu^0.25 scale
```

9.8 Example 9.7: Predictions and Inverse Predictions for Linear Regression

For linear or nonlinear regression models, working with the means is usually unimportant. At the same time, it is relevant to use the fitted model to make predictions, i.e., to derive the expected response of the predictor at a given level or, conversely, to derive the required predictor level to obtain a given response (inverse prediction). Both these statistics can be seen as linear or nonlinear combinations of model parameters, and they can be performed in R, using one of several available functions, such as the `predict()` function, as well as the other aforementioned `emmeans()`, `glht()`, and `gnlht()` functions.

As an example, we can consider the "Ammi94" data, relating to an experiment to define the relationship between the density of *Ammi majus* (an important weed for several spring crops in central Italy) in plants per square meter and the yield of sunflower in tons per hectare. Weed densities were established by sowing weed seeds by hand, while yield data represent the means of four replicates (Onofri and Tei 1994). The dataset is available in the `statforbiology` package. In Code Box 9.17, a simple linear regression model is fitted, and the two estimates (intercept and slope, i.e., β_0 and β_1) are retrieved and displayed.

Code Box 9.17

```
# Example 9.7
# Predictions and inverse predictions for linear regression
# Weed density/Yield relationship for Ammi majus

# Loading the packages
library(statforbiology)
library(multcomp)
library(emmeans)

# Loading the data
dataset <- getAgroData("Ammi94")
dataset
##   Density  Yield
## 1       0 2.4866
## 2      16 2.1806
## 3      21 1.8456
## 4      36 1.8412
## 5      49 1.6486

# Fitting a regression model
mod <- lm(Yield ~ Density, data = dataset)
```

```
summary(mod)
##
## Coefficients:
##              Estimate Std. Error t value Pr(>|t|)
## (Intercept)  2.402566   0.108697  22.103 0.000203 ***
## Density     -0.016477   0.003667  -4.494 0.020567 *
##
## Residual standard error: 0.138 on 3 degrees of freedom
## Multiple R-squared:  0.8707, Adjusted R-squared:  0.8275
## F-statistic: 20.19 on 1 and 3 DF,  p-value: 0.02057
```

The interest of these experiments is twofold:

1. Forecasting the yield with early measurements of weed densities (prediction)
2. Determining the density of weeds that provokes a certain level of yield loss (inverse prediction)

These estimates can be obtained as linear or nonlinear combinations. For example, let us imagine we want to determine the expected yield level with ten plants of *Ammi majus* per square meter. There are three possibilities:

1. Use the `glht()` function to fit a contrast $C = 1 \times \beta_0 + 10 \times \beta_1$, where the parameters β_0 and β_1 are, respectively, the intercept and slope from linear model fitting.
2. Use the `predict()` function and pass a dataframe (not a vector!) containing the dose level for prediction (`newdata` argument).
3. Use the `emmeans()` function, also passing a dataframe to the `at` argument.

All three possibilities are demonstrated in Code Box 9.18; the results are, obviously, totally equal.

Code Box 9.18

```
# Example 9.7 [continuation]

# Three methods for predictions

# 1.Fitting with 'glht()'#################
# Setting a contrast matrix
K <- matrix(c(1, 10), nrow = 1, ncol = 2)
summary(glht(mod, linfct = K))
##
## Linear Hypotheses:
##          Estimate Std. Error t value Pr(>|t|)
## 1 == 0  2.23779    0.08123   27.55 0.000105 ***
## ---
```

```
## Signif. codes:
## 0 '***' 0.001 '**' 0.01 '*' 0.05 '.' 0.1 ' ' 1
## (Adjusted p values reported -- single-step method)

# 2.Fitting with 'predict()' ################
predict(mod, newdata = data.frame(Density= c(10)), se.fit = T)
## $fit
##        1
## 2.237793
##
## $se.fit
## [1] 0.08123191
##
## $df
## [1] 3
##
## $residual.scale
## [1] 0.1380352

# 3.Fitting with 'emmeans()' ####################
emmeans(mod, ~Density, at = data.frame(Density= c(10)))
##  Density emmean     SE df lower.CL upper.CL
##       10   2.24 0.0812  3     1.98      2.5
##
## Confidence level used: 0.95
```

Now, let us imagine that there is an interest in estimating the level of weed density that provokes a 10% yield reduction. Considering that the weed-free yield is 2.403 tons per hectare (the intercept of the fitted model), a 10% yield reduction corresponds to obtaining a yield level equal to $2.403 - 0.1 \times 2.403 = 2.163$, which is equal to $(2.163 - \beta_0)/\beta_1$. This latter equation is intrinsically nonlinear; thus, the gnlht() function is to be used (Code Box 9.19).

Code Box 9.19

```
# Example 9.7 [continuation]

# Inverse prediction with gnlht()

gnlht(mod, func = list(~(21.53 - b0)/b1),
      parameterNames = c("b0", "b1"))
##                Form  Estimate       SE t-value   p-value
## 1 (21.53 - b0)/b1 -1160.835 263.7767 4.400825 0.0217523
```

9.9 Questions and Exercises

1. Consider the exercises from 5 to 7 in Chap. 4. For all these exercises, after having made sure whether a transformation is needed to meet the basic assumptions for linear models, perform MCT by adopting an appropriate correction for multiplicity.

References

Bretz F, Hothorn T, Westfall P (2011) Multiple Comparisons Using R. CRC Press, Boca Raton, FL

Chew V (1976) Comparing treatment means: a compendium. Hortscience 11(4):348–357

Cousens R (1988) Misinterpretetion of results in weed research through inappropriate use of statistics. Weed Res 28:281–289

Hsu JC (1996) Multiple Comparisons: Theory and Methods. Chapman & Hall, London

Lenth RV (2016) Least-squares means: the *R* package **lsmeans**. J Stat Softw 69(1). https://doi.org/10.18637/jss.v069.i01. http://www.jstatsoft.org/v69/i01/, bibtex: lenth2016_LeastSquaresMeansPackage

Onofri A, Tei F (1994) Competitive ability and threshold levels for three broadleaf weed species in sunflower. Weed Res 34:471–479

Onofri A, Carbonell EA, Piepho HP, Mortimer AM, Cousens RD (2010) Current statistical issues in Weed Research. Weed Res 50(1):5–24

Piepho HP (2004) An algorithm for a letter-based representation of all-pairwise comparisons. J Comput Graph Stat 13(2):456–466

Weisberg S (2005) Applied Linear Regression, 3rd edn. Wiley, Hoboken

Chapter 10
Putting Everything Together

Statisticians, like artists, have the bad habit of falling in love with their models

—G. Box

Abstract In this chapter, five real-life examples are presented, which relate to field experiments in agriculture. A work plan is proposed as a guide to produce reliable results and reach correct conclusions, which are fully supported by the data at hand. These examples are about a genotype experiment in a Randomized Complete Block Design (RCBD), a Latin square experiment to compare adjuvants, a two-factor factorial RCBD experiment to compare genotypes at different N levels, a nested design to compare maize crosses, and a germination experiment repeated in two different ovens. R codes are given, as well as several hints of general interest that might be easily transferred to other experiments in other situations.

The time has come to assemble all the tools presented in the previous chapters and develop a work plan to perform correct data analyses, produce reliable results, and reach correct conclusions that are fully supported by the data at hand. The proposed work plan should not be taken too strictly: It is just one of the possible approaches to data analyses, and it is only meant as a starting point for beginners. The work plan is as follows:

1. Load the data in R and transform the variables as needed.
2. Describe the data by calculating, at least, the means and standard deviations for each experimental group; use graphs, as necessary, to unveil the main traits of the dataset at hand, discover patterns, and spot outliers: **Let the data speak for themselves, and "listen" to what they have to say**. This preliminary step is referred to as Exploratory Data Analysis (EDA) and is a fundamental part of data analyses, before model fitting, inference, and hypothesis testing.
3. Select a suitable model to describe the cause-effect relationships under study according to the objectives of the research project. Fit this model to the observed data.

A. Onofri, *Field Research Methods in Agriculture*,
https://doi.org/10.1007/978-3-032-08199-5_10

4. Ensure that the model provides an accurate description of the observed data and that all the basic assumptions for model fitting are met. If necessary, adopt the appropriate correcting measures and refit the model.
5. Calculate standard errors and/or confidence intervals, and add them to all point estimates. Test the significance of all effects by way of variance partitioning and F-ratios.
6. Use linear or nonlinear combinations of model parameters or means to test further hypotheses of interest, and answer all the research questions.
7. Present the results in the form of graphs and tables, being concise and ensuring that you reveal all the key characteristics of interest for the dataset at hand.

In this chapter, examples are provided of how this work plan can be put into practice.

10.1 Example 10.1: A Genotype Experiment in Blocks

Let us consider a field experiment comparing eight winter wheat genotypes, laid out in three complete blocks, in the hills of central Italy during the 2002 sowing season (Ciriciofolo, 2004; published in Belocchi et al. 2003). The response variable is the yield (in tons per hectare), and the dataset is available as "WinterWheat2002," in the `statforbiology` package. The "block" variable needs to be transformed into a factor before analysis; otherwise, R would incorrectly fit a regression model. The genotype variable may also be transformed into a factor, although this is optional,[1] as the genotypes are represented by a character vector.

The EDA reveals that the genotypes, except for Simeto, are relatively similar in terms of mean yield. At the same time, some differences exist in terms of standard deviation, which may warrant a careful examination for possible heteroscedasticity (Code Box 10.1).

Code Box 10.1

```
# Example 10.1
# A genotype experiment in blocks

# Loading the packages
library(statforbiology)
library(MASS)
library(car)
library(emmeans)
library(multcomp)
```

[1] At least until R version 4.5.1, released on June 13, 2025.

```
# Loading the 'WinterWheat2002' dataset and performing an EDA
dataset <- getAgroData("WinterWheat2002")
head(dataset)
##   Plot Block Genotype Yield
## 1   57     A COLOSSEO  4.31
## 2   61     B COLOSSEO  4.73
## 3   11     C COLOSSEO  5.64
## 4   60     A    CRESO  3.99
## 5   10     B    CRESO  4.82
## 6   42     C    CRESO  4.17
dataset$Block <- factor(dataset$Block)
dataset$Genotype <- factor(dataset$Genotype)

with(dataset, data.frame(Mean = tapply(Yield, Genotype, mean),
                         SD = tapply(Yield, Genotype, sd)))
##              Mean        SD
## COLOSSEO 4.893333 0.6798774
## CRESO    4.326667 0.4366158
## DUILIO   4.240000 0.1400000
## GRAZIA   4.340000 0.3764306
## IRIDE    4.963333 0.1892969
## SANCARLO 4.503333 0.2250185
## SIMETO   3.340000 0.3915354
## SOLEX    4.790000 0.2645751
```

A model with two nominal predictors can be fitted to the observed yields, as shown in Example 4.3 in Chap. 4. The graphical analyses of residuals show some slight signs of heteroscedasticity (Fig. 10.1, left side) but no clear evidence of a lack of normality. The `leveneTest()` function, as shown in Chap. 8, cannot be used with data from RCBDs, although we can use a modified form based on the absolute residuals from model fit (Code Box 10.2; Bhandary and Dai 2013); this test is not significant, and the Box-Cox graph (not shown) confirms that no transformation is needed. Consequently, we conclude that there are no dramatic deviations from the basic assumptions and proceed to inspect the ANOVA table. A preliminary check of the degrees of freedom confirms that there are no problems with model misspecification (i.e., the numbers of DF are equal, respectively, to the number of blocks minus one and to the number of genotypes minus one), and, based on the P-value, the null hypothesis of no significant differences between genotypes can be rejected (Code Box 10.2).

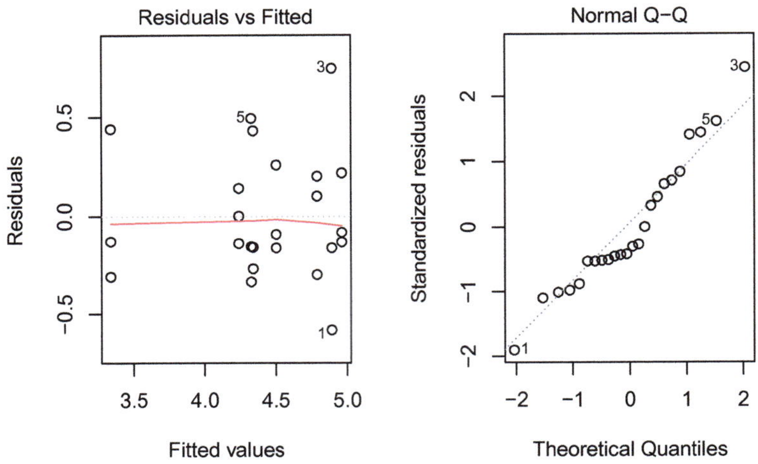

Fig. 10.1 Graphical analyses of residuals for the genotype experiment in blocks (Example 10.1)

Code Box 10.2

```
# Example 10.1 [continuation]

# Model fitting with two nominal predictors
mod <- lm(Yield ~ Block + Genotype, data = dataset)

# Inspection of plots
par(mfrow=c(2,2))
plot(mod, which = 1)
plot(mod, which = 2)
boxcox(mod)

# Levene test (modified version for RCBDs)
leveneTest(abs(residuals(mod)) ~ Genotype, data = dataset)
## Levene's Test for Homogeneity of Variance
 (center = median)
##       Df F value Pr(>F)
## group  7  0.7932 0.6037
##       16

# Variance partitioning
anova(mod)
## Analysis of Variance Table
##
```

```
## Response: Yield
##            Df Sum Sq Mean Sq F value    Pr(>F)
## Block       2 0.7977 0.39883  3.8502 0.0465178 *
## Genotype    7 5.6305 0.80436  7.7651 0.0006252 ***
## Residuals 14 1.4502 0.10359
```

The estimates of model parameters are relatively uninteresting in this case, while pairwise comparisons may be helpful for varietal recommendations. With eight genotypes and, thus, $(8 \times 7)/2 = 28$ contrasts, a multiplicity correction is in order. Apart from pairwise differences with confidence intervals, we report a table of means in decreasing yield order, augmented with the compact letter display (Code Box 10.3). The conclusion is that Simeto was significantly worse than all the other genotypes except for Duilio.

Code Box 10.3

```
# Example 10.1 [continuation]

# Multiple comparisons
meds <- emmeans(mod, ~Genotype)
confint(contrast(meds, method = "pairwise"))
## contrast             estimate    SE df lower.CL upper.CL
## COLOSSEO - CRESO       0.5667 0.263 14  -0.3606    1.494
## COLOSSEO - DUILIO      0.6533 0.263 14  -0.2740    1.581
## COLOSSEO - GRAZIA      0.5533 0.263 14  -0.3740    1.481
## COLOSSEO - IRIDE      -0.0700 0.263 14  -0.9973    0.857
## COLOSSEO - SANCARLO    0.3900 0.263 14  -0.5373    1.317
## COLOSSEO - SIMETO      1.5533 0.263 14   0.6260    2.481
## COLOSSEO - SOLEX       0.1033 0.263 14  -0.8240    1.031
## CRESO - DUILIO         0.0867 0.263 14  -0.8406    1.014
## CRESO - GRAZIA        -0.0133 0.263 14  -0.9406    0.914
## CRESO - IRIDE         -0.6367 0.263 14  -1.5640    0.291
## CRESO - SANCARLO      -0.1767 0.263 14  -1.1040    0.751
## CRESO - SIMETO         0.9867 0.263 14   0.0594    1.914
## CRESO - SOLEX         -0.4633 0.263 14  -1.3906    0.464
## DUILIO - GRAZIA       -0.1000 0.263 14  -1.0273    0.827
## DUILIO - IRIDE        -0.7233 0.263 14  -1.6506    0.204
## DUILIO - SANCARLO     -0.2633 0.263 14  -1.1906    0.664
## DUILIO - SIMETO        0.9000 0.263 14  -0.0273    1.827
## DUILIO - SOLEX        -0.5500 0.263 14  -1.4773    0.377
## GRAZIA - IRIDE        -0.6233 0.263 14  -1.5506    0.304
## GRAZIA - SANCARLO     -0.1633 0.263 14  -1.0906    0.764
```

```
## GRAZIA - SIMETO          1.0000 0.263 14   0.0727    1.927
## GRAZIA - SOLEX          -0.4500 0.263 14  -1.3773    0.477
## IRIDE - SANCARLO         0.4600 0.263 14  -0.4673    1.387
## IRIDE - SIMETO           1.6233 0.263 14   0.6960    2.551
## IRIDE - SOLEX            0.1733 0.263 14  -0.7540    1.101
## SANCARLO - SIMETO        1.1633 0.263 14   0.2360    2.091
## SANCARLO - SOLEX        -0.2867 0.263 14  -1.2140    0.641
## SIMETO - SOLEX          -1.4500 0.263 14  -2.3773   -0.523
##
## Results are averaged over the levels of: Block
## Confidence level used: 0.95
## Conf-level adjustment: tukey method for comparing a family
     of 8 estimates

# Letter display
cld(meds, Letters = LETTERS, reverse = T)
## Genotype emmean    SE df lower.CL upper.CL .group
## IRIDE       4.96 0.186 14     4.56     5.36  A
## COLOSSEO    4.89 0.186 14     4.49     5.29  A
## SOLEX       4.79 0.186 14     4.39     5.19  A
## SANCARLO    4.50 0.186 14     4.10     4.90  A
## GRAZIA      4.34 0.186 14     3.94     4.74  A
## CRESO       4.33 0.186 14     3.93     4.73  A
## DUILIO      4.24 0.186 14     3.84     4.64  AB
## SIMETO      3.34 0.186 14     2.94     3.74   B
```

10.2 Example 10.2: Comparing Adjuvants on a Latin Square

Three adjuvants for the rimsulfuron herbicide were compared in maize by using a Latin square design with four replicates. The results are available in the "adjuvantsLS" dataset, in the `statforbiology` package. In this example, the observed yields will be considered as the response variable, the adjuvants will be the nominal predictor, while the rows and columns of the Latin square grid will be the two blocking factors. These three independent variables will need to be transformed into factors before analysis, although this is strictly necessary only for the rows and columns, which are characterized by numerical coding. Instead of transforming the three variables one at a time (as in Code Box 10.1), we can use the `transform()` function by passing the dataframe as the first argument and providing the list of transformations to be performed within that dataframe (see Code Box 10.4).

The EDA is based on inspecting the arithmetic means and SDs for the adjuvants: The mean for the surfactant appears to be higher than the other means. At the same time, there are no apparent differences among the adjuvants in terms of SDs (Code Box 10.4).

Code Box 10.4

```
# Example 10.2
# Comparing adjuvants on a latin square

# Loading the packages
library(statforbiology)
library(MASS)
library(emmeans)
library(multcomp)

# Loading and transforming the data
dataset <- getAgroData("adjuvantsLS")
dataset <- transform(dataset,
                     Adjuvant = factor(Adjuvant),
                     Row = factor(Row),
                     Column = factor(Column))
head(dataset[,c(2, 6, 7, 24)])
##            Adjuvant Column Row Yield
## 1 AmmoniumSulphate      1   3 58.23
## 2 AmmoniumSulphate      2   1 47.98
## 3 AmmoniumSulphate      3   4 92.39
## 4 AmmoniumSulphate      4   2 85.97
## 5       MineralOil      1   2 73.99
## 6       MineralOil      2   4 92.97

# EDA
with(dataset, data.frame(Mean = tapply(Yield, Adjuvant, mean),
                         SD = tapply(Yield, Adjuvant, sd)))
##                      Mean       SD
## AmmoniumSulphate  71.1425 21.40518
## MineralOil       101.1475 23.00979
## None              80.5525 30.51889
## Surfactant       115.4250 20.69268
```

A suitable model for a Latin square design is

$$Y_{ijk} = \mu + \gamma_k + \beta_j + \alpha_i + \varepsilon_{ijk} \quad (10.1)$$

In this model, μ is the intercept, γ_k is the effect of the kth row, β_j is the effect of the jth column, and α_i is the effect of the ith adjuvant. The elements ε_{ijk} represent the individual random sources of experimental error, which are assumed to be Gaussian, with a mean of 0 and a standard deviation of σ.

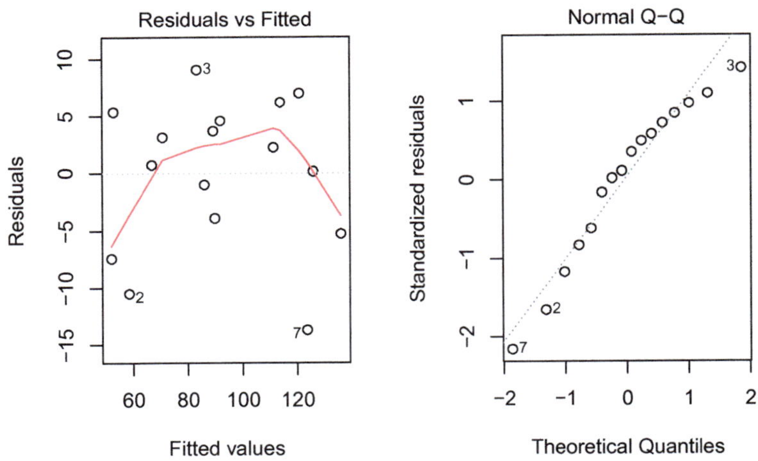

Fig. 10.2 Graphical analyses of residuals for the Latin square experiment to compare adjuvants (Example 10.2)

Model fitting with R requires the inclusion of all blocking factors (Jensen et al. 2018). After the fitting process, the residuals are extracted and checked using graphical analyses. Figure 10.2 shows no evident problems of any kind, while the Box-Cox graph confirms that no transformation is needed (not shown). Therefore, we can proceed to variance partitioning to test the significance of all experimental factors (Code Box 10.5).

Code Box 10.5

```
# Example 10.2 [continuation]

# Fitting the model and checking the residuals
mod <- lm(Yield ~ Adjuvant + Row + Column, data = dataset)
plot(mod, which = 1)
plot(mod, which = 2)
boxcox(mod)

# Variance partitioning
anova(mod)
## Analysis of Variance Table
##
## Response: Yield
##           Df Sum Sq Mean Sq F value   Pr(>F)
## Adjuvant   3 4793.9 1597.96 14.9051 0.003458 **
## Row        3  375.8  125.28  1.1685 0.396678
```

```
## Column     3 6022.6 2007.53 18.7253 0.001893 **
## Residuals  6  643.3  107.21
```

The difference between adjuvants is significant (P-value = 0.0035), and the multiple comparison procedure reveals that the surfactant significantly improved the performance of the herbicide used alone, while the yield with mineral oil was not significantly lower than that with the surfactant.

Code Box 10.6

```
# Example 10.2 [continuation]

# Multiple comparisons
avgs <- emmeans(mod, ~Adjuvant)
confint(contrast(avgs, method = "pairwise"))
## contrast                         estimate   SE df lower.CL upper.CL
## AmmoniumSulphate - MineralOil      -30.00 7.32  6   -55.35    -4.66
## AmmoniumSulphate - None             -9.41 7.32  6   -34.75    15.93
## AmmoniumSulphate - Surfactant      -44.28 7.32  6   -69.63   -18.94
## MineralOil - None                   20.59 7.32  6    -4.75    45.94
## MineralOil - Surfactant            -14.28 7.32  6   -39.62    11.07
## None - Surfactant                  -34.87 7.32  6   -60.22    -9.53
##
## Results are averaged over the levels of: Row, Column
## Confidence level used: 0.95
## Conf-level adjustment: tukey method for comparing a family of
        4 estimates

cld(avgs, Letters = LETTERS, reversed = TRUE)
## Adjuvant         emmean   SE df lower.CL upper.CL .group
## Surfactant        115.4 5.18  6    102.8    128.1  A
## MineralOil        101.1 5.18  6     88.5    113.8  AB
## None               80.6 5.18  6     67.9     93.2   BC
## AmmoniumSulphate   71.1 5.18  6     58.5     83.8    C
```

10.3 Example 10.3: Genotype by N Interactions

Fifteen winter wheat genotypes were compared at two different nitrogen fertilization levels, according to an RCBD, with three replicates. The experiment aimed to assess whether the ranking of genotypes and, thus, the recommendation of genotypes are affected by the level of N availability. The dataset was generated through Monte Carlo simulation, starting from the results reported in Stagnari et al. (2013), and is available as the "NGenotypeFull" dataset in the `statforbiology` package.

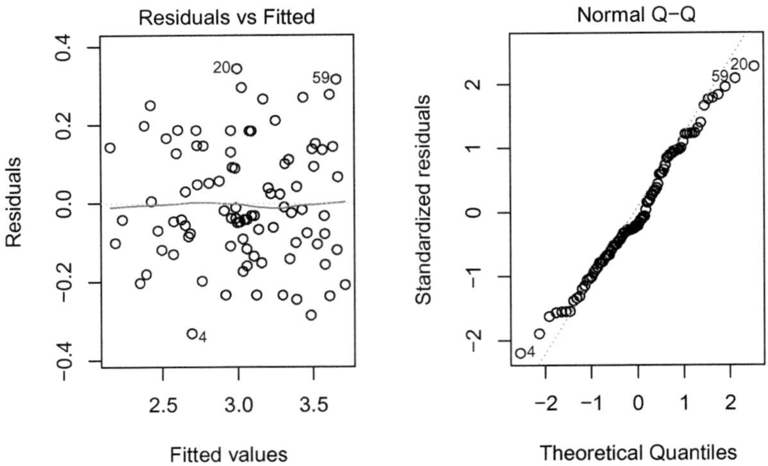

Fig. 10.3 Graphical analyses of residuals for the two-way "nitrogen by genotype" experiment (Example 10.3)

In this experiment, the yield response is determined by four effects:

1. Blocks
2. Genotypes
3. N levels
4. "Genotype × N" interaction

Accordingly, the model shown in Example 4.4 (Chap. 4) can be used by adding the block effect. To fit that model, we can load the data and transform the numeric predictors into factors. For this transformation, in Code Box 10.6, we use the `lapply()` function instead of the `transform()` function. With `lapply()`, the variables to be transformed are retrieved by indexing the columns; they are transformed using the `factor()` function (which is passed as the second argument) and reassigned to the same positions.

For brevity, the EDA is not shown; instead, model fitting is performed directly. A graphical check of model residuals yields the results shown in Fig. 10.3. We observe no evident deviations from the basic assumptions for linear models; therefore, we proceed to variance partitioning.

Code Box 10.6

```
# Example 10.3 [continuation]
# Genotype by Nitrogen Interactions

# Loading the packages
library(statforbiology)
```

```
library(MASS)
library(car)
library(emmeans)
library(multcomp)

# Loading and transforming the data
dataset <- getAgroData("NGenotypeFull")
dataset[,1:3] <- lapply(dataset[,1:3], factor)
head(dataset)
##   Block Genotype N Yield
## 1     1        A 1 2.146
## 2     2        A 1 2.433
## 3     3        A 1 2.579
## 4     1        A 2 2.362
## 5     2        A 2 2.919
## 6     3        A 2 2.912

# Model fitting
mod <- lm(Yield ~ Block + Genotype * N, data=dataset)

# Model checking
plot(mod, which = 1)
plot(mod, which = 2)
boxcox(mod)

# Variance partitioning
anova(mod)
## Analysis of Variance Table
##
## Response: Yield
##             Df  Sum Sq Mean Sq F value    Pr(>F)
## Block        2  0.0944 0.04721  1.3310 0.2721536
## Genotype    14 10.5408 0.75291 21.2297 < 2.2e-16 ***
## N            1  1.6246 1.62463 45.8092 7.175e-09 ***
## Genotype:N  14  1.6061 0.11472  3.2349 0.0008204 ***
## Residuals   58  2.0570 0.03547
```

Reading the P-levels for a two-way ANOVA requires some care. For the two main factors and their interaction, **it is fundamental to proceed from bottom to top** by exploring the significance of the interaction first. A significant crossover interaction may mask the effects of the main factors (see Chap. 4), and thus, **whenever the interaction is significant, we should always report and comment on the means for the combinations** of the experimental factor levels. On the other hand, **whenever the interaction is not significant, we are allowed to summarize the results by reporting and commenting the means for main effects.**

In this example, the interaction is significant, and the conclusion is that the genotype recommendation is not unique, but it depends on the level of N fertilization. Thus, it is necessary to report the genotype means for each N level separately.

Pairwise comparisons between genotypes can be done in two fashions:

1. Within and across N levels
2. Only within N levels

The first approach is very flexible, but it implies a high number of contrasts [$(10 \times 9)/2 = 45$ contrasts]; consequently, it also implies a strong adjustment of P-levels for multiplicity, decreased power, and higher risks of type II errors. Such an approach is to be recommended only if it is strictly necessary, and it is implemented in R using the `emmeans()` function and the interaction operator (i.e., `emmeans(mod,~Genotype:N)`).

The second approach is implemented by using the "conditioning operator" (i.e., `emmeans(mod,~Genotype|N)`). It implies a lower number of comparisons [$(2 \times [5 \times 4)/2 = 20$] and, in this example, appears to be of higher relevance from an agronomic perspective. In Code Box 10.7, the default multiplicity adjustment is performed. Due to the high number of comparisons, pairwise differences with their confidence intervals are not shown.

Code Box 10.7

```
# Example 10.3 [continuation]

# Pairwise comparisons within Nitrogen levels
GNmeans2 <- emmeans(mod, ~Genotype|N)
cld(GNmeans2, Letters=LETTERS)

## N = 1:
##  Genotype emmean    SE df lower.CL upper.CL .group
##  A          2.39 0.109 58     2.17     2.60  A
##  M          2.43 0.109 58     2.21     2.65  AB
##  C          2.53 0.109 58     2.32     2.75  ABC
##  G          2.61 0.109 58     2.39     2.83  ABCD
##  H          2.69 0.109 58     2.47     2.91  ABCD
##  I          2.77 0.109 58     2.55     2.99  ABCDE
##  B          2.92 0.109 58     2.70     3.13  ABCDEF
##  D          2.96 0.109 58     2.74     3.17   BCDEF
##  N          2.99 0.109 58     2.77     3.21    CDEFG
##  O          3.00 0.109 58     2.78     3.22    CDEFG
##  F          3.06 0.109 58     2.85     3.28    CDEFG
##  J          3.10 0.109 58     2.88     3.31     DEFG
```

```
##  E              3.26 0.109 58      3.04      3.47       EFG
##  K              3.40 0.109 58      3.18      3.61        FG
##  L              3.52 0.109 58      3.31      3.74         G
##
## N = 2:
##  Genotype emmean    SE df lower.CL upper.CL .group
##  C              2.19 0.109 58      1.97      2.41  A
##  I              2.63 0.109 58      2.41      2.85  AB
##  A              2.73 0.109 58      2.51      2.95  ABC
##  M              2.99 0.109 58      2.77      3.21   BCD
##  H              3.02 0.109 58      2.80      3.24   BCD
##  F              3.11 0.109 58      2.90      3.33   BCDE
##  G              3.13 0.109 58      2.91      3.34   BCDEF
##  B              3.24 0.109 58      3.02      3.46    CDEF
##  D              3.35 0.109 58      3.13      3.56     DEF
##  O              3.35 0.109 58      3.13      3.57     DEF
##  E              3.47 0.109 58      3.25      3.68     DEF
##  L              3.53 0.109 58      3.32      3.75     DEF
##  J              3.62 0.109 58      3.40      3.83      EF
##  K              3.62 0.109 58      3.40      3.83      EF
##  N              3.67 0.109 58      3.45      3.89       F
##
```

10.4 Example 10.4: Comparing Crosses in a Nested Design

Let us consider an experiment where three maize-pollinating inbred lines (A1, A2, and A3) were crossed with three different female inbred lines (A1 was crossed with B1, B2, and B3, A2 was crossed with B4, B5, and B6, and A3 was crossed with B7, B8, and B9) for a total of nine hybrids (Fig. 10.4). The experimental design is a nested factorial (the mothers are different for each father; see Chap. 2), and it was laid out in complete blocks with four replicates (36 observations, in total). The results are available as the "crosses" dataset in the `statforbiology` package.

The yield variation is determined by the causal effects of:

1. Block (γ)
2. "Father" (α)
3. "Mother" within each "father" (δ)

We cannot determine the overall "mother" effect because the female lines are different for each male line, and thus, the "mother" effect is nested within the "father" effect (Fig. 10.4). Likewise, we cannot determine the interaction between

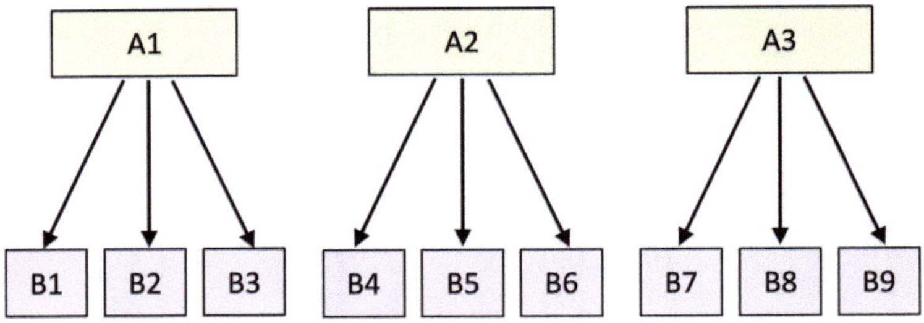

Fig. 10.4 Structure for a nested design

mother and father, as this would require a crossed design. The following model is reasonable:

$$Y_{ijk} = \mu + \gamma_k + \alpha_i + \delta_{ij} + \varepsilon_{ijk} \tag{10.2}$$

In this model, μ is the intercept, i.e., the expected yield for the first male crossed with the first female. The random component ε is assumed to be Gaussian and homoscedastic, with a mean of 0 and a standard deviation of σ.

In R, nested effects can be coded by using the "nesting" operator (/),[2] which means that the main effect of the nested treatment must be omitted (Code Box 10.8). The graphical analyses of residuals permit the exclusion of any significant deviations from the basic assumptions (not shown), and the ANOVA table shows that all the effects are significant, in particular, the female effect within males. MCP can be applied to compare the females within males, which is left as an exercise.

Code Box 10.8

```
# Example 10.4
# Comparing crosses in a nested factorial design

# Loading the packages
library(statforbiology)
library(MASS)

# Loading the data and fitting a model with a nested effect
dataset <- getAgroData("crosses")
dataset[,1:3] <- lapply(dataset[,1:3], factor)
head(dataset, 5)
```

[2] For example, A/B means that B is nested within A and expands to A + A:B. The behavior of the nesting operator changes slightly with numerical predictors in ANCOVA models (see Chap. 11).

```
##   Male Female Block     Yield
## 1   A1     B1     1  9.984718
## 2   A1     B1     2 13.932663
## 3   A1     B1     3 12.201312
## 4   A1     B1     4  1.916661
## 5   A1     B2     1  8.928465

# Model fitting and parameter estimation
mod <- lm(Yield ~ Block + Male/Female, data = dataset)

# Analyses of residuals
plot(mod, which = 1)
plot(mod, which = 2)
boxcox(mod)

# Variance partitioning
anova(mod)
## Analysis of Variance Table
##
## Response: Yield
##             Df Sum Sq Mean Sq F value    Pr(>F)
## Block        3 383.75 127.917  44.355 6.051e-10 ***
## Male         2 134.76  67.378  23.363 2.331e-06 ***
## Male:Female  6 575.16  95.860  33.239 1.742e-10 ***
## Residuals   24  69.21   2.884
```

10.5 Example 10.5: A Germination Experiment in Two Runs

The conclusions from a single experiment in agriculture are most often regarded as weak evidence despite being based on high precision and statistical significance. Indeed, a single experiment can be influenced by flaws of any kind, measurement errors, unexpected events, or intrusions, which can go unnoticed. Furthermore, a significant result may be specific to the conditions in which it was observed and may not be reproducible in other situations (see Chap. 1).

Therefore, testing the reproducibility of results by independently running confirmatory experiments is considered a fundamental key to scientific progress in agriculture, permitting sound generalizations (see White et al. 2025, for a definition of reproducibility). We cannot repeat agricultural field experiments under the same conditions; therefore, we need to perform independent runs at different sites, in different years, or with different vegetable materials, so that we can expect a greater or lesser degree of variability across runs. It is always beneficial to conduct a final pooled analysis of all the replicated experiments to test for the hypothesis that the runs do not differ significantly from one another.

Let us consider an experiment to compare the germination of three oilseed rape genotypes (Pace et al. 2012). The experimental units consisted of Petri dishes with 50 seeds each, and the assay was conducted in controlled conditions at 20 °C, with six replicates per genotype in six complete blocks, represented by different shelves of an oven. To confirm the results, the experiment was independently repeated in a different oven and, obviously, with different seeds, at the same temperature. In both experiments, the number of germinated seeds was counted 15 days after the beginning of the assay and expressed as the Final Proportion of Germinated seeds (FGP).

The results of these two experiments are available as the "FGP_rape" data in the `statforbiology` package; after loading the data, it is necessary to transform the numeric predictors (run and shelf) into factors (Code Box 10.9).

The EDA should include separate analyses for each run to explore their similarity and, in particular, to ensure that the data are good for all runs, with no outliers and dubious values. Furthermore, it is necessary to make sure that the residual mean squares for all experiments are comparable (homoscedasticity of within-run errors).

To facilitate within-run analyses, it is possible to simplify the coding by using the split-apply-combine strategy (Wickham 2011) based on the `by()` and `lapply()` functions.[3] The first function operates on subsets of the selected dataset, split according to a classification variable (the "run" variable, in this case). It produces a list with the results of the fitting function `lm()` applied to each subset. This list is explored using the `lapply()` function, which applies the `leveneTest()` and `shapiro.test()` functions to each linear model object in the list. Both the tests show no problems for either experiment.

We can perform a swift and simple test for the homoscedasticity of within-run errors using Hartley's F max test (Hartley 1950). It consists of calculating the ratio between the highest and lowest mean square values in the different runs (in this case, we only have two values, though); the sampling distribution for this ratio under the null hypothesis of homoscedasticity is given by the `pmaxFratio()` function in the `SuppDists` package (Wheeler 2024), and the P-value is not low enough for the null to be rejected (Code Box 10.9).

Code Box 10.9

```
# Example 10.5
# A germination experiment in two runs

# Loading packages
library(statforbiology)
```

[3] Powerful methods for the split-apply-combine strategy exist also in the `tidyverse` package.

```
library(car)
library(SuppDists)
library(MASS)
library(emmeans)
library(multcomp)

# Loading and transforming the data
dataset <- getAgroData("FGP_rape")
dataset[,1:5] <- lapply(dataset[,1:5], factor)
head(dataset)
##   Dish Run Shelf     Species Genotype  FGP
## 1    1   1     1 OilseedRape        A 0.81
## 2   13   1     1 OilseedRape        B 0.81
## 3   25   1     1 OilseedRape        C 0.74
## 4    2   1     2 OilseedRape        A 0.91
## 5   14   1     2 OilseedRape        B 0.92
## 6   26   1     2 OilseedRape        C 0.76

# Fitting linear models to the two runs, separately
lmFits <- by(dataset, dataset$Run,
      function(df) lm(FGP ~ Genotype + Shelf, data = df) )

# Check for within-experiments homoscedasticity
# Modified Levene's test for RCBDs (see Code box 10.2)
levTest <- by(dataset, dataset$Run,
      function(df)
        leveneTest(abs(residuals(lm(FGP ~ Genotype + Shelf,
                        data = df))), df$Genotype))
levTest
## dataset$Run: 1
## Levene's Test for Homogeneity of Variance (center = median)
##       Df F value Pr(>F)
## group  2  0.2779 0.7612
##       15
## ------------------------------------------------------------
## dataset$Run: 2
## Levene's Test for Homogeneity of Variance (center = median)
##       Df F value Pr(>F)
## group  2  1.5841 0.2376
##       15

lapply(lmFits, function(mods) shapiro.test(residuals(mods)))
## $`1`
##
##  Shapiro-Wilk normality test
##
## data:  residuals(mods)
```

```
## W = 0.990201, p-value = 0.06229
##
##
## $‘2‘
##
##  Shapiro-Wilk normality test
##
## data:  residuals(mods)
## W = 0.93221, p-value = 0.2124

# Check for homoscedasticity of errors across runs
# by the Hartley Fmax test
mses <- unlist(
  lapply(lmFits, function(mods) summary(mods)$sigma^2))
Fmax <- max(mses)/min(mses)
pmaxFratio(Fmax, 15, 2, lower.tail = FALSE)
## [1] 0.7404869

# Variance partitioning
lapply(lmFits, function(mods) anova(mods))
## $‘1‘
## Analysis of Variance Table
##
## Response: FGP
##           Df   Sum Sq   Mean Sq F value   Pr(>F)
## Genotype   2 0.033011 0.0165056 15.6864 0.000825 ***
## Shelf      5 0.019911 0.0039822  3.7846 0.034871 *
## Residuals 10 0.010522 0.0010522
##
## $‘2‘
## Analysis of Variance Table
##
## Response: FGP
##           Df   Sum Sq   Mean Sq F value    Pr(>F)
## Genotype   2 0.042544 0.0212722 16.9876 0.0006081 ***
## Shelf      5 0.001761 0.0003522  0.2813 0.9129498
## Residuals 10 0.012522 0.0012522
```

The EDA demonstrates that there are no problems with the basic assumptions in either of the two experiments. Besides, the treatment effect was significant in both runs, and the residual variances appear to be homogeneous.

For the pooled analyses, the dataset is similar to those from any other two-factor factorial experiment, with the only difference being that the block effect is **nested within runs**, as the shelves differ across different runs (ovens). Accordingly, the final model is

$$y_{ijk} = \mu + \gamma_{ik} + \alpha_i + \beta_j + \alpha\beta_{ij} + \varepsilon_{ijk} \tag{10.3}$$

In this model, y is the response for the ith run, jth treatment level, and kth shelf, μ is the intercept, γ_{ik} is the effect of the kth shelf in the ith run, α_i is the effect of the ith run, β_j is the effect of the jth treatment level, $\alpha\beta_{ij}$ is the "treatment by run" interaction effect, and ε_{ijk} is the residual random effect for each observation, which is assumed as normally distributed and homoscedastic [$\epsilon_{ijk} \sim N(0, \sigma_\varepsilon)$]. This model is fitted in Code Box 10.10.

Code Box 10.10

```
# Example 10.5 [continuation]

# Pooled analyses: model fitting
mod <- lm(FGP ~ Genotype * Run + Run:Shelf, data = dataset)

# model checking
plot(mod, which = 1)
plot(mod, which = 2)
boxcox(mod)

# Variance partitioning
anova(mod)
## Analysis of Variance Table
##
## Response: FGP
##              Df   Sum Sq  Mean Sq F value    Pr(>F)
## Genotype      2 0.074289 0.037144 32.2372 5.534e-07 ***
## Run           1 0.003025 0.003025  2.6254    0.1208
## Genotype:Run  2 0.001267 0.000633  0.5497    0.5856
## Run:Shelf    10 0.021672 0.002167  1.8809    0.1100
## Residuals    20 0.023044 0.001152
```

Inspecting the ANOVA table for a set of pooled experiments gives an idea of the reproducibility of results across runs. It is possible to encounter the following situations:

1. The "run by treatment" interaction is significant. In this case, the conclusion is that the effects of treatment levels and, possibly, their ranking varied across different runs. Consequently, pooling the results is not appropriate, and **we should only display and compare the means of treatment levels within each run**.

2. The interaction is not significant, but the main effect of the run is significant. The conclusion is that the treatment effect and the run effect were independent and additive; consequently, the means for treatment levels changed across runs, but the treatment effects were fully reproducible (White et al. 2025). It is up to the researcher to decide whether it is appropriate and meaningful to calculate and display the means for treatment levels.
3. Neither the interaction nor the main effects of the run are significant. The conclusion is that the results of the repeated experiments are fully reproducible, and it is usually appropriate to report only the means for treatment levels.

For our example, we see that the "run" and "run by treatment" effects are not significant, which means that the results are fully reproducible. Therefore, we pool the two runs and compare the genotypes across runs (Code Box 10.11).

Code Box 10.11

```
# Example 10.5 [continuation]

# Multiple comparison testing for pooled data

cld(emmeans(mod, ~ Genotype), Letters = LETTERS)
## Genotype  emmean     SE df  lower.CL upper.CL .group
##  C         0.781 0.0098 20     0.760    0.801  A
##  A         0.871 0.0098 20     0.850    0.891   B
##  B         0.882 0.0098 20     0.862    0.903   B
```

Before concluding, it is worth noting that the proposed method of data analysis for this example is always appropriate. However, in some circumstances, especially when the number of runs is very high, different methods of data analysis could be preferred, as will be exemplified in Chap. 12.

10.6 Exercises

For all these exercises, use the work plan proposed in this chapter, and try to reach sound conclusions. All datasets are available in the `statforbiology` package and can be accessed using the `getAgroData()` function. The name of the dataset is specified for each exercise.

1. An experiment was conducted with a completely randomized design to compare the yield of five wheat genotypes. The results (in bushels per acre) are reported in the table below. Determine the best genotype, and draw sound conclusions.

The example is taken from Le Clerg et al. (1962), and the dataset is available as "LeClerg."

	Replicate		
Variety	1	2	3
A	32.4	34.3	37.3
B	20.2	27.5	25.9
C	29.2	27.8	30.2
D	12.8	12.3	14.8
E	21.7	24.5	23.4

2. Cell cultures of tomato were grown using three types of media, which were prepared by adding a certain amount of either glucose or fructose or sucrose to the untreated check. The experiment was conducted using a completely randomized design with five replicates, and the growth of cells was recorded for each subject. Determine which growth media gave the highest cell growth, and comment on the results. The dataset is taken from Kuehl (2000), and it is shown in the table below. It is available as "sugarsMedia" in the `statforbiology` package.

Check	Glucose	Fructose	Sucrose
45	25	28	31
39	28	31	37
40	30	24	35
45	29	28	33
42	33	27	34

3. An experiment was conducted to assess the failure time for a heating system as affected by four different operating temperatures. The design was completely randomized with six replicates, and the number of hours before failure was measured. Regard the temperature as a factor, and determine the optimal operating temperature, which results in delayed failure. The results are shown below, and they are available as "failureTimes." *Hint: In this exercise, a stabilizing transformation is needed, which is not automatically recognized by the* `emmeans()` *function. Therefore, the back-transformation will require the process described for Example 9.6.*

Temp	1	2	3	4	5	6
1520	1953	2135	2471	4727	6134	6314
1620	1190	1286	1550	2125	2557	2845
1660	651	837	848	1038	1361	1543
1708	511	651	651	652	688	729

4. An entomologist counted the number of eggs laid by a *Lepidoptera* on three different substrates according to a completely randomized design with 15 replicates. Identify the substrate with the lowest oviposition. The results are reported below, and they are available as "lepidopteraEggs." *Hint: The response is a count variable, and possible deviations from the basic assumptions are to be expected. Perform a careful check and, if necessary, apply the most suitable stabilizing transformation.*

Rep	A	B	C
1	456	118	72
2	411	213	99
3	594	74	24
4	280	26	20
5	664	163	89
6	379	76	47
7	444	240	32
8	436	75	29
9	294	108	1
10	431	68	33
11	476	108	20
12	382	153	22
13	413	98	27
14	485	120	39
15	440	126	12

5. An irrigation experiment was conducted in an orange grove in southern Italy, comprising five irrigation systems in five complete blocks. The observed yields (in tons per hectare) are reported in the table below and are available as "orangeIrrigation." Which irrigation system offered the best performance? What is your sound conclusion?

Method	1	2	3	4	5
Localized	26.7	27.9	51.2	29.0	34.8
Surface	46.4	47.7	33.9	32.7	21.7
Sprinkler	38.5	29.1	33.6	11.8	27.6
Sprinkler + localized	41.3	33.9	31.3	5.8	12.1
Submersion	35.2	46.9	19.8	27.9	26.7

6. A fertilization trial was conducted according to a randomized complete block design with five replicates; however, due to unforeseen circumstances, one value is missing for the "50N" treatment in the second block. The observed data are percentage contents of P_2O_5 in leaf samples and are available as "missingVal."

Is it convenient to fertilize? Is it convenient to increase the N fertilization level to 100 kg/ha? Is the addition of P_2O_5 a convenient practice? *Hint: Consider the missing value, and make sure that the variance partitioning approach is appropriate, as indicated in Sect. 4.8*

Fertilization	1	2	3	4	5
100N	6.9	9.6	5.6	7.4	8.2
100N+75P	9.6	9.3	12.0	10.6	11.6
50N	7.3	NA	7.7	7.7	7.0
50N+75P	10.8	9.2	8.8	9.9	9.4
Unfertilized	5.6	6.1	5.3	5.9	7.4

7. A Latin square experiment was designed to evaluate the impact of four different fertilizers on lettuce yield. The observed data are available as "lettuceLS," and they are reported in the table below. Which is the best fertilizer?

Fertilizer	Row	Column	Yield
A	1	1	104
B	1	2	114
C	1	3	90
D	1	4	140
A	2	4	134
B	2	3	130
C	2	1	144
D	2	2	174
A	3	3	146
B	3	4	142
C	3	2	152
D	3	1	156
A	4	2	147
B	4	1	160
C	4	4	160
D	4	3	163

8. A pot experiment was planned to evaluate the best timing for herbicide application against rhizome *Sorghum halepense*. Five timings were compared (2-3, 4-5, 6-7, and 8-9 leaves), including a split treatment in two timings (3-4/8-9 leaves) and the untreated control. To determine whether the application is effective against plants originating from rhizomes of different sizes, this second factor was introduced in the experiment (2, 4, and 6 nodes). This experiment was a fully crossed two-way factorial, laid out as a completely randomized design with four replicates. The results (plant weights 3 weeks after the herbicide application)

are taken from Onofri and Tei (1994) and are available as "johnsongrass." At which timing was the herbicide treatment most effective? Is the split treatment convenient against the single treatments? Is the recommendation for farmers independent from rhizome size?

Sizes/timings	2-3	4-5	6-7	8-9	3-4/8-9	Untreated
2-nodes	34.03	0.10	30.91	33.21	2.89	41.63
	22.31	6.08	35.34	43.44	19.06	22.96
	21.70	3.73	24.23	44.06	0.10	52.14
	14.90	9.15	28.27	35.34	0.68	59.81
4-nodes	42.19	14.86	52.34	39.06	8.62	68.15
	51.06	36.03	43.17	61.59	0.05	42.75
	43.77	21.85	57.28	48.89	0.10	57.77
	31.74	8.71	29.71	49.14	9.65	44.85
6-nodes	20.84	11.37	55.00	41.77	9.80	43.20
	26.12	2.24	28.46	37.38	0.10	40.68
	35.24	14.17	21.81	39.55	1.42	34.11
	13.32	23.93	60.72	48.37	6.83	32.21

References

Belocchi A, Fornara M, Ciriciofolo E, Biancolatte E, Del Puglia S, Olimpieri G, Vecchiarelli V, Gosparini E, Piccioni C, Desiderio E (2003) Grano duro: Risultati 2002–03 della Rete Nazionale. Lazio e Umbria. L'Informatore Agrario 19(Suppl.1):41–44

Bhandary M, Dai H (2013) An alternative test for the equality of variances for several populations in randomised complete block design. Stat Methodol 11:22–35. https://doi.org/10.1016/j.stamet.2012.08.002. https://linkinghub.elsevier.com/retrieve/pii/S1572312712000482

Hartley HO (1950) The Maximum F-ratio as a short-cut test for heterogeneity of variance. Biometrika 37(3/4):308. https://doi.org/10.2307/2332383. https://www.jstor.org/stable/2332383?origin=crossref

Jensen SM, Schaarschmidt F, Onofri A, Ritz C (2018) Experimental design matters for statistical analysis: how to handle blocking: experimental design matters for statistical analysis. Pest Manag Sci 74(3):523–534. https://doi.org/10.1002/ps.4773. http://doi.wiley.com/10.1002/ps.4773

Kuehl RO (2000) Design of Experiments: Statistical Principles of Research Design and Analysis. Duxbury Press, Pacific Grove

Le Clerg EL, Leonard WH, Clark AG (1962) Field Plot Technique. Burgess Publishing Company, Minneapolis

Onofri A, Tei F (1994) Influence of application timing on the effectiveness of rimsulfuron against rhizome *Sorghum halepense* (L.) Pers. In: Tei F, Onofri A (eds) Weed Control in Sustainable Agriculture in the Mediterranean Area. Proceedings 5th EWRS Mediterranean Symposium, Università degli Studi di Perugia, Reprints, pp 105–111

Pace R, Benincasa P, Ghanem ME, Quinet M, Lutts S (2012) Germination of untreated and primed seeds in rapeseed (brassica napus var oleifera del.) under salinity and low matric potential. Exp Agricul 48(02):238–251. https://doi.org/10.1017/S0014479711001189. http://www.journals.cambridge.org/abstract_S0014479711001189

Stagnari F, Onofri A, Codianni P, Pisante M (2013) Durum wheat varieties in N-deficient environments and organic farming: a comparison of yield, quality and stability performances. Plant Breed 132:266–275

Wheeler B (2024) SuppDists: Supplementary Distributions. https://CRAN.R-project.org/package=SuppDists, r package version 1.1-9.8

White JW, Boote KJ, Kimball BA, Porter C, Salmeron M, Shelia V, Thorp KR, Hoogenboom G (2025) From field to analysis: strengthening reproducibility and confirmation in research for sustainable agriculture. npj Sustain Agricul 3(1):27. https://doi.org/10.1038/s44264-025-00067-z. https://www.nature.com/articles/s44264-025-00067-z

Wickham H (2011) The split-apply-combine strategy for data analysis. J Stat Softw 40(1):1–29. https://doi.org/10.18637/jss.v040.i01. http://www.jstatsoft.org/v40/i01/

Chapter 11
Extending Regression Models

Regression analysis is the hydrogen bomb of the statistics arsenal

—C. Wheelan

Abstract When the predictor is a quantitative variable, we may be interested in fitting the observed data to one of the so-called *regression models*, which take the form of continuous "dose-response" curves. In this chapter, the simple linear regression model presented in Chap. 4 is slightly extended to cover some everyday situations in agriculture research. Specifically, examples are given regarding regression models with grouping factors, ANCOVA models, and nonlinear regression models. For nonlinear regression in R, the `drc` package and its facilities are briefly introduced.

As anticipated in Chap. 4, the effects of quantitative factors are commonly studied in agriculture, for example, to quantify the response of yield to increasing rates of fertilizers or to determine the mortality of pests treated with different doses of a pesticide. To deal with quantitative factors, a simple linear regression model was introduced earlier in this book and used to analyze the data from an experiment with no replicates; unfortunately, such a simple model is most often insufficient for the needs posed by agriculture research, and in this chapter, several extensions are introduced, by using real-life examples.

11.1 Example 11.1: Linear Regression for a Randomized Block Design

In contrast to the data shown in Example 4.2, small plot experiments in agriculture typically contain true replicates and are designed in complete blocks. For example, let us consider the "NWheat" dataset from the `statforbiology` package, which comes from an experiment conducted in four complete blocks to investigate the

A. Onofri, *Field Research Methods in Agriculture*,
https://doi.org/10.1007/978-3-032-08199-5_11

relationship between nitrogen fertilization rate (four levels, ranging from 0 to 180 kg/ha) and wheat yield (in tons per hectare).

This dataset can be described by using a simple linear regression model, augmented with a term for the block effect, which is necessary to ensure the independence of residuals:

$$Y_{ij} = \gamma_j + \beta_0 + \beta_1 X_i + \varepsilon_{ij} \tag{11.1}$$

In this model, Y_{ij} is the yield for the ith dose in the jth block, γ_j is the effect of the jth block, under the usual constraint that $\gamma_1 = 0$, β_0 is the intercept for the first block, β_1 is the slope of the regression line (straight line), X_i is the fertilization dose, and ε_{ij} are the residuals, with a mean of 0 and a standard deviation of σ. In practice, the previous equation represents a yield response that decreases linearly with nitrogen dose, with a unique slope. At the same time, the intercept depends on the block level (i.e., four parallel straight lines, one for each block).

Considering that the dataset contains true replicates, it would also be possible to “transform” the quantitative predictor into a nominal factor and fit an alternative model with two nominal predictors, as shown in Example 4.3 (Chap. 4).

The comparison between these two models is of great interest: The second model always provides the best fit to the observed data because it only considers the responses at the selected dose levels without putting any constraints on what happens between a “dose” and the succeeding one. On the other hand, a linear regression model imposes a strong constraint, as the responses at increasing doses must be aligned; however, it is more realistic from a biological point of view, as it does not neglect the existence of a continuous “dose-response” curve, which is the primary focus of the study.

To understand the insights obtained from model comparison, we begin the analysis by transforming both the dose and block into nominal factors (please note that a new factor variable is created for the dose to retain the numeric variable for later use). Next, we fit a linear model with two nominal predictors (Code Box 11.1); the check for basic assumptions did not evidence any problems, and it is not shown for brevity. The residual sum of squares for this model is calculated (RSS_{pure} = 0.381) and stored for later analyses.

Code Box 11.1

```
# Example 11.1
# Linear regression for an RCBD

# Loading the packages
library(statforbiology)
library(emmeans)
library(multcomp)
```

```
# Loading and transforming the data
# The dose is recoded as a factor and a new variable is
  created
dataset <- getAgroData("NWheat")
dataset <- transform(dataset, DoseF = factor(Dose),
                     Block = factor(Block))
head(dataset)
##   Dose Block Yield DoseF
## 1    0     1 2.198     0
## 2    0     2 2.569     0
## 3    0     3 2.771     0
## 4    0     4 1.914     0
## 5   60     1 3.507    60
## 6   60     2 3.527    60

# Model 1: ANOVA model with two nominal predictors
mod.pure <- lm(Yield ~ DoseF + Block, data = dataset)

# Variance partitioning
anova(mod.pure)
## Analysis of Variance Table
##
## Response: Yield
##           Df  Sum Sq Mean Sq F value    Pr(>F)
## DoseF      3 17.2596  5.7532 136.005 8.172e-08 ***
## Block      3  0.2315  0.0772   1.824    0.2129
## Residuals  9  0.3807  0.0423

# Getting the RSS and storing it
RSSpure <- deviance(mod.pure)
RSSpure
## [1] 0.3807132
```

In the second instance, the regression model in Eq. (11.1) is fitted (Code Box 11.2); the residual sum of squares for this model is, as expected, higher than that of the previous model ($RSS_{reg} = 0.4723$), confirming that the model with the nominal dose fits better than the regression model.

Code Box 11.2

```
# Example 11.1 [continuation]

# Model 2. Regression model
# The dose is not transformed into a factor!
mod.reg <- lm(Yield ~ Block + Dose, data = dataset)
coef(summary(mod.reg))
##              Estimate Std.Err. t val.     Pr(>|t|)
## (Intercept)   2.32775 0.124752 18.659 1.123724e-09
## Block2        0.12975 0.146513  0.886 3.947884e-01
## Block3        0.19450 0.146513  1.328 2.112272e-01
## Block4       -0.11775 0.146513 -0.804 4.386038e-01
## Dose          0.01544 0.000772 19.997 5.352483e-10

# Residual sum of squares
RSSreg <- deviance(mod.reg)
RSSreg
## [1] 0.4722555
```

At this point, it is possible to compare the two models. Such a comparison cannot be made using indices like the R^2 value, which always favor the best-fitting model, regardless of its complexity. Indeed, comparing two models should be done by following Occam's razor principle (see Chap. 1), which keeps simplicity under due consideration. Thus, we can use the so-called **F-test for lack-of-fit**; this procedure is based on the idea that the residual sum of squares for the regression model always contains two possible types of errors:

1. *Pure error*, i.e., the discrepancy between each observed value and the mean of the group to which that observation belongs
2. *Lack-of-fit error*, i.e., the discrepancy between the group mean and the regression line, which is a measure of how "bad" the regression model is

Conversely, the residual sum of squares for the model with two nominal predictors only contains the "pure error"; hence, the lack-of-fit error can be obtained by subtraction ($SS_{lof} = SS_{reg} - SS_{pure} = 0.0915$).

The numbers of DF for the residual terms are, respectively, 11 for the regression model (16 individuals minus 5 estimated parameters) and 9 for the model with two nominal predictors (see Code Box 11.1); consequently, the number of DF for the lack-of-fit component is 2 (i.e., 11 − 9).

The mean squares for the lack-of-fit and pure error components are obtained by dividing the sum of squares for the respective degrees of freedom, i.e., $MS_{lof} = 0.09154/2 = 0.04577$ and $MS_{pure} = 0.38071/9 = 0.04230$. The F-ratio for lack-of-fit is

$$F_{LOF} = \frac{MS_{LOF}}{MS_{\text{pure}}} = \frac{0.4577}{0.4230} = 1.082 \tag{11.2}$$

With R, we can complete the task using the anova() function and passing both models as arguments (Code Box 11.3).

Code Box 11.3

```
# Example 11.1 [continuation]

# Test for lack-of-fit with R
anova(mod.reg, mod.pure)
## Analysis of Variance Table
##
## Model 1: Yield ~ Block + Dose
## Model 2: Yield ~ DoseF + Block
##   Res.Df     RSS Df Sum of Sq     F Pr(>F)
## 1     11 0.47226
## 2      9 0.38071  2  0.091542 1.082 0.3792
```

The null hypothesis is that the lack-of-fit component is not significant. Based on a P-value higher than 0.05, we fail to reject the null hypothesis and conclude that the regression model provides a good description of the observed data.

The ANOVA table for the regression model confirms that the causal effect of the dose on yield is highly significant (Code Box 11.4).

Code Box 11.4

```
# Example 11.1 [continuation]

# Test for goodness of fit with R
anova(mod.reg)
## Analysis of Variance Table
##
## Response: Yield
##           Df  Sum Sq Mean Sq  F value    Pr(>F)
## Block      3  0.2315  0.0772   1.7972    0.2058
## Dose       1 17.1680 17.1680 399.8863 5.352e-10 ***
## Residuals 11  0.4723  0.0429
```

At this point, it is necessary to derive the equation that describes the cause-effect relationship between N rate and yield. In the fitted model, the estimated intercept is block-specific (see Code Box 11.2), and it is usually necessary to calculate the average value, for example, for plotting and prediction purposes. The average intercept is obtained as the following linear combination of model parameters:

$$\begin{aligned} \beta_{0\cdot} &= \frac{\beta_{01}+(\beta_{01}+\gamma_2)+(\beta_{01}+\gamma_3)+(\beta_{01}+\gamma_4)}{4} = \\ &= \beta_{01} + \frac{1}{4}\gamma_2 + \frac{1}{4}\gamma_3 + \frac{1}{4}\gamma_4 \end{aligned} \quad (11.3)$$

In this equation, β_{01}, γ_2, γ_3, and γ_4 are the first four parameter estimates for the regression model in Code Box 11.2. Considering these estimates and their ordering, the matrix of coefficients for Eq. (11.3) is $K = [1\ 0.25\ 0.25\ 0.25\ 0]$. The linear combination can be fitted with the `glht()` function or, more easily, with the `emmeans()` function (Code Box 11.5).

Code Box 11.5

```
# Example 11.1 [continuation]

# Calculating the average intercept across blocks

# Fitting the contrast with 'glht()'
# Creating a matrix of coefficients
# with reference to the ordering of parameters
# in the model output. Please note the final 0,
# relating to the slope (see Code box 11.2)
K <- matrix(c(1, 1/4, 1/4, 1/4, 0),
            nrow = 1, ncol = 5)
row.names(K) <- c("b0_mean")
con <- glht(mod.reg, linfct = K)
summary(con)
##
## Linear Hypotheses:
##              Estimate Std. Error t value Pr(>|t|)
## b0_mean == 0  2.37937    0.08668   27.45 1.75e-11 ***

# Fitting the contrast with emmeans
emmeans(mod.reg, ~1, at = data.frame(Dose = 0))
##  1        emmean     SE df lower.CL upper.CL
##  overall    2.38 0.0867 11     2.19     2.57
```

The average slope is 2.379 (SE $= 0.0867$) t/ha, and it can be used, together with the slope, to draw a swift graph of the observed data, augmented with

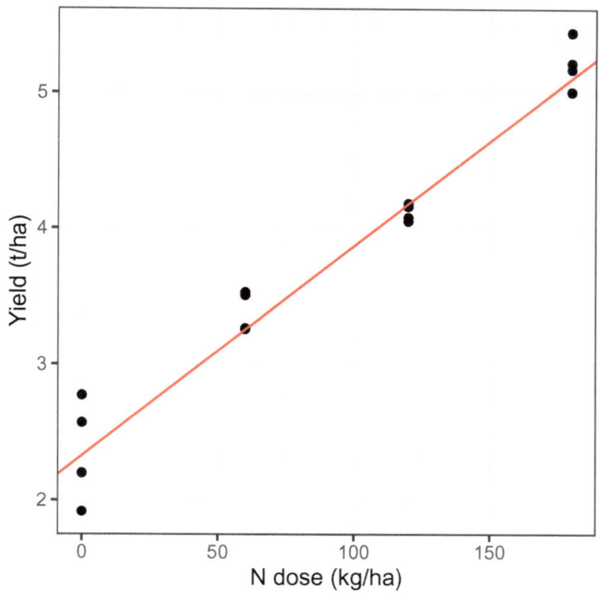

Fig. 11.1 Regression analysis for the "NWheat" data: The symbols show the observed yield, while the red line shows the fitted model

model predictions, e.g., by using the `geom_abline()` function in `ggplot2` (Code Box 11.6; Fig. 11.1).

Code Box 11.6

```
# Example 11.1 [continuation]

# Swift plot of observed yields and predictions
library(ggplot2)
ggplot(dataset) +
  geom_point(mapping = aes(x = Dose, y = Yield)) +
  geom_abline(mapping = aes(intercept = 23.8, slope = 0.154),
              col = "red") +
  labs(x = "N dose (kg/ha)", y = "Yield (q/ha)") +
  theme_bw()
```

Making predictions for regression models that contain block effects is slightly more complex than for simple linear regression models without blocks. For example, should we be interested in estimating the expected yields with 50 and 100 kg Na ha^{-1}, the easiest methods would consist of either:

1. Using `glht()` to fit two linear combinations $\beta_{01} + \frac{1}{4}\gamma_2 + \frac{1}{4}\gamma_3 + \frac{1}{4}\gamma_4 + \beta_1 \times 50$ and $\beta_{01} + \frac{1}{4}\gamma_2 + \frac{1}{4}\gamma_3 + \frac{1}{4}\gamma_4 + \beta_1 \times 100$ or more easily
2. Using `emmeans()` and passing a dataframe with the doses for prediction (Code Box 11.7)

An example of inverse prediction is also in order: What is the N fertilization rate to obtain, e.g., a yield of 3.5 tons per hectare? In this case, the nonlinear combination is

$$\frac{3.5 - (\beta_{01} + \frac{1}{4}\gamma_2 + \frac{1}{4}\gamma_3 + \frac{1}{4}\gamma_4)}{\beta_1} \tag{11.4}$$

This combination can be fitted with the `gnlht()` function (Code Box 11.7).

Code Box 11.7

```
# Example 11.1 [continuation]


# Making predictions for the NWheat data and determining
# the expected yield with N doses equal to 50 and 100 kg/ha

# Method 1. Fitting as linear contrast
C1 <- c(1, 1/4, 1/4, 1/4, 50)
C2 <- c(1, 1/4, 1/4, 1/4, 100)
K <- rbind(C1, C2)
summary(glht(mod.reg, linfct = K))
##
## Linear Hypotheses:
##          Estimate Std. Error t value Pr(>|t|)
## C1 == 0   3.15146    0.06031   52.25   <1e-10 ***
## C2 == 0   3.92354    0.05237   74.92   <1e-10 ***

# Method 2. Fitting with emmeans()
emmeans(mod.reg, ~Dose, at = data.frame(Dose = c(50, 100)))
##  Dose emmean     SE df lower.CL upper.CL
##    50   3.15 0.0603 11     3.02     3.28
##   100   3.92 0.0524 11     3.81     4.04

# Making inverse predictions
# Determining the N dose to obtain a yield of 5 tons per
  hectare
invPred <- gnlht(mod.reg,
  func = list(~(3.5 - (b0 + 1/4*gamma2 + 1/4*gamma3 +
```

```
                          1/4*gamma4))/b1),
    parameterNames = c("b0", "gamma2", "gamma3",
    "gamma4", "b1"))
  invPred$Form <- "Yield_3.5"
  invPred
  ##          Form Estimate       SE  t-value      p-value
  ## 1 Yield_3.5 72.57151 3.465948 20.93843 3.266002e-10
```

The results indicate that fertilizing with 50 and 100 Kg N ha^{-1} yields, respectively, 3.15 (SE $= 0.06$) and 3.92 (SE $= 0.05$) t ha^{-1}. Furthermore, a yield of 3.5 t ha^{-1} can be obtained by fertilizing with 72.6 (SE $= 3.47$) Kg N ha^{-1}.

11.2 Example 11.2: Herbicide Degradation in Different Conditions

In the previous example, the only element of interest was the overall effect of the dose, while blocking was only included to reduce the amount of unexplained variability and, thus, to improve the control of experimental errors. In other frequent cases, the experiment aims to compare regression lines across different experimental groups.

For example, let us consider an experiment to study the degradation of metamitron (M) in soil, either alone or in the presence of two co-applied herbicides, i.e., phenmedipham (P) and chloridazon (C). In all, the herbicide treatments consisted of four herbicide combinations (i.e., M, MP, MC, and MPC), which were used to enrich 96 independent soil samples (32 samples for each combination). Treated samples were stored in a climatic chamber at 20 °C; at eight different times (0, 7, 14, 21, 32, 42, 55, and 67 days after treatment), three random samples were collected for each herbicide combination and were stored in a refrigerator, until chemical analyses. At the end of the experiment, all soil samples were analyzed to determine the residual concentration of metamitron. This dataset was obtained through Monte Carlo simulation, starting from the data in Vischetti et al. (1996), and is available as "metamitron" in the `statforbiology` package.

Preliminarily, the new nominal predictor "TimeF" is created by transforming the original numeric "Time" variable (Code Box 11.8); afterword, a two-factor factorial model is fitted, as shown in Example 4.4 (Chap. 4); the check for basic assumptions shows clear signs of heteroscedasticity, and the Box-Cox technique suggests that a logarithmic transformation may represent a proper remedy (Fig. 11.2). Consequently, the model is refitted by using the logarithms of concentration as the response, and it is retained as a reference for further analyses.

Code Box 11.8

```
# Example 11.2
# Herbicide degradation in different conditions

# Loading the packages
library(statforbiology)
library(MASS)
library(emmeans)
library(multcomp)

# Loading and transforming the data
dataset <- getAgroData("metamitron")
dataset <- transform(dataset,
                     Herbicide = factor(Herbicide),
                     TimeF = factor(Time))
head(dataset)
##   Time Herbicide Rep ConcReal   Conc TimeF
## 1    0         M   1    92.00 101.52     0
## 2    0         M   2   118.64  95.77     0
## 3    0         M   3    89.58  92.43     0
## 4    7         M   1    59.32  53.05     7
## 5    7         M   2    62.95  80.31     7
## 6    7         M   3    62.95  67.39     7

# Fitting a model with two nominal predictors
model1 <- lm(Conc ~ Herbicide * TimeF, data = dataset)

# Graphical analyses of residuals
plot(model1, which = 1)
plot(model1, which = 2)
boxcox(model1)

# Working with log-transformed concentrations
# Re-fitting a model with two nominal predictors
model <- lm(log(Conc) ~ Herbicide * TimeF, data = dataset)
```

As the original aim of this experiment was to study the entire degradation kinetics, a second model is fitted, where the response (log-transformed metamitron concentration values) is assumed to decrease linearly with time, by following different kinetics, depending on the presence of co-applied herbicides. This model is fitted by using the same coding as in Code Box 11.8 but replacing the nominal

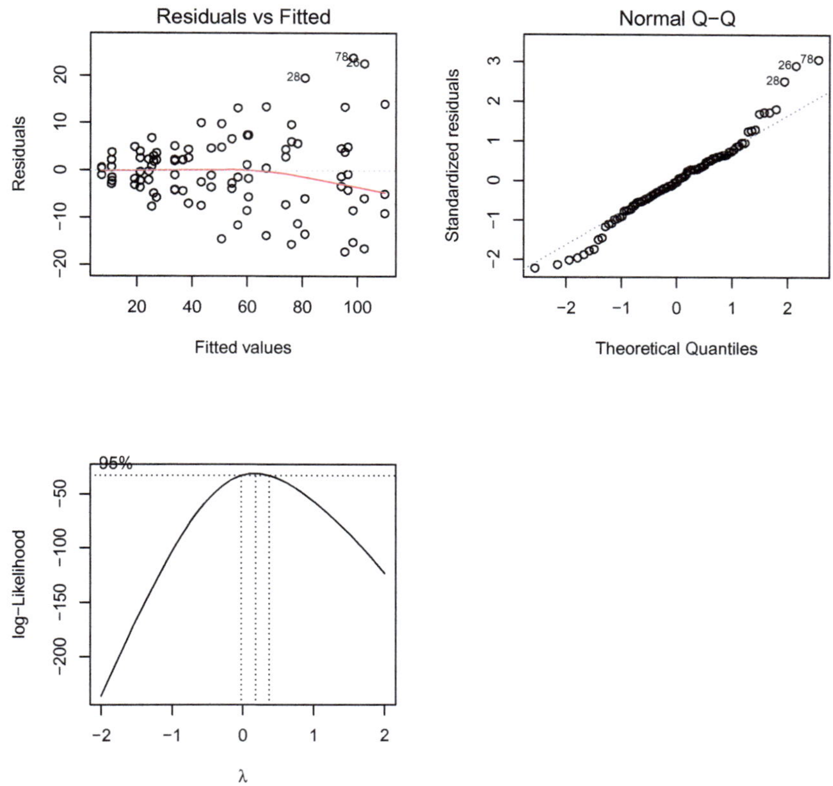

Fig. 11.2 Graphical analyses of residuals for the ANOVA model fitted to the untransformed data of Example 11.2 (top panels) and Box-Cox graph for the selection of the transformation parameter "lambda" (bottom panel)

variable "TimeF" with the original quantitative variable "Time." The estimated parameters in Code Box 11.9 represent, respectively, the intercept for the M herbicide, the differences between the intercepts for MC, MP, and MPC and the intercept for M, the slope of M, and the differences between the slopes for MC, MP, and MPC and the slope for M.

The F-test for lack-of-fit is not significant (P-value = 0.802), and thus, we conclude that the regression model provides a good description of the observed degradation kinetics. We can plot the observed and predicted concentrations against time using the `ggplot2` package, the `geom_smooth()` function (to draw the fitted lines), and the `facet_wrap()` function (to make separate panels for the herbicide treatments) (Code Box 11.9 and Fig. 11.3).

Code Box 11.9

```
# Example 11.2 [continuation]

# Fitting a regression model, with four straight lines
model.1 <- lm(log(Conc) ~ Herbicide * Time,
              data = dataset)
summary(model.1)
## Coefficients:
##                      Estimate Std. Error t value Pr(>|t|)
## (Intercept)          4.515911   0.057760  78.184  < 2e-16 ***
## HerbicideMC          0.024260   0.081685   0.297  0.76718
## HerbicideMP          0.114574   0.081685   1.403  0.16425
## HerbicideMPC         0.238786   0.081685   2.923  0.00440 **
## Time                -0.038617   0.001559 -24.778  < 2e-16 ***
## HerbicideMC:Time     0.015429   0.002204   7.000 4.84e-10 ***
## HerbicideMP:Time     0.006726   0.002204   3.051  0.00301 **
## HerbicideMPC:Time    0.015215   0.002204   6.903 7.54e-10 ***

# F-test for lack-of-fit
anova(model.1, model)
## Analysis of Variance Table
##
## Model 1: log(Conc) ~ Herbicide * Time
## Model 2: log(Conc) ~ Herbicide * TimeF
##   Res.Df    RSS Df Sum of Sq    F Pr(>F)
## 1     88 2.5057
## 2     64 1.9672 24    0.5385 0.73 0.8023

# Graph of model fits
library(ggplot2)
ggplot(data = dataset) +
  geom_point(mapping = aes(x = Time, y = log(Conc), col = Herbicide),
             show.legend = FALSE) +
  geom_smooth(mapping = aes(x = Time, y = log(Conc), col = Herbicide),
              method = "lm", se = FALSE, lwd = 0.5, show.legend = FALSE) +
  facet_wrap(~ Herbicide) +
  labs(x = "Time (days after treatment)", y = "Concentration [log(ng/g)]") +
  theme_bw()
```

At this stage, it may be relevant to derive the four intercepts and the four slopes using linear combinations of model parameters. It is also possible to compare both the intercepts and the slopes of the herbicide treatments with the corresponding parameter of metamitron alone. These linear combinations can be fitted by the `emmeans()` and `emtrends()` functions, as displayed in Code Box 11.10. However, it is necessary to remember that the data were log-transformed before analysis, and thus, the intercepts are expressed as logarithms (Fig. 11.3). Hence, it may be necessary to back-transform them to the original concentration scale.[1] Considering

[1] I have used `regrid = "response"` instead of `type = "response"` so that the back-transformation is performed before multiple comparison testing. This way, differences are

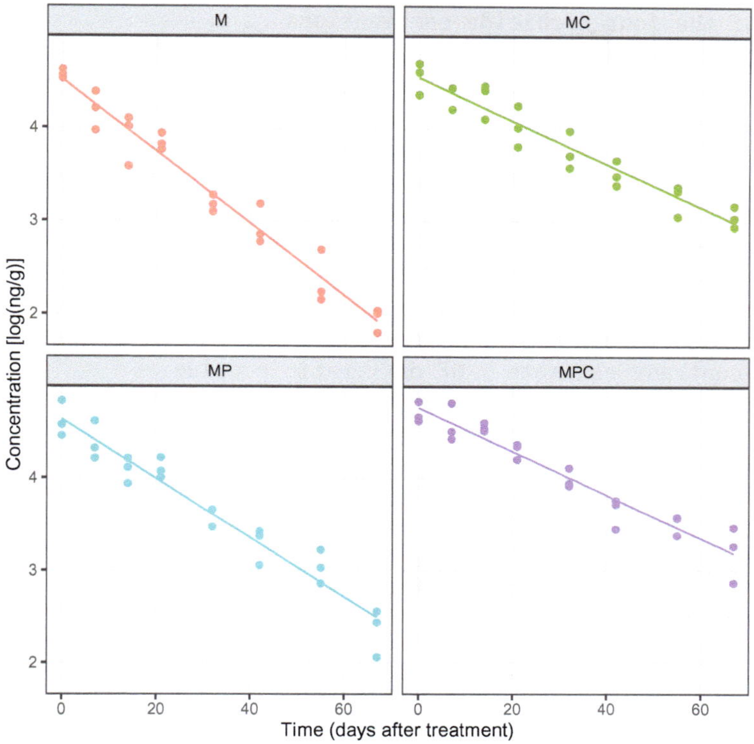

Fig. 11.3 Regression analysis for the data in Example 11.2: The symbols represent the observed concentrations (as logarithms) for the different herbicide combinations (see the text for further details), while the solid lines represent the fitted models

the results of data analyses, it is possible to conclude that the presence of all co-applied herbicides significantly increased the degradation rate of metamitron, as indicated by the absolute values of regression slopes. Otherwise, the intercept was significantly affected only for the MPC combination (Code Box 11.10).

Code Box 11.10

```
# Example 11.2 [continuation]

# Linear and nonlinear contrasts for the 'metamitron' data

# Deriving and comparing the back-transformed intercepts
```

---

calculated and tested on the concentration scale. This is not necessarily the best approach; see the vignettes for the emmeans package for further explanations.

```
# of the four herbicide combinations
intcp <- emmeans(model.1, ~Herbicide, at = c(Time = 0),
                 regrid = "response")
intcp
## Herbicide response   SE df lower.CL upper.CL
##  M               91.5 5.28 88     81.0      102
##  MC              93.7 5.41 88     83.0      104
##  MP             102.6 5.92 88     90.8      114
##  MPC            116.1 6.71 88    102.8      129
#
contrast(intcp, method = "dunnett")
## contrast estimate   SE df t.ratio p.value
##  MC - M       2.25 7.56 88   0.297  0.9642
##  MP - M      11.10 7.94 88   1.399  0.3702
##  MPC - M     24.67 8.54 88   2.889  0.0137 *

# Deriving and comparing the slopes (degradation rates) for
# the four herbicide combinations
slp <- emtrends(model.1, ~Herbicide, var="Time")
slp
## Herbicide Time.trend      SE df lower.CL upper.CL
##  M           -0.0386 0.00156 88  -0.0417  -0.0355
##  MC          -0.0232 0.00156 88  -0.0263  -0.0201
##  MP          -0.0319 0.00156 88  -0.0350  -0.0288
##  MPC         -0.0234 0.00156 88  -0.0265  -0.0203

contrast(slp, method = "dunnett")
## contrast estimate     SE df t.ratio p.value
##  MC - M   0.01543 0.0022 88   7.000  <.0001 ***
##  MP - M   0.00673 0.0022 88   3.051  0.0086 **
##  MPC - M  0.01522 0.0022 88   6.903  <.0001 ***
```

It is also relevant to calculate the half-life of metamitron alone and in the presence of co-applied herbicides (i.e., the time required for the concentration of metamitron to drop to 50% of the initial concentration). These values can be estimated by fitting four nonlinear combinations of model parameters in the form $T_{1/2_j} = \log(0.5)/b_j$, where b_j are the slopes for the different herbicide combinations (Code Box 11.12). With simple math, it is also possible to derive expressions to calculate the differences between the half-life of metamitron alone and those of metamitron in the presence of co-applied herbicide. t-tests (see Chap. 7) can be used to assess whether these differences are significant, as shown in Code Box 11.11.

Code Box 11.11

```
# Example 11.2 [continuation]

# Determining the half-lives of metamitron alone and
# in the three combinations

coefs <- coef(model.1)
nameParms = c("k1", "k2", "k3", "k4",
              "k5", "k6", "k7", "k8")
funList <- list(~log(0.5)/k5,
                ~log(0.5)/(k5 + k6),
                ~log(0.5)/(k5 + k7),
                ~log(0.5)/(k5 + k8))
halflf <- gnlht(model.1, func = funList,
                parameterNames = nameParms)
row.names(halflf) <- c("M", "MC", "MP", "MPC")
halflf[,-1]
##     Estimate        SE  t-value      p-value
## M   17.94951 0.7244276 24.77750 1.893736e-41
## MC  29.89266 2.0091805 14.87803 9.469304e-26
## MP  21.73499 1.0622066 20.46212 3.289632e-35
## MPC 29.61995 1.9726890 15.01501 5.296090e-26

# Differences between the half-lives
funList <- list(~ -k6*log(0.5)/(k5*(k5+k6)),
                ~ -k7*log(0.5)/(k5*(k5+k7)),
                ~ -k8*log(0.5)/(k5*(k5+k8)))
halfdf <- gnlht(model.1, func = funList,
                                 parameterNames = nameParms)
row.names(halfdf) <- c("MC - M", "MP - M", "MPC - M")
halfdf[,-1]
##          Estimate       SE  t-value      p-value
## MC - M  11.943149 2.135791 5.591910 2.491422e-07
## MP - M   3.785487 1.285721 2.944253 4.140136e-03
## MPC - M 11.670445 2.101499 5.553391 2.933644e-07
```

11.3 Example 11.3: Dose-Response Curves for an Herbicide Bioassay

With few changes, the same approach can be used with curvilinear equations that are nonlinear in the parameters (Draper and Smith 1998); first of all, the minimization of the residual sum of squares may have no closed-form solution, and, in this case, it is necessary to resort to numerical optimization methods (nonlinear least squares; Bates and Watts 1988). Two possible options in R are the `nls()` function in the `stats` package (R Development Core Team 2024) and the `drm()` function in the `drc` package (Ritz et al. 2019). In this book, the use of this latter function is proposed, as it has numerous service functions and methods tailored to the needs of agriculture research. For the interested readers, thorough information about `nls()` can be found in Ritz and Streibig (2008).

Apart from the use of a different fitting function, nonlinear regression, compared to linear regression, poses two additional difficulties: (i) selecting the most appropriate model for a given dataset and (ii) providing initial guesses for model parameters, as required by the optimization procedure. The selection of a model is typically made by using literature information or in a purely empirical fashion, i.e., examining at the shape of the response and selecting an equation that matches that shape. In this respect, Fig. 11.4 provides simple guidance for matching the shape of data and the nonlinear function; other helpful information can be found in Landsberg (1977), Ratkowsky (1990), and Miguez et al. (2018).

The second problem can be solved by using self-starting functions that do not require starting values for model parameters, as they contain algorithms for an automatic selection. A list of self-starters for the models in Fig. 11.4 is reported in Appendix B; these self-starters are available in the `statforbiology` and `drc` packages, while other self-starters can be found in the `MASS` package (Venables and Ripley 2002). Further information can also be found in several pages of the accompanying blog for this book.[2]

Let us consider an experiment where plants of *Tripleurospermum inodorum* were treated with a sulphonylurea herbicide (tribenuron-methyl) at a range of increasing doses, and the fresh weight of treated plants per pot was recorded 3 weeks after treatment. The experiment was completely randomized with three replicates, and it was carried out at the Department of Integrated Pest Management, University of Aarhus, Denmark (Pannacci et al. 2010). The results are available as `Tripleuspermum` in the `statforbiology` package.

For nonlinear regression models fitted with the `drm()` function, there is no need to start the analyses by transforming the "dose" into a nominal predictor, as the F-test for lack-of-fit is already incorporated in the `modelFit()` function (see later). Thus, we ignore this step and proceed to nonlinear regression model fitting.

[2] Go to https://www.statforbiology.com/tags/nonlinear_regression/.

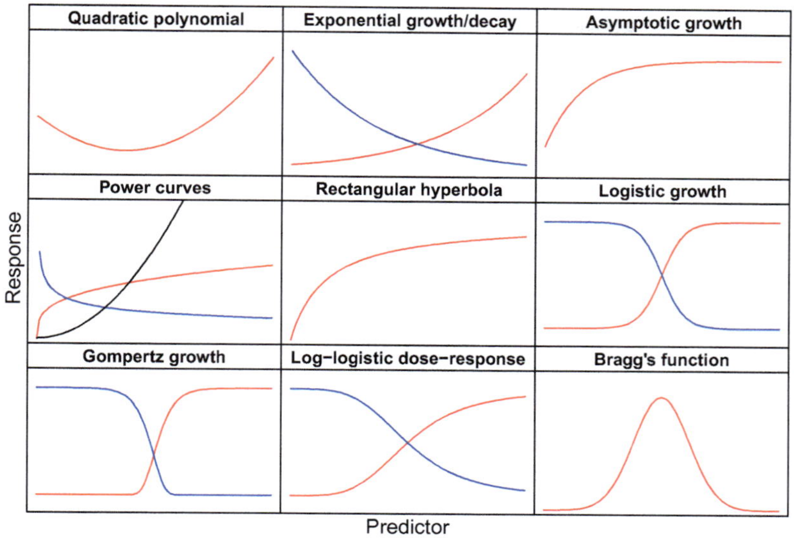

Fig. 11.4 Empirical selection of a model for nonlinear regression. The curves of different colors can be obtained by changing the values of certain model parameters (see Ratkowsky 1990). The equations for these (and other) models can be found, e.g., in Appendix B and on the accompanying website for this book

According to the literature information (Finney 1979; Streibig 1988), a good candidate model is the log-logistic equation:

$$Y_i = c + \frac{d - c}{1 + \exp\left\{b\left[\log\left(X_i\right) + \log\left(e\right)\right]\right\}} + \varepsilon_i \tag{11.5}$$

The corresponding curve has a sigmoidal shape (Fig. 11.4), and on a log-dose scale, it is symmetric around the inflection point. In this model, Y_i is the response for the ith individual, X_i is the herbicide dose with which that individual has been treated, c is the lower asymptote (the response at very high herbicide doses), d is the upper asymptote (response on the untreated control), b is the slope of the curve around the inflection point, while e is the dose giving a response half-way between c and d. As usual, the residuals ε_i are assumed to be Gaussian and homoscedastic.

Parameter estimates indicate that c has a large standard error and is not significantly different from 0; therefore, it is possible to remove it and refit the model (please note the shift from `LL.4()` to `LL.3()` in Code Box 11.12).

Code Box 11.12

```
# Example 11.3
# Dose response curve for a herbicide bioassay

# Loading the packages
library(statforbiology)

# Loading the data
dataset <- getAgroData("Tripleuspermum")
head(dataset)

##   Dose FreshWeight
## 1 0.00      115.83
## 2 0.00      102.90
## 3 0.00      114.35
## 4 0.25       91.60
## 5 0.25      103.23
## 6 0.25      133.97

# Fitting a log-logistic model
mod <- drm(FreshWeight ~ Dose, fct = LL.4(),
           data = dataset)
summary(mod)

## Parameter estimates:
##
##                  Estimate Std. Error t-value   p-value
## b:(Intercept)   3.97552    3.71014  1.0715 0.3068793
## c:(Intercept)  16.80741   21.34746  0.7873 0.4477233
## d:(Intercept) 110.53618    7.49870 14.7407 1.369e-08 ***
## e:(Intercept)   1.00496    0.17122  5.8696 0.0001078 ***

# Reducing the model
mod <- drm(FreshWeight ~ Dose, fct = LL.3(),
           data = dataset)
summary(mod)

## Parameter estimates:
##
##                  Estimate Std. Error t-value   p-value
## b:(Intercept)   2.69273    0.78369  3.4360  0.004931 **
## d:(Intercept) 112.31710    6.84338 16.4125 1.383e-09 ***
```

```
## e:(Intercept)    1.14902    0.14154  8.1181 3.235e-06 ***
#
# Test F for lack-of-fit
modelFit(mod)

## Lack-of-fit test
##
##           ModelDf    RSS Df F value p value
## ANOVA          10 3183.6
## DRC model      12 3258.3  2  0.1174  0.8904
```

Graphical analyses of residuals can be performed similarly to those for linear models but using different R functions. The `plotRes()` function in `statforbiology` produces a plot of residuals against fitted values and a QQ-plot of standardized residuals. Additionally, the `boxcox()` function generates the Box-Cox graph, which allows for the selection of the optimal λ value for the Box-Cox transformation (see Chap. 8). For the example under study, these graphs do not show any relevant deviations from the basic assumptions (not shown, for brevity).[3]

Code Box 11.13

```
# Example 11.3 [continuation]

# Graphical analyses of residuals and model fit
# in nonlinear regression

par(mfrow = c(1,3))
plotRes(mod, which = 1)
plotRes(mod, which = 2)
boxcox(mod)
```

The F-test for lack-of-fit is not significant (Code Box 11.12), and the graph of the observed responses against the predictor levels, augmented with model predictions, confirms that the log-logistic three-parameter model provides a good fit to this dataset (Fig. 11.5). We could produce this plot using the `plot()` method, although in Code Box 11.14 the `ggplot2` package is used, which is preferable for publication

[3] In the event that a transformation is necessary, it must be managed using the Transform-Both-Sides approach, which is discussed later in this section.

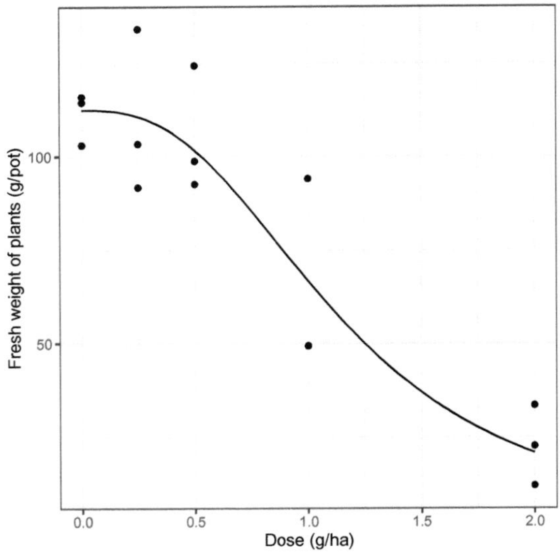

Fig. 11.5 Nonlinear regression analysis for the "Tripleuspermum" data. The symbols show the observed data, while the solid line shows the fitted model

purposes; the data for plotting can be retrieved from the `drc` object using the `getPlotData()` function in the `statforbiology` package.

Code Box 11.14

```
# Example 11.3 [continuation]

# Plotting the fitted model with ggplot()

library(ggplot2)
plotData <- getPlotData(mod, type = "all")

ggplot() +
  geom_point(data = plotData$plotPoints,  aes(x = Dose, y = FreshWeight)) +
  geom_line(data = plotData$plotFits,   aes(x = Dose, y = FreshWeight)) +
  labs(x = "Dose (g/ha)", y = "Fresh weight of plants (g/pot)") +
  theme_bw()
```

After having demonstrated that the fitted model provides a good description of the observed cause-effect relationship, we can use the model to retrieve some relevant information, such as the Effective Dose (ED) levels, i.e., the doses causing some particular level of damage on the test organisms (e.g., 50% or 90%; see Code Box 11.14), that are regarded as relevant indicators of phytotoxicity. These ED levels can be expressed as nonlinear combinations of model parameters and can be easily fitted using the `ED()` function in `drc`.

Code Box 11.15

```
# Example 11.3 [continuation]

# Retrieving the effective doses from model fit
ED(mod, respLev = c(50, 90))
##
## Estimated effective doses
##
##          Estimate Std. Error
## e:1:50   1.14902    0.14154
## e:1:90   2.59840    0.66311
```

Before concluding this brief introduction to nonlinear regression, it is worth mentioning a few issues with this method of data analysis. If the residuals do not appear to comply with the basic assumptions, transforming the response may not be an appropriate solution for regression models because it also alters the shape of the response (e.g., a linear response may become curvilinear when it is log-transformed). For this reason, transformations in both linear and nonlinear regression must be managed with the Transform-Both-Sides (TBS) approach, which consists of transforming both the response and the model (i.e., $Y^\lambda = [f(X)]^\lambda$). By doing so, parameter estimates retain their original measurement units. Such an approach is implemented in the `boxcox()` function for the `drc` object, which finds the optimal λ value and refits the model using the TBS approach with that optimal value. If you want to select the λ value by yourself, you can specify your selection through the `bcVal` argument in the `drm()` function call (see Ritz et al. 2019 for further detail). For example, in Code Box 11.6 the optimal λ value was 0.75, but I preferred to employ $\lambda = 0.5$, which is easier to understand.

Code Box 11.16

```
# Example 11.3 [continuation]

# Re-fitting the model after applying a TBS approach,
# with the optimal lambda value (selected by the function)
newMod <- boxcox(mod, plotit = F)
summary(newMod)
# Model fitted: Log-logistic (ED50 as parameter) with lower limit at 0
   (3 parms)
#
# Parameter estimates:
#
#                  Estimate Std. Error t-value   p-value
```

```
# b:(Intercept)   2.61202    0.64589  4.0441  0.001628 **
# d:(Intercept) 112.45184    7.48427 15.0251 3.813e-09 ***
# e:(Intercept)   1.13902    0.13732  8.2945 2.592e-06 ***
#
# Non-normality/heterogeneity adjustment through Box-Cox transformation
#
# Estimated lambda: 0.75
# Confidence interval for lambda: [0.142,1.437]


# Employing a user-defined lambda value (e.g., 0.5) for the TBS approach
newMod2 <- drm(FreshWeight ~ Dose, fct = LL.3(),
           data = dataset, bcVal = 0.5)
summary(newMod2)

# Model fitted: Log-logistic (ED50 as parameter) with lower limit at 0
 (3 parms)
#
# Parameter estimates:
#
#                Estimate Std. Error t-value   p-value
# b:(Intercept)   2.55753    0.57584  4.4414 0.0008049 ***
# d:(Intercept) 112.56858    8.49544 13.2505 1.591e-08 ***
# e:(Intercept)   1.12568    0.14136  7.9634 3.941e-06 ***
#
# Non-normality/heterogeneity adjustment through Box-Cox transformation
#
# Specified lambda: 0.5
```

A second issue relates to the possible presence of additional nominal factors apart from the quantitative predictor (similar to Example 11.1 or 11.2, but when the relationship between the quantitative predictor and the response is nonlinear). Treatment and grouping factors can be managed in `drm()` by using the `curveid` argument, as shown in Ritz et al. (2019). In practice, model parameters are allowed to take different values for each level of the specified factor. If necessary the `pmodels` argument can be used to specify which parameters should change between groups and which should remain constant across groups. Block effects, for example, can be accounted for by using this technique, as shown in the associated blog.[4]

Grouping factors in nonlinear regression can also be managed within the frame of mixed models, which will be discussed in the next chapter.

11.4 Exercises

1. An RCBD experiment was conducted to evaluate the effect of increasing densities of a weed (*Sinapis arvensis*) on sunflower yield (tons per hectare).

[4] Go to https://www.statforbiology.com/2020/stat_nlmm_designconstraints/.

The observed results are taken from Onofri and Tei (1994) and are presented in the table below. They are also available as “Sinapis” in the `statforbiology` package. Assuming that the yield response is linear, parameterize the model, check the goodness of fit, and find the economic threshold level of weed density (i.e., the weed density that causes a damage equal to the cost of weed control), taking into account that the yield is valued at 150 euros per ton, compared with a herbicide treatment cost of 40 euros per hectare.

Density	1	2	3	4
0	36.63	36.11	38.35	36.740
14	29.73	34.72	32.16	32.566
19	32.12	30.12	31.72	29.570
28	30.61	30.80	28.69	33.663
32	27.70	26.53	25.88	28.751
38	27.43	27.60	28.43	27.114
54	24.79	23.31	30.26	24.664

2. An experiment was conducted in a citrus grove in Sicily (Southern Italy) to determine the species-area relationship for the local weed community. In this study, a nested-plot survey was employed, where the number of weed species was counted in a 1 m^2 plot and the sampling area was progressively doubled, with the number of new weed species counted at each increment Muller-Dumbois and Ellenberg (1974). The data are taken from Cristaudo et al. (2015) and available as “citrusGrove” in the `statforbiology` package (see also the table below). Parameterize a power curve $Y = a\,X^b$, and check for lack-of-fit.

Area	Species
1	4
2	5
4	7
8	8
16	10
32	14
64	19
128	22
256	22

3. Crop growth can often be described by using a logistic growth model, with the form $Y = d/\{1 + \exp[-b(X - e)]\}$. The data reported in the table below refer to an experiment where sugar beet was grown either weed-free or weed-infested (Covarelli and Onofri 1998), and the weight of the crop per unit area (in kg/ha) was measured at six different timings (in Days After Emergence (DAE)). The

experiment was conducted by using a completely randomized design with three replicates, and the results are available as "beetGrowth" in the `statforbiology` package. Parameterize two logistic growth models (one for the weed-free crop and one for the infested crop), and, by way of t-tests, evaluate which of the parameters are significantly influenced by the competition.

DAE	Infested	WeedFree
21	6	7
21	6	8
21	11	7
27	20	34
27	20	40
27	21	25
38	213	232
38	303	172
38	127	122
49	613	1178
49	576	1362
49	778	1215
65	1705	3311
65	2248	2496
65	1266	3466
186	2151	3883
186	2626	2784
186	2768	3772

References

Bates DM, Watts DG (1988) Nonlinear Regression Analysis & Its Applications. Wiley, Hoboken

Covarelli G, Onofri A (1998) Effects of timing of weed removal and emergence in sugarbeet. In: Proceedings 6th EWRS Mediterranean Symposium, Montpellier, 13–15 May 1998, EWRS, pp 65–72

Cristaudo A, Restuccia A, Onofri A, Giudice VL, Gresta F (2015) Species-area relationships and minimum area in citrus grove weed communities. Plant Biosyst 149(2):337–345

Draper NR, Smith H (1998) Applied Regression Analysis. Some Chapters Are on Linear Models Shelf, 3rd edn. Wiley, Hoboken

Finney DJ (1979) Bioassay and the practice of statistical inference. Int Stat Rev 47:1–12

Landsberg JJ (1977) Some useful equations for biological studies. Exp Agricul 13:273–286

Miguez F, Archontoulis S, Dokoohaki H, Glaz B, Yeater KM (2018) Chapter 15: Nonlinear regression models and applications. In: ACSESS Publications, American Society of Agronomy, Crop Science Society of America, and Soil Science Society of America, Inc.. https://doi.org/10.2134/appliedstatistics.2016.0003. https://dl.sciencesocieties.org/publications/books/abstracts/acsesspublicati/appliedstatistics/401

Muller-Dumbois D, Ellenberg H (1974) Community sampling: the relevè method. In: Aims and methods of vegetation ecology. Species/Area curves: John Wiley & Sons, Inc, pp 45–66

Onofri A, Tei F (1994) Competitive ability and threshold levels for three broadleaf weed species in sunflower. Weed Res 34:471–479

Pannacci E, Mathiassen S, Kudsk P (2010) The effect of adjuvants on the rainfastness and performance of tribenuron-methyl on broadleaf weeds. Weed Biol Manag 10:126–131

R Development Core Team (2024) R: A Language and Environment for Statistical Computing. R Foundation for statistical Computing. http://www.R-project.org (ISBN 3-900051-00-3)

Ratkowsky DA (1990) Handbook of Nonlinear Regression Models. Dekker, New York City

Ritz C, Streibig JC (2008) Nonlinear Regression with R. Springer, New York

Ritz C, Jensen SM, Gerhard D, Streibig JC (2019) Dose-Response Analysis Using R. CRC Press, Boca Raton

Streibig JC (1988) Herbicide bioassay. Weed Res 28(28):479–484

Venables WN, Ripley BD (2002) Modern Applied Statistics with S. Statistics and Computing, 4th edn. Springer, New York

Vischetti C, Marini M, Businelli M, Onofri A (1996) The effect of temperature and co-applied herbicides on the degradation rate of phenmedipham, chloridazon and metamitron in a clay loam soil in the laboratory. In: Re AD, Capri E, Evans SP, Trevisan M (eds) The Environmental Fate of Xenobiotics, Proceedings X Symposium on Pesticide Chemistry, Piacenza, La Goliardica Pavese, Piacenza, pp 287–294

Chapter 12
A Brief Intro to Mixed Models

Mixed-effects models provide a powerful and flexible framework for analyzing data with multiple sources of variability, capturing both fixed effects of interest and random effects that represent individual differences

—D. Bates

Abstract Mixed models have recently become one of the most important classes of linear and nonlinear models. Although such a topic is too advanced to be treated in this introductory book, it seemed fundamental to mention how mixed models can be used to analyze data from several important types of experiments that are widely prevalent in agricultural research. Six real-life examples are presented, relating to a split-plot design, a strip-plot design, a genotype experiment with subsampling, a genotype experiment with random blocks, a multiyear genotype experiment, and a multiyear experiment with a perennial crop. For these case studies, the use of the `lme4` package is proposed, and the differences between fixed-effects model fitting and mixed model fitting are pointed out and discussed.

So far, this book has covered some of the so-called **fixed models**, containing only *fixed effects* and the residual random error term. Fixed effects relate to fixed factors that are identified by the following characteristics:

1. The levels are purposely selected (not sampled).
2. The levels are repeatable (we could make a new experiment with the very same levels).
3. The expected effects are deterministic and meaningfully expressed for each factor level as differences (increases or decreases) with respect to a baseline value.

Apart from fixed factors, models in agriculture and biology may require the inclusion of *random factors* that have the following characteristics:

A. Onofri, *Field Research Methods in Agriculture*,
https://doi.org/10.1007/978-3-032-08199-5_12

1. The levels are not interesting in themselves, but they are sampled from a broader population of possible levels.
2. The levels are not repeatable, in the sense that if the experiment is repeated, other levels might be selected with no loss of biological meaning.
3. The expected effects are random, and they change at each sampling effort.
4. The levels may represent randomization units that receive the allocation of treatment factors through a randomization process (e.g., the plots).

As a consequence of the previous items, the primary interest for random factors is not to estimate the effects of each level included in the experiment but to estimate the overall amount of variance (*variance component*) that they induce in the experimental response.

For example, in the case of the random element ε in all the models described earlier in this book, there is no interest in the exact value of each residual, since these values occur randomly and, when the experiment is repeated, different values will appear. Indeed, residuals are only determined to derive their variance, which is used for several purposes, such as in the denominator of F-ratios. Another example is when several fields are randomly selected within a macro-environment, and the same experiment is repeated in all fields. In this case, the "fields" are not specifically interesting, and they are sampled to quantify the variability of yield within the whole macro-environment.

The field factor in the previous example would be an example of a so-called grouping factor (see Chap. 2); other examples include the blocks in randomized complete block designs, the rows and columns in Latin square designs, and the main-plots in split-plot designs. All these grouping factors often create problems because they are rarely interesting in themselves, and thus, they are sometimes forgotten at the stage of data analysis. Neglecting the grouping factors is a wrong practice because their effects remain in the residuals. Consequently, the residuals belonging to the same group will share the same group effect and will be more similar to one another than those belonging to different groups. In other words, residuals will be correlated (*intra-class correlation*), which will break the independence assumption (see Chap. 8) and invalidate all inferences and hypothesis testing.

Provided that the grouping factors need to be included in the model, the question is do we need to regard blocking factors as fixed or random? In most cases, the decision is up to the researcher, who should give convincing reasons to support that; in other cases, as mentioned earlier, a **blocking factor needs to be random, i.e., whenever its levels become randomization units and receive the allocation of the levels of a factor or a combination of factors, by way of a randomization process** (Piepho et al. 2003). Consider the following examples:

1. In an RCBD the blocks group the plots based on their positioning along a fertility gradient; however, they are not randomization units in the sense that the treatment levels are allocated to the plots within each block, not to the blocks themselves. Consequently, the block factor can be regarded as random or fixed, depending on the circumstances.

2. In a split-plot design, main-plots group several subplots, but they are also randomization units because they receive the allocation of the levels of the main factor. Consequently, the main-plot factor must be random.

The reason why main-plots and other randomization units need to be regarded as random factors relates to their role in the experiment: According to Ronald Fisher, the difference between the experimental units treated alike is the most appropriate measure of experimental error. Consequently, the difference between, e.g., main-plots treated alike can be regarded as a measure of experimental error, implying that the main-plot effect is, indeed, random.

Considering the previous premises, it follows that several common experiments in agriculture, such as split-plot, strip-plot, repeated measures, and subsampling designs, contain grouping factors and may need the inclusion of random effects in the model, in addition to the residual error term. Models that contain more than one random term along with fixed terms and the residual error term are named **mixed models**. Since the 1980s, they have become a very widespread class of models.

Providing details about mixed models is far beyond the scope of this book, and interested readers are referred to the book by Gałecki and Burzykowski (2013). For all other readers, the following real-life examples demonstrate how mixed models can be applied to analyze data from split-plot, strip-plot, and other common types of experiments in agricultural research.

12.1 Example 12.1: A Split-Plot Tillage Experiment

This experiment has already been presented in Chap. 2 as an example of split-plot design (Bianchi, unpublished data); three types of tillage (minimum tillage = MIN, shallow plowing = SP, and deep plowing = DP) and two types of chemical weed control methods (broadcast = TOT and in-furrow = PART) were compared in four complete blocks with three main-plots per block, split into two subplots per main-plot; the three types of tillage were randomly allocated to the main-plots in each block, while the two weed control treatments were randomly allocated to the subplots within each main-plot (see Fig. 2.9). The results of this experiment are available as "beet," in the `statforbiology` package.

This experiment contains two blocking factors (the blocks and the main-plots within each block), and both should be included in the model. A suitable option is

$$Y_{ijk} = \mu + \gamma_k + \alpha_i + \theta_{ik} + \beta_j + \alpha\beta_{ij} + \varepsilon_{ijk} \tag{12.1}$$

In this model, γ_k is the effect of the kth block, α_i is the effect of the ith tillage, β_j is the effect of the jth weed control method, $\alpha\beta_{ij}$ is the interaction between the ith tillage method and jth weed control method, and θ_{ki} is the effect of the main-plot identified by the kth block and the ith tillage method (see Fig. 2.9). The main-plots can be labeled in any other way as long as each one is uniquely identified.

Finally, ε_{ijk} is the subplot residual error, assumed as Gaussian with a mean of 0 and a standard deviation of σ.

The block factor does not reference any randomization units, and its effect could be regarded as either fixed or random. We will consider as fixed, as we have done so far in this book (but see later). Otherwise, the main-plots are randomization units, and their effects must be regarded as random with a mean of 0 and a standard deviation of σ_θ.

Fitting a mixed model in R is not very different from fitting a fixed-effects model. First, we need to create a new variable to uniquely identify the main-plots, which can be done either by using numeric coding or, more easily, by creating a new factor that combines the levels of block and tillage, as mentioned earlier (Code Box 12.1). Afterward, model fitting requires one of the R functions for mixed models; in this book, the `lmer()` function in the `lme4` package is proposed (Bates et al. 2015), and the `lmerTest` package (Kuznetsova et al. 2017) is also recommended to improve the readability of the ANOVA table.

The syntax of the `lmer()` function is similar to that of the `lm()` function. The random main-plot effect is entered by using the `1|` operator, and it is put in brackets, in order to better distinguish it from fixed effects (Code Box 12.1). In this chapter, the use of the "pipe" operator (`|>`) is also introduced to write clearer code. Such an operator "takes" the value returned by the previous function and passes it to the succeeding function as the first argument (Code Box 12.1; see also Appendix A.15).

Code Box 12.1

```
# Example 12.1
# A split-plot tillage experiment

# Loading the packages
library(statforbiology)
library(lme4)
library(lmerTest)

# Loading and transforming the data
dataset <- getAgroData("beet") |>
  transform(Tillage = factor(Tillage),
            WeedControl = factor(WeedControl),
            Block = factor(Block),
            mainPlot = factor(Block):factor(Tillage))

# Mixed-Model fitting
mod.split <- lmer(Yield ~ Block + Tillage * WeedControl +
                  (1|mainPlot), data=dataset)
```

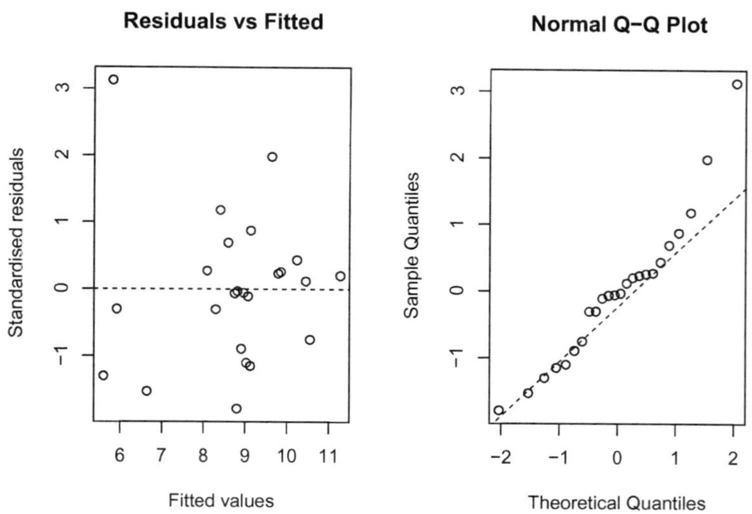

Fig. 12.1 Graphical analyses of residuals for the split-plot experiment in Example 12.1, where model fitting was performed with the `lmer()` function

Similar to all other models, mixed models must be inspected for their basic assumptions. When the `lmer()` function is used for fitting, the `plot()` method only returns the plot of "residuals against expected values," while the "which" argument does not work. Therefore, a QQ-plot should be produced using the generic `qqnorm()` and `qqline()` functions (Code Box 12.2). These two graphs exhibit some slight deviations from normality and homoscedasticity, which may be attributed to a few outlying observations (Fig. 12.1). However, the Shapiro-Wilk test does not seem to raise any particular concerns, and we can proceed to variance partitioning.

Code Box 12.2

```
# Example 12.1 [continuation]

# Check for the basic assumptions for the 'beet' data

# Graphical analyses
plot(mod.split) # Analogous to 'which = 1' for linear models
qqnorm(resid(mod.split)) # QQ-plot
qqline(resid(mod.split), lty = 2)

# Shapiro-Wilk's test
shapiro.test(residuals(mod.split))
```

```
#   Shapiro-Wilk normality test
#
# data:  residuals(mod.split)
# W = 0.93838, p-value = 0.1501
```

With `lmer()`, the `fixef()` function must be used in place of the `coef()` function to retrieve the estimated parameters. Variance partitioning can be produced by the usual `anova()` function, although it is necessary to select a method to approximate the degrees of freedom, which are not as easy to calculate as in linear models. We suggest the use of the "Kenward-Roger" approximation, which is usually recognized as more reliable than the default "Sattertwhaite" approximation (Kuznetsova et al. 2017).

Code Box 12.3

```
# Example 12.1 [continuation]

# Variance partitioning for the 'beet' data

anova(mod.split, ddf = "Kenward-Roger")
## Type III Analysis of Variance Table with Kenward-Roger's method
##                      Sum Sq Mean Sq NumDF DenDF F value  Pr(>F)
## Block                3.6596  1.2199     3     6  0.6521  0.610
## Tillage             23.6565 11.8282     2     6  6.3228  0.033 *
## WeedControl          3.3205  3.3205     1     9  1.7750  0.216
## Tillage:WeedControl 19.4641  9.7321     2     9  5.2023  0.032 *
```

The interaction between tillage and weed control is significant; thus, we can explore the means for the combinations, using the usual `emmeans()` function, which is left as an exercise.

12.2 Example 12.2: A Strip-Plot Recropping Experiment

A two-factor factorial experiment to determine the recropping interval for a sulphonylurea herbicide was described in Chap. 2. Rimsulfuron was applied at the recommended rate on bare soil, and untreated plots were included for comparison. Forty days after the treatment, sugar beet, rape and soybean were sown on treated and untreated plots, and the weight of the plants was determined 4 weeks after sowing. The experiment was laid out as a strip-plot in complete blocks (Fig. 2.10); in each block, the herbicide treatments (rimsulfuron and the untreated control) were randomly allocated to each of the two columns, while the three crops were randomly allocated to each of the three rows (Onofri, unpublished data). The dataset for this experiment, with four replicates, is available as “recropS” in the `statforbiology` package.

In this experiment, there are three blocking factors:

1. The blocks
2. The rows within each block (three rows per block)
3. The columns within each block (two columns per block)

The rows and columns are also randomization units, as they received the experimental treatments through a randomization process, analogous to the main-plots in Example 12.1.

Data analyses begin by loading the data and transforming all explanatory variables into factors. Two new variables need to be created to reference the randomization units. We can do so, considering that each row is uniquely identified by one specific crop and one specific block, while each column is uniquely identified by one specific herbicide and one specific block (see Code Box 12.4).

Code Box 12.4

```
# Example 12.2
# A strip-plot recropping experiment

# Loading packages
library(statforbiology)
library(lme4)
library(lmerTest)

# Loading and transforming the data
dataset <- getAgroData("recropS") |>
  transform(Herbicide = factor(Herbicide),
            Crop = factor(Crop),
            Block = factor(Block),
            Rows = factor(Crop):factor(Block),
            Columns = factor(Herbicide):factor(Block))
```

A good candidate model for this dataset is

$$Y_{ijk} = \mu + \gamma_k + \alpha_i + \theta_{ik} + \beta_j + \zeta_{jk} + \alpha\beta_{ij} + \varepsilon_{ijk}$$

In this model, μ is the intercept, γ_k are the block effects, α_i are the crop effects, θ_{ik} are the row effects, β_j are the herbicide effects, ζ_{jk} are the column effects, $\alpha\beta_{ij}$

are the "crop by herbicide" interaction effects, and ε_{ijk} are the residual random error terms. The block effect is regarded as fixed (although it could also be considered random), while the row and column effects need to be regarded as random, because the rows and the columns are randomization units. The three random effects (row, column, and residual term) are assumed to be Gaussian, with means of zero and standard deviations of, respectively, σ_θ, σ_ζ, and σ.

Model fitting is illustrated in Code Box 12.5, while model checking can be performed as in the previous example and is left as an exercise. The ANOVA table shows that only the crop effect is significant, while there is no difference between herbicide treatments (treated vs. untreated) within each crop. Thus, phytotoxic effects can be regarded as insignificant.

Code Box 12.5

```
# Example 12.2 [continuation]

# Model fitting

mod.strip <- lmer(CropBiomass ~ Block + Herbicide*Crop +
    (1|Rows) + (1|Columns), data = dataset)

# Variance partitioning
anova(mod.strip, ddf = "Kenward-Roger")
## Type III Analysis of Variance Table with Kenward-Roger's
method
##                 Sum Sq Mean Sq NumDF  DenDF F value  Pr(>F)
## Block            21451  7150.3     3 4.1367  2.5076 0.19387
## Herbicide          148   147.9     1 3.0000  0.0519 0.83450
## Crop             43874 21936.9     2 6.0000  7.6932 0.02208*
## Herbicide:Crop   12549  6274.4     2 6.0000  2.2004 0.19198
```

12.3 Example 12.3: A Genotype Experiment with Random Blocks

Let us reconsider Example 10.1, which describes a field experiment comparing eight winter wheat genotypes laid out in three complete blocks in the hills of central Italy in 2002 (Belocchi et al. 2003). Although the blocks do not represent randomization units, it is sometimes suggested that they are regarded as random. This practice is appropriate for recovering the inter-block information with incomplete block designs (Dixon 2016), and thus, it is not convenient in this case since the experiment is in complete blocks, and there is no inter-block information to recover. However, it might be helpful to show the R code for fitting a model with random blocks, as an example for the cases where the recovery of inter-block information may be required (Code Box 12.6).

Code Box 12.6

```
# Example 12.3
# A genotype experiment with random blocks

# Loading the packages
library(statforbiology)
library(lme4)
library(emmeans)
library(multcomp)

# Loading and transforming the data
dataset <- getAgroData("WinterWheat2002") |>
  transform(Block = factor(Block),
            Genotype = factor(Genotype))

# Model fitting (with random blocks)
modmix <- lmer(Yield ~ (1|Block) + Genotype, data = dataset)
meds <- emmeans(modmix, ~Genotype)
cld(meds, Letters = LETTERS, reverse = T)
## Genotype emmean    SE   df lower.CL upper.CL .group
##  IRIDE      4.96 0.216 10.8     4.49     5.44  A
##  COLOSSEO   4.89 0.216 10.8     4.42     5.37  A
##  SOLEX      4.79 0.216 10.8     4.31     5.27  A
##  SANCARLO   4.50 0.216 10.8     4.03     4.98  A
##  GRAZIA     4.34 0.216 10.8     3.86     4.82  A
##  CRESO      4.33 0.216 10.8     3.85     4.80  A
##  DUILIO     4.24 0.216 10.8     3.76     4.72  AB
##  SIMETO     3.34 0.216 10.8     2.86     3.82   B
```

12.4 Example 12.4: An RCBD with Subsampling

Subsampling may occur in field experiments whenever several random samples or multiple random measurements are taken in each plot. These subsamples cannot be regarded as true replicates because they received the experimental treatment altogether, and consequently, they are not independent (they are sub-replicates).

Let us consider the "TKW" data resulting from an experiment with 30 genotypes in three blocks, where the thousand kernel weight (TKW) was recorded in three subsamples of grain yield per plot (Ciriciofolo, unpublished data). The dataset is available in the `statforbiology` package.

Upon loading the data, the predictors need to be transformed into factors ("Genotype," "Block," and "Plot"); please note that this dataset includes the "Plot" variable that uniquely identifies all plots and acts as a grouping factor for the three subsamples within each plot. For comparison, a "naive" model is fitted in Code Box 12.7, which makes no distinction between true replicates and sub-replicates. Consequently, this analysis wrongly regards the design as a randomized complete block with nine replicates. The root mean square error is 2.71, the F-test for the genotypes is highly significant, and there are 225 significant pairwise comparisons among the 30 genotypes.

Code Box 12.7

```
# Example 12.4
# A RCBD with sub-sampling

# Loading the packages
library(statforbiology)
library(nlme)
library(car)
library(emmeans)
library(lme4)
library(lmerTest)

# Loading and transforming the data
TKW <- getAgroData("TKW") |>
  transform(Plot = factor(Plot),
            Block = factor(Block),
            Genotype = factor(Genotype))
head(TKW)
##   Plot Block  Genotype Sample  TKW
## 1    1     1 Meridiano      1 28.6
## 2    2     1     Solex      1 33.3
## 3    3     1  Liberdur      1 22.3
## 4    4     1  Virgilio      1 28.1
## 5    5     1   PR22D40      1 26.7
## 6    6     1    Ciccio      1 34.2

# WRONG ANALYSIS!!!!
# no distinction is made between true replicates and
  sub-replicates
```

```
# Fitting a 'naive' model
mod <- lm(TKW ~ Block + Genotype, data=TKW)
anova(mod)
## Analysis of Variance Table
##
## Response: TKW
##            Df Sum Sq Mean Sq F value    Pr(>F)
## Block       2  110.3  55.169   7.510 0.0006875 ***
## Genotype   29 7224.7 249.129  33.913 < 2.2e-16 ***
## Residuals 238 1748.4   7.346

# Residual standard deviation
summary(mod)$sigma
## [1] 2.710373

# Number of significant pairwise comparisons between genotype
  means
pairwise <- as.data.frame(pairs(emmeans(mod, ~Genotype)))
sum(pairwise$p.value < 0.05)
## [1] 225
```

The analysis in Code Box 12.7 is straightforward and tempting, but it breaks the basic assumption of independent residuals. Indeed, the residuals in the same plot are more alike than the residuals in different plots because they share the same "origin." Furthermore, the degree of precision is too high: The three subsamples are correlated, and they do not contribute three whole pieces of information.

A correct model must make the distinction between replicates and sub-replicates by including an extra term for the plots, which are the "grouping" units:

$$Y_{ijs} = \mu + \alpha_i + \gamma_j + \delta_{ij} + \varepsilon_{ijs} \quad (12.2)$$

In this model, Y_{ijs} is the thousand kernel weight for the ith genotype, jth block, kth plot, and sth subsample, α_i is the effect of the ith genotype, γ_j is the effect of the jth block, δ_{ij} is the effect of the plot identified by the ith genotype and jth block, and ε_{ijs} is the effect of the sth subsample, in the plot identified as previously mentioned. The presence of the δ element accounts for the plot-to-plot differences, thereby restoring the independence of model residuals.

The difference between plots (for a given genotype and block) must be regarded as purely random, as well as the difference between subplots within each plot. Consequently, this is a mixed model: The two variance components are σ_δ^2 and σ^2, and the latter is smaller, as it does not account for some relevant sources of experimental error, such as the variability due to the soil or cropping practices. The first component should be given the proper weight when building the correct error term to test for the genotypes.

This mixed model can be fitted by using the `lmer()` function in the `lme4` package (Code Box 12.8). The check for basic assumptions does not reveal any possible deviations; therefore, the variance components and the ANOVA table can be displayed. It is confirmed that the genotype effect is significant. However, the SEMs are higher than those obtained with the previous naive analysis (1.75 vs. 0.903), and the number of significant comparisons has decreased to 91. For the sake of brevity, the graphs of model residuals and the full results of pairwise comparisons are omitted.

Code Box 12.8

```
# Example 12.4 [continuation]

# CORRECT ANALYSES!!!
# True replicates and sub-replicates are parted


# Fitting a mixed model with the random 'plot' term
mod.mix <- lmer(TKW ~ Block + Genotype + (1|Plot), data=TKW)

# Check for basic assumptions
plot(mod.mix)
qqnorm(resid(mod.mix)) # QQ-plot
qqline(resid(mod.mix), lty = 2)

leveneTest(lm(residuals(mod.mix) ~ Genotype, data=TKW))
## Levene's Test for Homogeneity of Variance
   (center = median)
##        Df F value Pr(>F)
## group  29  1.0143 0.4507
##       240

shapiro.test(residuals(mod.mix))
##
##  Shapiro-Wilk normality test
##
## data:  residuals(mod.mix)
## W = 0.99277, p-value = 0.2141

# Printing the variance components
print(VarCorr(mod.mix), comp = "Variance")
##  Groups   Name        Variance
```

```
## Plot      (Intercept) 8.89201
## Residual              0.84526

# Variance partitioning
anova(mod.mix, ddf = "Kenward-Roger")
## Type III Analysis of Variance Table with Kenward-Roger's
   method
##            Sum Sq Mean Sq NumDF DenDF F value    Pr(>F)
## Block       3.389  1.6944     2    58  2.0046    0.1439
## Genotype 221.892  7.6515    29    58  9.0522 9.944e-13 ***

# Number of significant pairwise comparisons between genotype
  means
pairwise <- as.data.frame(pairs(emmeans(mod.mix, ~Genotype)))
sum(pairwise$p.value < 0.05)
## [1] 91
```

The method of data analysis in Code Box 12.8 is strongly recommended. However, when the number of subsamples is the same for all plots, correct results can also be obtained by a two-step analysis: In the first step, the means of subsamples for each plot is calculated, and, in the second step, these means are submitted to model fitting, by considering the genotype and the block as fixed factors. Code Box 12.9 shows that two-step fitting yields the same results without the need for a mixed model software.

Code Box 12.9

```
# Example 12.4 [continuation]

# Fitting in two-steps without a mixed model
# Only correct when the number of sub-samples is the
# same for all plots!

# First step
TKWm <- aggregate(TKW ~ Block + Genotype, data = TKW, mean)

# Second step
mod2step <- lm(TKW ~ Genotype + Block, data = TKWm)
anova(mod2step)
## Analysis of Variance Table
##
## Response: TKW
```

```
##              Df  Sum Sq Mean Sq F value    Pr(>F)    
## Genotype     29 2408.24  83.043  9.0522 9.943e-13 ***
## Block         2   36.78  18.390  2.0046    0.1439    
## Residuals    58  532.08   9.174                      
```

12.5 Example 12.5: A Multiyear Winter Wheat Experiment

The importance of repeating experiments has already been mentioned in Sect. 10.5. For genotype trials, multiyear or multisite experiments are widespread and often involve a wide range of research units across countries or continents. These research units typically employ a common core of genotypes and the same experimental design (e.g., randomized complete blocks with 3–4 replicates), while innovative genotypes are progressively introduced each year, and the old ones are abandoned (Annichiarico 2002).

Let us consider a field experiment to compare eight winter wheat genotypes laid out in complete blocks with three replicates. The experiment was repeated in 7 years to provide varietal recommendations for farmers. The results are taken from Onofri and Ciriciofolo (2007) and are available as "WinterWheat" in the `statforbiology` package.

A suitable model for this dataset is

$$y_{ijk} = \mu + \gamma_{ik} + \alpha_i + \beta_j + \alpha\beta_{ij} + \varepsilon_{ijk} \tag{12.3}$$

In this equation, y is the response for the ith year, jth treatment level, and kth replicate, μ is the intercept, γ_{ik} is the effect of the kth block in the ith year, α_i is the effect of the ith year, β_j is the effect of the jth genotype, $\alpha\beta_{ij}$ is the "genotype x year" interaction effect, and ε_{ijk} is the residual random effect for each observation, which we assume to be Gaussian and homoscedastic [$\epsilon_{ijk} \sim N(0, \sigma_\varepsilon)$].

What is peculiar about experiments repeated over several years, locations, environments, or more generally, runs is that it is necessary to decide the nature of the "run" effect, whether it is "fixed" or "random." Such a decision is specific to each experiment, and it is up to the researcher, who should provide solid reasons to support it. As a rule of thumb, the following suggestions can be made:

1. Whenever the experiment is repeated in a small number of "runs" (e.g., 2 or 3), the "run" effect could be preferably taken as fixed, as in Example 10.5; indeed, a reliable estimation of variance components requires that the number of levels for the random factor is sufficiently high (at least 4, approximately).
2. With field experiments repeated in a relatively high number of years, this latter effect could be reasonably considered as random for, at least, one good reason: Although the years are not sampled (we cannot sample years, and we can only

take them in the same order as they come), the effects they produce are not repeatable and thus random.

3. With field experiments repeated in a relatively high number of locations, the nature of this latter effect is more dubious. In some cases, locations are fixed because they are intentionally selected and represent an element of interest in themselves. In other instances, the locations are randomly selected to represent a macro-environment.

When the "run" effect is taken as random, "runs" become a sort of "iper-replicates" defining an additional source of variability. In practice, the yield changes from run to run and from plot to plot within each run. Parting these two sources of variability is relevant for, e.g., breeding purposes.

In the "WinterWheat" data, the number of years is relatively high; considering that the year effect is intrinsically random and unrepeatable, it would make no sense to condition the varietal recommendation on specific years; thus, the year effect can be assumed to be random and Gaussian, with a mean of 0 and a standard deviation of σ_E:

$$\alpha_i \sim N(0, \sigma_E) \tag{12.4}$$

The corresponding variance (σ_E^2) is referred to as the "variance component" for the year effect. If the year is random, also, the "genotype x year" and "block within year" effects are random, and they are defined as

$$\alpha\beta_{ij} \sim N(0, \sigma_{GE}) \tag{12.5}$$

$$\gamma_{ik} \sim N(0, \sigma_{EB}) \tag{12.6}$$

The analysis is displayed in Code Box 12.10. Once the dataset is loaded and the necessary transformations are performed (i.e., the "Block," "Year," and "Genotype" variables are transformed into factors), a careful EDA is in order, implying a thorough examination of each single experiment, to make sure that the data from all years are good, and the variances of within-year residuals are in comparable scale (see also Example 10.5). In Code Box 12.10, formal tests of homoscedasticity and normality do not reveal any significance, while graphical analyses of residuals for each year are omitted for brevity.

Code Box 12.10

```
# Example 12.5
# A multi-year winter wheat experiment

# Loading the packages
library(statforbiology)
library(nlme)
```

```
library(car)
library(emmeans)
library(multcomp)
library(lme4)
library(lmerTest)
library(SuppDists)

# Loading and transforming the data
WinterWheat <- getAgroData("WinterWheat") |>
  transform(Block = factor(Block),
            Year = factor(Year),
            Genotype = factor(Genotype))

# Model fitting for each year
fits <- by(WinterWheat, WinterWheat$Year,
   function(group) lm(Yield ~ Block + Genotype,
                      data = group))

# Levene's test for each year: fit a reduced model with
# only the Genotype in each year and use the 'leveneTest' function
# Levene's test for each year: fit a reduced model with
# only the Genotype in each year and use the 'leveneTest' function
fits2 <- by(WinterWheat, WinterWheat$Year,
   function(group) leveneTest(residuals(lm(Yield ~ Block + Genotype,
                      data = group)) ~ Genotype, data = group ))
lev.test <- unlist( lapply(fits2, function(mod) mod$`Pr(>F)`[1] ))
lev.test
##    1996    1997    1998    1999    2000    2001    2002
## 0.96062 0.92277 0.82724 0.76156 0.94008 0.88759 0.73620

# Shapiro-Wilks' test for each year
norm.tests <- unlist( lapply(fits, function(mod)
  shapiro.test(residuals(mod))$p.value ))
norm.tests
##     1996      1997     1998      1999      2000      2001      2002
## 0.432388 0.2436310.701038 0.988207 0.857077 0.469858 0.033229

# Retrieve the residual variance for each year
mses <- unlist( lapply(fits, function(mod) summary(mod)$sigma^2) )
mses
##     1996     1997     1998     1999     2000     2001     2002
## 0.161781 0.201840 0.071983 0.101168 0.126209 0.275060 0.103586

# Hartley's Fmax test
Fmax <- max(mses)/min(mses)
pmaxFratio(Fmax, 15, 7, lower.tail = F)
## [1] 0.1573404
```

Before fitting a mixed model, it may be a good idea to fit a fixed model (Code Box 12.11) for a preliminary evaluation of residuals and to compare the results with those of a mixed model fit.

Code Box 12.11

```
# Example 12.5 [continuation]

# Pooled analyses: fitting a preliminary fixed model
modfix <- lm(sqrt(Yield) ~ Year/Block + Genotype * Year,
             data = WinterWheat)

# Checking the residuals
plot(modfix, which= 1)
plot(modfix, which = 2)
boxcox(modfix)

# No problems with the assumptions, thus proceed to ANOVA
anova(modfix)
## Analysis of Variance Table
##
## Response: sqrt(Yield)
##               Df Sum Sq Mean Sq  F value    Pr(>F)
## Year           6 6.8527 1.14212 192.5546 < 2.2e-16 ***
## Genotype       7 0.4760 0.06799  11.4633 1.488e-10 ***
## Year:Block    14 0.1657 0.01183   1.9949   0.02568 *
## Year:Genotype 42 1.1627 0.02768   4.6671 1.804e-10 ***
## Residuals     98 0.5813 0.00593
```

The previous box confirms that there are no problems with heteroscedastic and non-normal residuals, and the ANOVA table shows that the “genotype by year” interaction is significant, which would only permit year-specific (and, thus, rather useless) varietal recommendations. On the contrary, recommendations for a specific site should be made across the entire range of weather conditions that might occur.

Thus, we fit a mixed model with random years using the `lmer()` function; the variance components are estimated by the REstricted Maximum Likelihood (REML) method (Pinheiro and Bates 2000), and they can be displayed using the `VarCorr()` function (Code Box 12.12).

These variance components show that the overall yield variability is mainly due to the year effect (year to year variability: $\sigma_E^2 = 1.07$), followed by the genotype by year interaction ($\sigma_{GE}^2 = 0.170$), by the within-year plot-to-plot variability (residual error term $\sigma^2 = 0.149$) and, finally, by the block to block variability within years ($\sigma_{EB}^2 = 0.016$). These components are used to build F-tests and standard errors.

Code Box 12.12

```
# Example 12.5 [continuation]

# Pooled analyses: fitting a mixed model with random years
modmix <- lmer(Yield ~ (1|Year) + (1|Year:Block) + Genotype +
                 (1|Year:Genotype),
               data = WinterWheat)

# Variance components
print( VarCorr(modmix), comp=c("Variance", "Std.Dev.") )
##  Groups        Name        Variance Std.Dev.
##  Year:Genotype (Intercept) 0.170341 0.41272
##  Year:Block    (Intercept) 0.016418 0.12813
##  Year          (Intercept) 1.073146 1.03593
##  Residual                  0.148804 0.38575

# ANOVA table
anova(modmix, ddf = "Kenward-Roger")
## Type III Analysis of Variance Table with Kenward-Roger's
   method
##          Sum Sq Mean Sq NumDF DenDF F value  Pr(>F)
## Genotype 2.6033  0.3719     7    42  2.4993 0.03058 *
```

The ANOVA table indicates that the F-ratio remains significant, although it is smaller than that of the fixed model fit. Indeed, in the denominator, apart from the residual error term, it is also necessary to consider the specific variability of each genotype across years (Annichiarico 2002).

Finally, the overall means of genotypes are derived and compared, but no significant differences between genotypes are evidenced. Indeed, mixed models permit to consider all possible sources of yield variability (within years and across years), allowing inferences across the entire population of possible years (broad-space inference).

Code Box 12.13

```
# Example 12.5 [continuation]

# Multiple comparisons for a mixed model with random years
cld(emmeans(modmix, ~Genotype), Letters = letters)
##  Genotype emmean    SE   df lower.CL upper.CL .group
```

```
## SIMETO      5.93 0.431 8.23     4.94     6.91  a
## CRESO       5.97 0.431 8.23     4.99     6.96  a
## GRAZIA      6.08 0.431 8.23     5.09     7.07  a
## SANCARLO    6.22 0.431 8.23     5.23     7.21  a
## SOLEX       6.23 0.431 8.23     5.24     7.22  a
## COLOSSEO    6.41 0.431 8.23     5.43     7.40  a
## DUILIO      6.59 0.431 8.23     5.60     7.58  a
## IRIDE       6.70 0.431 8.23     5.71     7.68  a
##
## Degrees-of-freedom method: kenward-roger
## Confidence level used: 0.95
## P value adjustment: tukey method for comparing a family of
   8 estimates
```

12.6 Example 12.6: Repeated Measures in Perennial Crops

With perennial crops, measures are taken repeatedly in the same plots across years. For this reason, even though the dataset appears very much similar to that of Example 12.5, it must be analyzed in a completely different manner.

In particular, we should not neglect that, unlike the winter wheat example, the observations are not independent but are grouped within the same plots. The situation is similar to that of an experiment with subsampling (see Example 12.4) with a relevant difference. Indeed, subsamples are taken at random within each plot, with the sole aim of assessing the intra-plot variability; on the other hand, repeated measures are specifically taken to elucidate the course of the response over time.

It is also helpful to highlight the similarity with split-plot experiments since the "Time" factor can be regarded as the subplot factor (a split-plot in time). The notable difference with split-plot designs is that, with repeated measures, the subplot factor cannot be randomized, but it is always in systematic order (see also Chap. 2)

Let us consider a genotype experiment with alfalfa, laid out with an RCBD with four replicates. Yield measurements are taken annually for three consecutive years from the same plots. The dataset is taken from Ligabue et al. (2009), and it is available as "alfalfa3years" in the `statforbiology` package.

In Code Box 12.4, the dataset is loaded, and some necessary transformations are performed. The plots are uniquely identified in the "plot" variable, although, if required, they could also be identified by combining the genotype and block levels.

Code Box 12.14

```
# Example 12.6
# Repeated measures in a perennial crop
```

```
# Loading the packages
library(statforbiology)
library(lme4)
library(lmerTest)
library(emmeans)
library(multcomp)

# Loading and transforming the data
dataset <- getAgroData("alfalfa3years") |>
  transform(Block = factor(Block),
            Genotype = factor(Genotype),
            Year = factor(Year))
head(dataset)
##   Plot Block Genotype Year    Yield
## 1    1     1 4cascine 2006 6.631775
## 2   25     2 4cascine 2006 6.705397
## 3   60     3 4cascine 2006 6.499588
## 4   63     4 4cascine 2006 7.087686
## 5    7     1 casalina 2006 8.033558
## 6   33     2 casalina 2006 8.265165

# Reference the plots (not necessary in this instance)
# dataset$Plot <- dataset$Block:dataset$Genotype
```

For repeated measures designs, models can be built by using the rules proposed by Piepho et al. (2004):

1. Consider one single year, and build the treatment model (i.e., the model for the treatment factors).
2. Consider one single year, and build the block model (i.e., the model for the grouping factors).
3. Include the year factor in the model, and combine the year with all the effects in the treatment model by crossing or nesting as appropriate.
4. Consider that the "plot" factor in the block model references the randomization units, i.e., those units that received the genotypes through a randomization process. Assign to the plot factor a random effect.
5. Excluding the terms for randomization units, nest the year in all the other terms in the block model.
6. Combine random effects for randomization units with the repeated factor by using the colon (:) operator, to derive the correct error terms for accommodating correlation structures.

Accordingly, the model for Example 12.6 is built as follows (with R notation):

1. Treatment model (for 1 year): YIELD ~ GENOTYPE
2. Block model (for 1 year): YIELD ~ BLOCK + BLOCK:PLOT
3. Treatment model (including the year): YIELD ~ GENOTYPE * YEAR
4. Block model (set the plot as random): YIELD ~ BLOCK + (1|BLOCK:PLOT)
5. Block model (include the year): YIELD ~ BLOCK + BLOCK:YEAR + (1|BLOCK:PLOT)
6. Block model (complete): YIELD ~ BLOCK + BLOCK:YEAR + (1|BLOCK:PLOT) + (1|BLOCK:PLOT:YEAR)

In this case, considering that alfalfa lasts, on average, for 3 years and follows a specific pattern of yield across these years, we can take the block, year, and genotype effects as fixed. Hence, the final model, with R notation, is
YIELD ~ BLOCK + BLOCK:YEAR + GENOTYPE * YEAR + (1|BLOCK:PLOT) + (1|BLOCK:PLOT:YEAR)

The last term represents the residuals and does not need to be included in R, as it is fitted by default.

Code Box 12.15

```
# Example 12.6 [continuation]

# Mixed model analysis for the 'alfalfa3years' dataset
mod <- lmer(Yield ~ Block + Block:Year + Genotype*Year +
            (1|Block:Plot),
           data = dataset)
anova(mod, ddf = "Kenward-Roger")
## Type III Analysis of Variance Table with Kenward-Roger's method
##                Sum Sq Mean Sq NumDF DenDF   F value    Pr(>F)
## Block            3.96    1.32     3    57    2.1389  0.105316
## Genotype        54.00    2.84    19    57    4.6024  3.75e-06 ***
## Year          2602.53 1301.27     2   114 2107.3223 < 2.2e-16 ***
## Block:Year      14.14    2.36     6   114    3.8176  0.001667 **
## Year:Genotype   31.83    0.84    38   114    1.3563  0.111546

# Multiple comparisons
cld(emmeans(mod, ~Genotype), Letters = LETTERS, reverse = TRUE)
## Genotype          emmean    SE df lower.CL upper.CL .group
##  casalina          12.46 0.315 57    11.83     13.1  A
##  FDL0101           12.22 0.315 57    11.59     12.9  A
##  LaBellaCampagnola 12.17 0.315 57    11.54     12.8  A
##  PicenaGR          12.12 0.315 57    11.49     12.8  A
##  Selene            12.11 0.315 57    11.48     12.7  A
##  robot             12.11 0.315 57    11.48     12.7  A
##  Zenith            11.94 0.315 57    11.31     12.6  A
##  prosementi        11.79 0.315 57    11.15     12.4  A
##  marina            11.76 0.315 57    11.13     12.4  A
##  garisenda         11.76 0.315 57    11.13     12.4  A
##  dimitra           11.75 0.315 57    11.12     12.4  A
```

```
## PR57Q53             11.70 0.315 57     11.07       12.3  A
## classe              11.59 0.315 57     10.96       12.2  AB
## 4cascine            11.59 0.315 57     10.96       12.2  AB
## PR56S82             11.56 0.315 57     10.93       12.2  AB
## LaTorre             11.36 0.315 57     10.73       12.0  ABC
## linfa               11.23 0.315 57     10.60       11.9  ABC
## Palladiana          10.89 0.315 57     10.26       11.5  ABC
## RivieraVicentina     9.98 0.315 57      9.35       10.6   BC
## costanza             9.89 0.315 57      9.26       10.5    C
##
## Degrees-of-freedom method: kenward-roger
## P value adjustment: tukey method for comparing a family of 20
   estimates
```

The genotype by year interaction is not significant, so the overall means of genotypes across years can be derived and compared (Code Box 12.15). The group of the best, on average of the 3 years, contains all genotypes except Riviera Vicentina and Costanza.

Before concluding, it is necessary to reinforce the idea that if this dataset is analyzed as in Example 12.5, all inferences and hypothesis tests would be invalid because the basic assumption of independence would be broken, as is the case whenever grouping factors are not included in the model.

Another caveat is that the mixed model analysis proposed earlier in Code Box 12.15 regards the design as a "split-plot in time," which is not necessarily correct. Indeed, such an analysis assumes that the within-plot correlation remains the same for all pairs of observations, regardless of their temporal distance. Indeed, it would be reasonable to expect that the correlation is higher for measures that are very close in time and drops for measures taken at high time distances. Therefore, especially when the number of years is high, further analyses might be necessary to assess whether the adoption of serial correlation structures is warranted (Piepho et al. 2004). However, this aspect is beyond the scope of this introductory book; useful information can be found in Littell et al. (2006).

Lastly, it is worth noting that designs can be found where measurements are not repeated over time but rather over space, such as in different positions (see Chap. 2) or at varying depths. Although the term "split-plot in time" may not be appropriate for these situations, the resulting dataset can still be analyzed using the same methods as shown in this example.

12.7 Grouping Factors in Regression Models

It was anticipated (Chap. 11) that grouping factors (blocks, main-plots, plots, and so forth) need to be adequately referenced in the model, which is also true for regression models. For these latter models, especially when the shape is nonlinear, it is often best to regard the effect of grouping factors as random, assuming that all model parameters (or part of them) change randomly from one group to the other. For example, for simple linear regression models, it is possible to define random intercept models, random slope models, or models with both random intercept and slope.

To fit nonlinear mixed models, we need to shift to a different fitting function, such as the `medrm()` function in the `medrc` package (Gerhard and Ritz 2018) or the `nlme()` function in the `nlme` package (Pinheiro and Bates 2000).

Accounting for the experimental design in linear or nonlinear regression models is a frequently overlooked aspect, and, thus, it seemed appropriate to mention it here, although it is also far too advanced for an introductory book. The interested reader is referred to Pinheiro and Bates (2000) for further information. Also, several posts are devoted to this aspect in the accompanying blog for this book.[1]

12.8 Exercises

1. Six faba bean genotypes were tested at two sowing times using a split-plot design with four complete blocks. Sowing times were randomized to main-plots within blocks, and genotypes were randomized to subplots within main-plots and blocks. The results are derived from Stagnari et al. (2007) by Monte Carlo simulation. They are available as "SowingTime" in the `statforbiology` package, and they are displayed below. Is the genotype recommendation consistent across sowing time? If not, what is the best genotype(s) for autumn sowing? And for spring sowing?

Sowing time	Genotype	1	2	3	4
Autumn	Chiaro	4.36	4.00	4.23	3.83
	Collameno	3.01	3.32	3.27	3.40
	Palombino	3.85	3.85	3.68	3.98
	Scuro	4.97	3.98	4.39	4.14
	Sicania	4.38	4.01	3.94	2.99
	Vesuvio	3.94	4.47	3.93	4.21
Spring	Chiaro	2.76	2.64	2.25	2.38
	Collameno	2.50	1.79	1.57	1.77
	Palombino	2.24	2.21	2.50	2.05
	Scuro	3.45	2.94	3.12	2.69
	Sicania	3.24	3.60	3.16	3.08
	Vesuvio	2.34	2.44	1.71	2.00

[1] See, e.g., https://www.statforbiology.com/2020/stat_nlmm_designconstraints/.

2. Four crops were sown in soil 20 days after the application of three herbicide treatments to evaluate possible carryover effects of herbicide residues. The untreated check was also included in the design, and the weight of the plants was measured 4 weeks after sowing. The experiment was laid out as a split-plot design, and within each block, the herbicides were randomized to main-plots, while the crops were randomized to subplots (Onofri, unpublished data). What crops could be safely sown 20 days after the application of imazethapyr, primisulfuron, and rimsulfuron? The weights of plants are reported below, and the dataset is available as "recrop" in the `statforbiology` package. (*Hint: In this case, stabilizing a transformation might be needed. To assess the type of transformation, you can fit a linear model with no grouping factors (i.e., a simple two-factor factorial in complete blocks, as in Example 10.3) and explore this model object with the* `boxcox()` *function. Derive the optimal* λ *value for the transformation, and use it for the mixed model fit.*)

Block	Herbicide	Grain-sorghum	Rape	Soybean	Sunflower
1	Check	180	157	199	201
1	Imazethapyr	47	10	193	51
1	Primisulfuron	271	8	335	379
1	Rimsulfuron	403	238	226	290
2	Check	236	111	257	358
2	Imazethapyr	43	1	113	4
2	Primisulfuron	182	0.1	201	201
2	Rimsulfuron	227	169	195	494
3	Check	287	217	346	435
3	Imazethapyr	0.1	20	187	13
3	Primisulfuron	283	22	206	307
3	Rimsulfuron	400	364	257	397
4	Check	350	170	211	327
4	Imazethapyr	3	21	122	15
4	Primisulfuron	147	24	240	337
4	Rimsulfuron	171	134	137	180

3. Consider the dataset "oats" in the `MASS` package, which reports the results of a split-plot experiment in a randomized complete block design with six replicates. Genotypes were allocated to main-plots, and nitrogen rates were allocated to subplots. The variables are B = blocks, V = genotypes, N = nitrogen doses, and Y = yield. Fit the correct model for this dataset, retrieve the estimated parameters, and assess the significance of all effects, by looking at the ANOVA table. Based on the observed data, what is your recommendation in terms of genotype and fertilization? (*Hint: To open the dataset, load the* `MASS` *package, and use the* `data(oats)` *command.*)
4. Consider the dataset "pea_MultiLoc," which reports the results of a field experiment comparing pea genotypes. This experiment was repeated in 12 locations,

using an RCBD in all locations. Considering the location and block effects as fixed, perform the ANOVA with R, and evaluate the significance of all the effects. Compare the genotypes in each location, and decide which are the winning genotypes [*HINT: Consider that the blocks, despite the same numbering, are different in each location, and, therefore, the block effect is nested within the locations*].

References

Annichiarico P (2002) Genotype x Environment Interactions - Challenges and Opportunities for Plant Breeding and Cultivar Recommendations, Plant Production and Protection Paper, vol 1. FAO, MET

Bates D, Mächler M, Bolker B, Walker S (2015) Fitting linear mixed-effects models using lme4. J Stat Softw 67(1):1–48. https://doi.org/10.18637/jss.v067.i01

Belocchi A, Fornara M, Ciriciofolo E, Biancolatte E, Del Puglia S, Olimpieri G, Vecchiarelli V, Gosparini E, Piccioni C, Desiderio E (2003) Grano duro: Risultati 2002-03 della Rete Nazionale. Lazio e Umbria. L'Informatore Agrario 19(Suppl. 1):41–44

Dixon P (2016) Should blocks be fixed or random? In: Conference on Applied Statistics in Agriculture. https://doi.org/10.4148/2475-7772.1474. https://newprairiepress.org/agstatconference/2016/proceedings/4

Gałecki A, Burzykowski T (2013) Linear Mixed-Effects Models Using R: A Step-by-Step Approach. Springer, Berlin

Gerhard D, Ritz C (2018) medrc: Mixed effect dose-response curves. https://github.com/doseResponse/medrc, r package version 1.1-0, commit bc36df514ad68d6e3f29ec4c740a563605231819

Kuznetsova A, Brockhoff PB, Christensen RHB (2017) lmerTest package: Tests in linear mixed effects models. J Stat Softw 82(13):1–26. https://doi.org/10.18637/jss.v082.i13

Ligabue M, Onofri A, Ruozzi F (2009) Le migliori varietà di erba medica da seme. Agricoltura 84:82–84

Littell RC, Milliken GA, Stroup WW, Wolfinger RD, Schabanberger O (2006) SAS for Mixed Models, 2nd edn. Books. SAS Publishing, Cary

Onofri A, Ciriciofolo E (2007) Using R to perform the AMMI analysis on agriculture variety trials. R News 7:14–19. http://www.r-project.org

Piepho HP, Büchse A, Emrich K (2003) A Hitchhiker's Guide to mixed models for randomized experiments. J Agron Crop Sci 189(5):310–322. https://doi.org/10.1046/j.1439-037X.2003.00049.x

Piepho HP, Büchse A, Richter C (2004) A mixed modelling approach for randomized experiments with repeated measures. J Agron Crop Sci 190(4):230–247. http://dx.doi.org/10.1111/j.1439-037X.2004.00097.x

Pinheiro JC, Bates DM (2000) Mixed-Effects Models in S and S-Plus. Springer-Verlag Inc. edn. Springer, New York

Stagnari F, Onofri A, Jemison J, Monotti M (2007) Improved multivariate analyses to discriminate the behaviour of faba bean varieties. Agron Sustain Develop 27(4):387–397

Appendix A
A Gentle Introduction to R

All is well that ends well.

—W. Shakespeare

This book is intended for beginners and does not require any prior knowledge of statistics or programming. However, there is a core of general information about R that does not fit into the topic of this book but is nonetheless essential to tackle the proposed exercises. This introductory information is summarized in this appendix in the form of a list of FAQs. It is intended for those who are total beginners in R or need some refreshment in this powerful language. A more comprehensive and advanced guide to R programming is provided by Wickham et al. (2023).

A.1 What Is R?

R is a programming language and environment mainly used for statistical computing, data handling, and visualization (R Core Team, 2025). It is open source, and it works under the GNU General Public License. It is very powerful, but it lacks a graphical interface; therefore, it is necessary to write code using a relatively simple object-oriented language. Although the R environment is self-sufficient, this language is typically used within the RStudio environment (RStudio Team, 2020), which provides additional facilities to write better code and enhance the coding experience.

Both R and RStudio can be installed by the respective websites.[1] Depending on your operating system, additional software tools may be necessary, and they are listed on the download page.

[1] The download pages are https://cloud.r-project.org and https://posit.co/products/open-source/rstudio/ (accesses June 27, 2025).

A. Onofri, *Field Research Methods in Agriculture*,
https://doi.org/10.1007/978-3-032-08199-5

A.2 What Do I Have to Know Before Starting?

After installing both R and Rstudio (in this order), you need to know that the working environment in RStudio consists of four panes, even though, at the beginning, you may only need two of them, namely (1) SOURCE and (2) CONSOLE. The basic principle is to write code in the SOURCE pane and send it to the CONSOLE pane by hitting "ctrl-R" or "ctrl-Return" ("cmd-Return" in macOS X). The SOURCE pane is a text editor, and you can save script files by using the ".R" extension. The CONSOLE pane is where the code is processed to return the results.

Before you start, there are a few essential things that you should keep in consideration to save yourself a few headaches:

1. R is case-sensitive and, for example, "A" is not the same as "a." Please note that most errors in R are due to minor typos, which can be very difficult to spot.
2. Code written in the SOURCE pane **MUST BE** sent to the console pane; otherwise, it is not executed. It is like writing a "WhatsApp" message: Your mate cannot read it until you send it away to them! Likewise, if you correct a line of code, you need to send it again to the console, so that it is re-executed.
3. Spaces can be used to write clearer code, and they are usually allowed, except within variable names, function names, and some operators that consist of more than one character.
4. While coding, it is helpful to add a few comments here and there so that, in future times, you can remember what you intended to do when writing that piece of code. Every line preceded by a hash symbol (#) is not executed, and it is regarded as a comment.

A.3 What Is the Main Activity in R?

The main activity in R consists of "creating" data objects, which must be assigned a name so that they can be stored in memory and easily recalled. For example, in Code box A.1, value 3 is assigned the name "y," i.e., it is stored in memory with that name, from where it can be recalled.

Code Box A.1

```
# Example of an assignment
y <- 3
y
## [1] 3
```

A.4 What Types of Data Can We Use?

In R, as in most programming languages, it is possible to deal with different data types, such as:

1. Numeric (real numbers)
2. Integer (natural numbers)
3. Character (use quotation marks, e.g., "apple" or "peach")
4. Logic (boolean): TRUE or FALSE

A.5 What Types of Objects Can We "Create"?

Depending on their type, data can be stored in specific objects. Working through this book, you will use the following objects:

1. Vectors
2. Matrices
3. Dataframes

A lot of other objects exist, but you do not need to know them right now.

A.6 What Is a "Vector"?

A **vector** is an essential object in R, and it is a unidimensional array storing data of the same type (either numeric or integer or logic... you cannot mix!). For example, the following box shows a vector of character strings and a vector of numeric values. We see that the vector is created by the `c()` function, and the elements are separated by commas.

Code Box A.2

```
# Example of a character vector

sentence <- c("this", "is", "an", "array", "of",
   "characters")
x <- c(12, 13, 14)
```

The factor differs from a character vector as it is used to store character values belonging to a predefined set of levels. The variables for the experimental treatment are usually stored as factors (the experimental factors, as we called them in Chap. 2). The code below shows a character vector that is transformed into a factor by using the `factor()` function.

Code Box A.3

```
# Example of a factor

treat  <-  c("A", "A", "B", "B", "C", "C")
treat
## [1] "A" "A" "B" "B" "C" "C"

factor(treat)
## [1] A A B B C C
## Levels: A B C
```

By now, you have already used a couple of functions; you may have noted that they are characterized by a name followed by a pair of round brackets (e.g., `c()` or `factor()`). The arguments are placed inside the brackets, but more details will be provided later.

A.7 What Is a Matrix?

Vectors are unidimensional arrays, while matrices are bidimensional arrays with rows and columns. Analogous to the vector, the matrix object can be used to store data of the same type, and it is created by using the `matrix()` function. The first argument to this function is a vector of values, the second argument is the number of rows, and the third one is the number of columns. The fourth argument is logical, specifying whether the matrix is to be populated by row ("byrow = TRUE") or by column ("byrow = FALSE").

Code Box A.4

```
# Example of a matrix

z  <-  matrix(c(1, 2, 3, 4, 5, 6, 7, 8),
              2, 4, byrow=TRUE)
z
##      [,1] [,2] [,3] [,4]
```

```
## [1,]    1    2    3    4
## [2,]    5    6    7    8
```

A.8 What Is a Dataframe?

The dataframe is also a table (like a matrix), but its columns can contain data of different types. It is the most common way to store experimental data, and it should be organized in a "tidy" manner, with one experimental unit per row and all the traits of each unit in separate columns. The code below creates three vectors and combines them in a dataframe.

Code Box A.5

```
# Example of a dataframe

plot  <-  c(1, 2, 3, 4, 5, 6)
treat  <-  factor(c("A", "A", "B", "B", "C", "C"))
yield  <-  c(12, 15, 16, 13, 11, 19)
dataset  <-  data.frame("Plot" = plot,
                        "Treatment" = treat,
                        "Yield" = yield)
dataset
##   Plot Treatment Yield
## 1    1         A    12
## 2    2         A    15
## 3    3         B    16
## 4    4         B    13
## 5    5         C    11
## 6    6         C    19
```

A.9 How Do I Work with All These Objects?

Suppose you have created several objects and stored them in memory. In that case you may be interested in viewing them or accessing some of their elements. Objects can be viewed by using their name, as shown below:

Code Box A.6

```
# Inspecting an object

z
##      [,1] [,2] [,3] [,4]
## [1,]    1    2    3    4
## [2,]    5    6    7    8
```

With objects containing more than one value (vectors, matrices, or dataframes), you can use indexing to retrieve an element in a specific position. Indexing is performed by using square brackets containing the index or a list of indices for multidimensional objects.

Code Box A.7

```
# Examples of indexing

x[1] # First element in a vector
## [1] 12

z[1, 3] # Element in first row and third column,
        # in a dataframe or matrix
## [1] 3

dataset[ ,1] # First Column of a dataframe/matrix
## [1] 1 2 3 4 5 6

dataset[1, ] # First Row of a dataframe/matrix
##   Plot Treatment Yield
## 1    1         A    12
```

Column vectors in dataframes can also be accessed by using their name and the "dollar" sign, as shown below:

Code Box A.8

```
# Using the '$' extractor with dataframes
```

```
dataset$Plot
## [1] 1 2 3 4 5 6
```

It is also helpful to ask for information about objects, which can be done by using two functions:

1. `str()` tells us the structure of an object.
2. `summary()` summarizes the main traits of an object.

Code Box A.9

```
str(dataset)
## 'data.frame':    6 obs. of  3 variables:
##  $ Plot     : num  1 2 3 4 5 6
##  $ Treatment: Factor w/ 3 levels "A","B","C": 1 1 2 2 3 3
##  $ Yield    : num  12 15 16 13 11 19

summary(dataset)
##       Plot       Treatment      Yield
##  Min.   :1.00   A:2        Min.   :11.00
##  1st Qu.:2.25   B:2        1st Qu.:12.25
##  Median :3.50   C:2        Median :14.00
##  Mean   :3.50              Mean   :14.33
##  3rd Qu.:4.75              3rd Qu.:15.75
##  Max.   :6.00              Max.   :19.00
```

A.10 What Is the Difference Between Expressions and Functions?

Expressions are simple programming structures that return results and permit the assignment of these results to new variables. Functions are more complex structures characterized by a name and a list of arguments in brackets.

Code Box A.10

```
# An expression returns a result
2 * y
```

```
## [1] 6

# Assigning the result of an expression
f  <-  2 * y
f
## [1] 6

# A function has brackets and arguments inside the brackets
log(5)
## [1] 1.609438
```

Very often, functions use multiple arguments, and you need to pay some attention to how to supply them. You can either:

1. Supply them in the exact order with which R expects them or
2. Use argument names

Code Box A.11

```
# Example of the use of the 'log()' function
# The two arguments are the value and the base for logarithm

# Arguments are supplied with their names
log(x = 100, base = 2)
## [1] 6.643856

# The names can be omitted, but arguments need to be supplied
# in the right order
log(100, 2)
## [1] 6.643856

# When the argument are supplied with names, their ordering is
  irrelevant
log(base = 2, x = 100)
## [1] 6.643856

# When the arguments have no names, changing the ordering
  produces
# wrong results
log(2, 100)
## [1] 0.150515
```

The list of arguments for each function and their ordering can be found by using the R help, which is invoked by a question mark followed by the function name, as shown in the example below:

Code Box A.12

```
# Getting help

?log
```

A.11 Which Functions Should I Learn Before Reading This Book?

Several functions are helpful for the management of the experimental data. For example, it is important to be able to create sequences of values by using the `seq()` function.

Code Box A.12

```
# Crating a sequence from 1 to 10, with an increment of 1
plot  <-  seq(from = 1, to = 10, by = 1)
plot
##  [1]  1  2  3  4  5  6  7  8  9 10
```

Likewise, we need to be able to save time by repeating vectors or vector elements by using the `rep()` function.

Code Box A.13

```
# Repeating a vector for three times
treat <- c("A", "B", "C")
rep(treat, times = 3)
## [1] "A" "B" "C" "A" "B" "C" "A" "B" "C"

# Repeating each element of a vector for three times
rep(treat, each = 3)
## [1] "A" "A" "A" "B" "B" "B" "C" "C" "C"
```

Several vectors can be combined in one single vector by using the `c()` function:

Code Box A.14

```
# Combining two vectors
y <- c(1,2,3)
z <- c(4,5,6)
c(y, z)
## [1] 1 2 3 4 5 6
```

During our R session, objects are created and written to the workspace (environment). At the end of a session (or at the beginning of a new one), we could clean the workspace by using the `rm()` function, as shown below. The same function can be used to remove specific objects.

Code Box A.15

```
# Remove all objects from the workspace
rm(list=ls())

# Remove two specific objects
rm(y, z)
```

A.12 What Is an "Extractor"?

As mentioned earlier for dataframes, functions may return several objects, which are allocated to different slots. To extract these objects, we use the $ operator. For example, the `eigen()` function calculates the eigenvector and eigenvalues of a matrix, and these results are saved into the same variable but in different slots. We can extract the results as shown below:

Code Box A.16

```
# Defining a matrix
MAT  <-  matrix(c(2,1,3,4),2,2)
MAT
##       [,1] [,2]
```

```
## [1,]    2    3
## [2,]    1    4

# Calculating the eigenvectors and eigenvalues
ev  <-  eigen(MAT)
ev
## eigen() decomposition
## $values
## [1] 5 1
##
## $vectors
##            [,1]       [,2]
## [1,] -0.7071068 -0.9486833
## [2,] -0.7071068  0.3162278

# Extracting the slot 'values'
ev$values
## [1] 5 1

# Extracting the slot 'vectors'
ev$vectors
##            [,1]       [,2]
## [1,] -0.7071068 -0.9486833
## [2,] -0.7071068  0.3162278
```

A.13 What Is a Package?

The R language is modular in the sense that its functionalities can be greatly extended by using external packages, which can be installed using the command `install.packages("LibraryName")`. A package is installed just once, but it needs to be loaded at every R session whenever we need to use it. To load a package we use the command `library("LibraryName")`.

Alternatively, it is possible to invoke a function located in an external package without explicitly loading that package. To this aim we use the `::` extractor. For example, the code `libName::funName()` permits to invoke the function `funName()` in the external package `libName`.

Prior to studying this book, the readers will need to install the following extension packages (in alphabetical order): `car` (Fox and Weisberg, 2019), `drc` (Ritz et al., 2019), `emmeans` (Lenth, 2024), `ggplot2` (Wickham, 2016), `lme4` (Bates et al., 2015), `lmerTest` (Kuznetsova et al., 2017), `MASS` (Venables and Ripley, 2002), `multcomp` (Hothorn et al., 2008), `multcompView` (Graves et al.,

2024), statforbiology (Onofri, 2025), and SuppDists (Wheeler, 2025). It is also worth noting that there are many other useful packages, such as dplyr and other packages in the tidyverse, which are particularly useful for data management tasks (Wickham et al., 2019). These packages were not necessary for the simple data management tasks in this introductory book; still, students who wish to acquire more advanced skills will need to learn them.

It is also worth mentioning that this book and its associated website are written in RMarkdown (Xie et al., 2018) using the bookdown (Xie, 2024) and blogdown (Xie et al., 2017) packages, which can be very useful for writing presentations, reports, and scientific manuscripts.

A.14 How Do I Enter Data into R?

R is not always the right tool for entering the experimental data; most often, we enter the data using a spreadsheet, such as Microsoft Excel. This data can be stored as ".xls" or ".xlsx" files or, as is often the case in this book, as ".csv" files. While the former file types are specific to Excel, ".csv" files are a type of cross-platform text data that does not store information about formatting (such as bold, italic, or background colors) but can be opened by all programs and operating systems.

To open ".csv" data, we can use the read.csv() function, which allows us to read local files or files in external repositories. For example, the code below reads a ".csv" file from the web repository of this book.

Code Box A.17

```
# Loading a 'csv' file from an internet repository
fileName <- "https://www.statforbiology.com/_data/
             WeedPop.csv"
dataset <- read.csv(fileName)
dataset
##   Code POLLA CHEPO ECHCG AMARE XANST POLAV
## 1    A   0.1    33    11     0   0.1   0.1
## 2    B   0.1     3     3     0   0.1   0.0
## 3    C   7.0    19    19     4   7.0   1.0
## 4    D  18.0     3    28    19  12.0   6.0
## 5    E   5.0     7    28     3  10.0   1.0
## 6    F  11.0     9    33     7  10.0   6.0
## 7    G   8.0    13    33     6  15.0  15.0
## 8    H  18.0     5    33     4  19.0  12.0
## 9    I   6.0     6    38     3  10.0   6.0
```

Suppose you want to read a ".csv" (or Excel) file from your local hard disk. In that case, you may need to set the working directory to point R to the directory where the file to be read is located. You can do this by using the menu entry "Session/Set working directory/Choose directory" and then selecting the desired directory on the selection form.

Suppose you want to read an Excel file. In that case, you need to download, install, and load an additional package (`readxl`) and use the `read_xls()` or the `read_xlsx()` functions (depending on the format of the file), passing the arguments for the name of the file and the name of the sheet to be loaded (if the data table does not start from the "A1" cell in the Excel worksheet, we may need to supply also the range of cells to be read).

Code Box A.18

```
# Reading an EXCEL file

# install.packages("readxl") # install the package: only at first instance
library(readxl) # Load the package: at the beginning of each session

dataset  <-  read_xls("fileName", sheet = "nameOfSheet") # Open XLS file
dataset  <-  read_xlsx("fileName", sheet = "nameOfSheet") # Open XLSX file
```

If you do not intend to set the working directory to the location where the file is stored, you can use the filename together with its full path in place of "fileName"; alternatively, you can use the `file.choose()` function, which shows a selection form, from where you can select the file to be opened [for instance, `read.csv(file.choose())`].

A.15 What About Data Handling?

Data handling is a crucial task in R, but you will not need to perform it while working through this book. If you are interested, you are advised to read specific books for this, such as "R for data Science" by Hadley Wickham et al., which is available at https://r4ds.hadley.nz.

However, there is one operator for data handling that is worth introducing here. It is the so-called `pipe` operator (|>), which we will use in this book. Pipes have become very popular in R because they permit us to write code in a way that closely resembles how humans think about solving problems. For example, suppose you need to take the values from 1 to 4, multiply them by "3," extract the square root of the result, take its logarithm, calculate the mean, and exponentiate it; you might use the traditional coding at the beginning of Code Box A.19. The same expression, by using the "pipe" operator, is longer but more readable. To grasp the meaning of the pipe operator, we can translate it into the following statement: "Take the value of the previous function and feed it into the next function as the first argument."

Code Box A.19

```
# Expression in traditional style

exp(mean(log(sqrt(1:4))))
## [1] 1.487738

# Same expression, by using the pipe operator

c(1:4) |>
  sqrt() |>
  log() |>
  mean() |>
  exp()
## [1] 1.487738
```

Appendix B
Models

See Tables B.1 and B.2.

Table B.1 Summary of the main linear models to describe the results of common experiments in agriculture. Each model is presented together with the proposed R function for fitting and the corresponding coding. "Y" is the response variable, "F1" and "F2" are the names of two experimental factors (nominal variables), while "X1" is the name of a continuous variable. "B" is a generic variable for the blocks (factor), "ENV" is the variable for environments (factor), and "MAIN," "ROW," and "COL" are, respectively, the variables (factors) for the main-plots in a split-plot design and the rows/columns in a strip-plot design

Model	Design	R functions for fitting	Model specification
One-way	CRD	lm()	$Y \sim F_1$
One-way	RCBD	lm()	$Y \sim F_1 + B$
Two-ways	CRD	lm()	$Y \sim F_1 * F_2$
Two-ways	RCBD	lm()	$Y \sim F_1 * F_2 + B$
Two-ways	Split-plot CRD	lmer()	$Y \sim F_1 * F_2 + (1\|\mathrm{MAIN})$
Two-ways[a]	Split-plot RCBD	lmer()	$Y \sim F_1 * F_2 + B + (1\|\mathrm{MAIN})$
Two-ways	Strip-plot CRD	lmer()	$Y \sim F_1 * F_2 + (1\|\mathrm{ROW}) + (1\|\mathrm{COL})$
Two-ways[a]	Strip-plot RCBD	lmer()	$Y \sim F_1 * F_2 + B + (1\|\mathrm{ROW}) + (1\|\mathrm{COL})$
One-way	One-way CRD, two environments	lm()/lmer()	$Y \sim F_1 * \mathrm{ENV}$
One-way	One-way RCBD, two environments	lm()/lmer()	$Y \sim \mathrm{ENV{:}B} + F_1 * \mathrm{ENV}$
Linear Regression	CRD	lm()	$Y \sim X_1$
Linear Regression	RCBD	lm()	$Y \sim X_1 + F_1$

[a] For split-plot and strip-plot designs in blocks, the main-plot, row, and column effects are nested within the blocks. With fixed blocks, the correct coding, for example, for a split-plot would be $Y \sim F_1 * F_2 + B + (1|\mathrm{B{:}MAIN})$. However, explicitly nesting the randomization factor within the blocks is not necessary if all the main-plots/rows/columns have been uniquely identified, as shown in Examples 12.1 and 12.2

A. Onofri, *Field Research Methods in Agriculture*,
https://doi.org/10.1007/978-3-032-08199-5

Table B.2 Summary of the main curvilinear regression models to describe the results of experiments in agriculture, together with the equation and self-starter function for the `drm()` fitting function. Y is the response variable, X is the predictor, and all the other letters represent model parameters to be estimated

Model	Equation	Self-starter
Quadratic polynomial[a]	$Y = a + b\,X + c\,X^2$	'DRC.poly2()'
Exponential	$Y = a\ \exp(\pm k\ X)$	'DRC.expoGrowth()' 'DRC.expoDecay()'
Asymptotic growth	$Y = a - (a - b)\ \exp(-cX)$	'DRC.asymReg()'
Power curve	$Y = a\ X^b$	'DRC.powerCurve()'
Rectangular hyperbola	$Y = \frac{a\,X}{b+X}$	'DRC.YL()'
Logistic equation	$Y = \frac{d}{1+\exp(-b(X-e))}$	'L.2()', 'L.3('), 'L.4()'
Gompertz equation	$Y = c + (d - c)\exp\{-\exp[-b\,(X - e)]\}$	'G.2()' 'G.3()' 'G.4()'
Log-Logistic equation	$Y = \frac{d}{1+exp(-b(\log(X)-\log(e)))}$	'LL.2()', 'LL.3('), 'LL.4()'
Bragg's equation	$Y = c + (d - c)\ \exp\left[-b(X - e)^2\right]$	'DRC.bragg.3()' 'DRC.bragg.4()'

[a] The quadratic polynomial function is a linear model, and it should preferably be fitted with the `lm()` function

Appendix C
Datasets

All the exercises and examples throughout this book use "`.csv`" datasets that are available in a web repository. To facilitate easier access to these datasets, the `statforbiology` package provides the `getAgroData()` function, which accepts the dataset name as an argument, as illustrated in several code boxes along the book. The list of the available datasets is presented below; for each dataset, a brief description is provided, along with a list of all the variables included.

C.1 `adjuvantsLS`

An experiment to compare three adjuvants (ammonium sulfate, mineral oil, and nonionic surfactant) and a control with no adjuvant for Rimsulfuron, which is an herbicide for weed control in maize. The experiment was designed as a Latin square with five replicates (Onofri, 1990; unpublished), and the resulting dataset was slightly modified to make it more suitable for teaching purposes.

- Herbicide (character): herbicide name
- Adjuvant (character): adjuvant name
- Dose (character): dose of the herbicide + adjuvant
- Code (character): code for the adjuvants
- Plot (numerical coding): code for the plots
- Column (numerical coding): code for the column in the Latin square grid
- Row (numerical coding): code for the row in the Latin square grid
- Columns 8–23 (character): Each column is a weed (identified by the respective Bayer code), and the values represent the abundances (Braun-Blanquet codes).
- Yield (numeric): crop yield (100 kg per hectare)
- Height (numeric): crop height (cm)

A. Onofri, *Field Research Methods in Agriculture*,
https://doi.org/10.1007/978-3-032-08199-5

C.2 `alfalfa3years`

A genotype experiment in alfalfa (Ligabue et al., 2009) to compare 20 genotypes in central Italy (medium Tiber Valley). The experiment was laid out as an RCBD with four replicates, and the total yearly forage yield (sum of 3–4 cuts per year) was measured in each plot over 3 years (from 2006 to 2008).

- Plot (numeric): code for the plot
- Block (numeric): code for the block
- Genotype (character): name of the genotype
- Year (numeric): year when yield was measured
- Yield (numeric): total yearly forage yield (sum of 3–4 cuts per year; in tons per hectare of dry matter)

C.3 `Ammi94`

A field experiment to evaluate the effect of different densities of *Ammi majus* on the achene yield of sunflower (Onofri and Tei, 1994a). The values represent the means of four replicates.

- Density (numeric): number of weed plants per square meter
- Yield (numeric): sunflower yield in tons per hectare

C.4 `beet`

A split-plot tillage experiment in sugar beet, where three types of tillage (minimum tillage = MIN, shallow plowing = SP, and deep plowing = DP) and two types of chemical weed control methods (broadcast = TOT and in-furrow = PART) were compared in four complete blocks with three main-plots per block, split into two subplots per main-plot; the three types of tillage were randomly allocated to the main-plots in each block, while the two weed control treatments were randomly allocated to the subplots within each main-plot (Bianchi, 1992; unpublished data).

- Tillage (character): tillage method
- WeedControl (character): weed control method
- Block (numeric): code for the block
- Yield (numeric): sugar beet root yield in tons per hectare

C.5 `beetGrowth`

An experiment in which sugar beet was grown either weed-free or weed-infested (Covarelli and Onofri, 1998). Crop weight per unit area (in kg/ha) was measured at six different timings (in days after emergence; DAE), using destructive methods from independent plots. The experiment was conducted using a completely randomized design with three replicates.

- DAE (numeric): days after emergence
- Infested (numeric): crop dry weight in weed-infested plots (kg/ha)
- WeedFree (numeric): crop dry weight in weed-free plots (kg/ha)

C.6 `citrusGrove` or `speciesArea`

An experiment was conducted in a citrus grove in Sicily (Southern Italy) to determine the species-area relationship for the local weed community. In this study, a nested-plot survey was employed (Muller-Dumbois and Ellenberg, 1974) where the number of weed species was counted in a plot of 1 m^2 surface and the sampling area was progressively doubled in size. At each step, the number of new weed species was counted. The dataset is taken from Cristaudo et al. (2015).

- Area (numeric): sampled area (in square meters)
- numSpecies (numeric): count of the number of species

C.7 `crosses`

An experiment to compare nine maize hybrids, obtained from three pollinating inbred lines (A1, A2, and A3), each one crossed with three different female inbred lines (A1 was crossed with B1, B2, and B3, A2 was crossed with B4, B5, and B6, while A3 was crossed with B7, B8, and B9). The experiment was laid out as complete blocks with four replicates (36 subjects in total). The dataset was generated through Monte Carlo simulation.

- Male (character): pollinating line
- Female (character): female line
- Block (numeric): code for the blocks
- Yield (numeric): maize yield (in tons per hectare)

C.8 failureTimes

An experiment to record the failure time of heating systems as affected by four different operating temperatures. The design was completely randomized with six replicates, and the number of hours before failure was measured. The dataset is taken from Nelson (1972).

- Temp (numeric): testing temperature (in °F)
- Hours_to_failure (numeric): number of hours before failure

C.9 FertilizationTiming

A field experiment to evaluate the effect of fertilization timing (early, optimal, late) on two genotypes (A and B). The experiment was laid out as an RCBD, and the response represents the amount of absorbed nitrogen by the plant (simulated data).

- Timing (character): timing of fertilization (early, optimal, late)
- Genotype (character): genotype
- Block (numeric): code for the block
- Nabs (numeric): amount of absorbed nitrogen

C.10 FGP_rape

An experiment where the germination of three genotypes of oilseed rape was assessed in controlled conditions, at 20 °C, according to an RCBD with six replicates. One replicate per genotype, consisting of a Petri dish with 50 seeds, was put in each of six shelves inside the oven. The number of germinated seeds was counted 15 days after the start of the assay and expressed as the Final Proportion of Germinated seeds (FGP). The assay was repeated twice in different and independent ovens with the same experimental design. The dataset is taken from Pace et al. (2012).

- Dish (numeric): code for the Petri dish
- Run (numeric coding): code for the run
- Shelf (numeric): code for the shelf
- Species (character): plant species
- Genotype (character): genotype
- FGP (numeric): Final Germinated Proportion in each dish

C.11 heights

Highly unbalanced dataset, containing the height (cm) and yield (t/ha) of 20 maize plants belonging to four different genotypes. The dataset was generated through Monte Carlo simulation.

- Id (numeric): code for the plot
- var (character): code for the genotype
- height (numeric): crop height (cm)
- yield (numeric): crop yield (t/ha)

C.12 insects

An experiment in which tobacco plants were treated with three different insecticides was conducted using a completely randomized design with five replicates (resulting in a total of 15 plants). The number of insects over the surface of leaves in each plant was counted 3 weeks after the treatments.

- Insecticide (character): code for the insecticide
- Rep (numeric): code for the replicate (not blocks)
- Count (numeric): count of insects

C.13 johnsongrass

A pot experiment to evaluate the best timing for herbicide application against *Sorghum halepense* originated by rhizomes. Five timings were compared including a split treatment (2-3, 4-5, 6-7, 8-9, and 3-4/8-9 leaves), and an untreated check was added for comparison. Treatments were repeated on plants originating from rhizomes of different lengths (2, 4, and 6 nodes). The design was a fully crossed two-way factorial, laid out as completely randomized with four replicates. The dataset is taken from Onofri and Tei (1994b).

- Length (character): length of rhizomes at the beginning of the experiment
- Timing (character): crop stage at spraying
- RizomeWeight (numeric): weight of rhizomes four weeks after spraying (in grams per pot)

C.14 `LeClerg`

A genotype experiment in a completely randomized design, with five genotypes and four replicates. The dataset is modified from Le Clerg et al. (1962).

- Variety (character): code for the genotype
- Yield (numeric): crop yield in bushels per acre

C.15 `LepidopteraEggs`

An entomologist counted the number of eggs laid by a species of moth, on three different substrates using a completely randomized design with 15 replicates. This dataset was modified from Kuehl (2000).

- Substrate (character): code for the substrate
- No_of_eggs (numeric): count of the number of eggs

C.16 `lettuceLS`

An experiment to assess the effect of four different fertilizers on lettuce yield. The experiment was laid out as a Latin square with four replicates. The dataset was generated through Monte Carlo simulation.

- Fertilizer (character): code for the fertilizer
- Row (numeric): code for the row in the Latin square grid
- Column (numeric): code for the column in the Latin square grid
- Yield (numeric): lettuce yield (in kg per hectare $\times$ 100)

C.17 `metamitron`

An experiment to study the degradation of the herbicide metamitron (M) in soil, either alone or in the presence of two co-applied herbicides, i.e., phenmedipham (P) and chloridazon (C). Ninety-six independent soil samples were treated with four herbicide combinations (i.e., M, M+P, M+C, and M+P+C, 32 samples per combination) and stored in a climatic chamber at 20 °C. Three random soil samples were collected for each herbicide combination at eight different time points (0, 7, 14, 21, 32, 42, 55, and 67 days after treatment). They were stored in a refrigerator until chemical analyses. At the end of the experiment, all soil samples were analyzed to determine the residual concentration of metamitron. This dataset is taken from

Vischetti et al. (1996), and it has been modified through Monte Carlo simulation, to make it more suitable for teaching purposes.

- Time (numeric): the time at sampling (in days after the treatment)
- Herbicide (character): code for the herbicide combination
- Rep (numeric): code for the replicate (not blocks; the experiment was fully randomized)
- Conc (numeric): the concentration of metamitron in % of the initial value

C.18 `missingVal`

A fertilization trial was conducted according to a randomized complete block design with five replicates; however, due to unforeseen circumstances, one value is missing for the "50N" treatment in the second block.

- Fert (character): fertilization treatment
- Block (numeric): code for the block
- P2O5 (numeric): content of P_2O_5 in leaves (%)

C.19 `mixture`

A pot experiment to compare weed control efficacy of two herbicides used alone and in a mixture. A control was also added as a reference, and thus, the four treatments were (i) Metribuzin, (ii) Rimsulfuron, (iii) Metribuzin + Rimsulfuron, and (iv) the untreated control. Sixteen uniform pots were prepared and sown with *Solanum nigrum*. When the plants reached the 4-true-leaf stage, the pots were sprayed with the above herbicide solution following a completely randomized design with four replicates. Three weeks after the treatment, the plants in each pot were harvested and weighed: The lower the weight, the higher the efficacy of herbicides. The dataset is taken from Onofri et al. (1995).

- Treat (character): herbicide treatment
- Weight (numeric): dry weight of weed plants (grams per pot)

C.20 `NGenotype` and `NGenotypeFull`

Fifteen genotypes of durum wheat were compared under two different N fertilization strategies (in the dataset "NGenotype" the number of genotypes has been reduced to 5). The dataset was generated through Monte Carlo simulation that started from the original data in Stagnari et al. (2013).

- Block (numeric): code for the block
- Genotype (character): code for the genotype
- Nitrogen (numeric): code for the fertilization strategy
- Yield (numeric): wheat yield in tons per hectare

C.21 `NWheat`

An N fertilization experiment was conducted in wheat using a randomized complete block design, with four N doses and four replicates. The dataset was generated through Monte Carlo simulation.

- Dose (numeric): N fertilization rate (Kg/ha)
- Block (numeric): code for the block
- Yield (numeric): crop yield in tons per hectare

C.22 `Oat1L`

A field experiment was laid out as a CRD with three replicates to compare five genotypes of oat in one location. The data were generated through Monte Carlo simulation.

- Genotype (character): code for the genotype
- Yield (numeric): oat yield in tons per hectare

C.23 `Oat2L`

The same experiment as for "Oat1L" was repeated in a second location, also with a completely randomized layout. Also the data for the second location were generated through Monte Carlo simulation.

- Location (character): code for the location
- Genotype (character): code for the genotype
- Yield (numeric): oat yield in tons per hectare

C.24 `orangeIrrigation`

An irrigation experiment was conducted in an orange grove in Southern Italy, comprising five irrigation systems in five complete blocks. The dataset was simulated by Monte Carlo methods.

- Method (character): irrigation systems
- Block (numeric): code for the block
- Yield (numeric): orange yield in tons per hectare

C.25 `pea_MultiLoc`

A multilocation genotype experiment in field pea, to compare 17 genotypes in 12 locations. In each location, the experiment was laid out as an RCBD, with four blocks. The dataset was generated through Monte Carlo simulation, starting from the data in Monotti et al. (2009).

- Id (numeric): code for the plot
- Loc (character): code for the location
- Var (character): code for the genotype
- Block (character): code for the block
- Yield (numeric): pea yield in tons per hectare

C.26 `Rainfall2022`

Daily rainfall amounts (mm) in central Italy in 2022 from a local meteorological station.

- DOY (numeric): Day Of the Year
- PRP (numeric): amount of daily rainfall (mm per day)

C.27 `recropS`

Rimsulfuron was applied at the recommended rate on bare soil, and untreated plots were included for comparison. Forty days after the treatment, sugar beet, rape, and soybean were sown on treated and untreated plots, and the weight of the plants was determined 4 weeks after sowing. The experiment was laid down as a strip-plot in complete blocks: In each block, the herbicide treatments (Rimsulfuron and the untreated control) were randomly allocated to each of the two columns, while the three crops were randomly allocated to each of the three rows (Onofri, unpublished data).

- Herbicide (Character): name of the herbicide treatment
- Crop (character): name of the crop
- Block (numeric): code for the block
- CropBiomass (numeric): weight of crop biomass four weeks after sowing

C.28 `rimsulfuron`

An herbicide experiment where Rimsulfuron was used with different timings and in different mixtures and compared to several other herbicide solutions for weed control in maize. At the end of the crop cycle, herbicide efficacy was assessed by measuring the coverage of weeds (%) and the yield of maize (in 100 kg per hectare).

- Herbicide (character): name of the herbicide treatment
- Plot (numeric): code for the plot
- Code (numeric): code for the herbicide
- Block (numeric): code for the block
- Column (numeric): code for the column within each block
- WeedCover (numeric): coverage of weeds (in %)
- Yield (numeric): maize yield (in 100 kg per hectare)

C.29 `Sinapis`

A study was conducted to evaluate the effect of increasing densities of a weed (*Sinapis arvensis*) on sunflower yield (tons per hectare). The dataset was taken from Onofri and Tei (1994a).

- Density (numeric): weed density in plants per square meter
- Block (numeric): code for the block
- Yield (numeric): sunflower grain yield in tons per hectare

C.30 `SowingTime`

Six faba bean genotypes were tested at two sowing times using a split-plot design in four complete blocks. Sowing times were randomized to main-plots within blocks, and genotypes were randomized to subplots within main-plots and blocks. The dataset was taken from Stagnari et al. (2007).

- Plot (numeric): code for the plot
- SowingTime (character): sowing season
- Genotype (character): name of the genotype
- Block (numeric): code for the block
- Yield (numeric): crop grain yield in tons per hectare

C.31 `sugarsMedia`

Plant tissues of tomato were grown in tissue cultures using three types of media, each based on the addition of a specific amount of either glucose or fructose or sucrose to the control. The experiment was conducted using a completely randomized design with five replicates, and the growth of cells was recorded for each subject. The dataset was generated through Monte Carlo simulation, starting from the original data in Kuehl (2000).

- Sugar (character): type of substrate
- Growth (numeric): tissue growth in mm

C.32 `Timings_77490`

A field experiment with maize in which Rimsulfuron was used postemergence in maize at four different timings and compared to the untreated unweeded control. The aim was to assess the selectivity of the herbicide for the crop, depending on the moment of intervention. One value is missing due to an unforeseen event. The dataset is taken from Onofri (unpublished data).

- Plot (numeric): code for the plot
- Timing (character): timing of weed control as the number of maize leaves
- Block (numeric): code for the block
- Height_30 (numeric): height of maize (cm) on 30 June (cm)
- Weight_30 (numeric): average weight of maize plants (g per plant) on 30 June
- FinalYield (numeric): grain yield of maize in kg/ha $\times$ 100

C.33 `TKW`

An experiment with 30 winter wheat genotypes in three blocks, where the Weight of Thousand Kernels (TKW) was recorded in three subsamples per plot (Ciriciofolo, unpublished data)

- Plot (numeric): code for the plot
- Block (numeric): code for the block
- Genotype (character): name of the genotype
- Sample (numeric): code for the subsample in each plot
- TKW (numeric): weight of 1000 wheat kernels (g)

C.34 `Tripleuspermum`

Plants of *Tripleuspermum inodorum* were treated with a sulphonylurea herbicide (tribenuron-methyl) at increasing doses, and the fresh weight of the treated plants per pot was recorded 3 weeks after treatment. The experiment was completely randomized with three replicates and conducted at the Department of Integrated Pest Management, University of Aarhus, Denmark (Pannacci et al., 2010).

- Dose (numeric): dose of tribenuron-methyl (in g/ha)
- FreshWeight (numeric): weight of plants 3 weeks after the treatment (in grams per pot)

C.35 `WeedCounts`

Counts of three weed species (CHEAL: *Chenopodium album*, CHEHY: *C. hybridum*, and CHEPO: *C. polyspermum*) in 20 random quadrats in a field of central Italy (Onofri, unpublished data).

- Species (character): the weed species, identified by its Bayer code
- Rep (numeric): code for the quadrat
- Count (numeric): count of the number of plants per quadrat

C.36 `WeedCover`

Results of a survey, where the yield of maize was determined, as affected by the early determined covering of weeds. The dataset was simulated by Monte Carlo methods.

- WeedCover (numeric): ground covering of weeds (%)
- Yield (numeric): yield of maize in tons per hectare

C.37 `WinterWheat` and `WinterWheat2002`

A multiyear experiment was conducted to compare eight winter wheat genotypes, with an RCBD with three replicates in the hills of central Italy and repeated for 7 years (Onofri and Ciriciofolo, 2007). The dataset "WinterWheat2022" only contains the data from the 2002 season.

- Plot (numeric): code for the plot
- Block (numeric): code for the block within each year
- Genotype (character): name of the genotypes
- Yield (numeric): grain yield in tons per hectare
- Year (numeric): the year in which the yield was measured

Appendix D
Answers to Questions and Exercises

D.1 Chapter 1

1. The fundamental traits of a valid experiment are (i) control, (ii) replication, and (iii) randomization. See Sect. 1.3 for details.
2. Galileo's research method is summarized in Fig. 1.1.
3. Systematic errors tend to occur repeatedly with similar extents and signs, while random errors relate to unknown, unpredictable, and episodic events and tend to occur with random extents and random signs. Examples are given in Sect. 1.1. Systematic errors are particularly concerning, because they may produce the so-called confounding, which is discussed in Sect. 1.3.3.
4. True replicates must have independently received the whole manipulation process to allocate the experimental treatments. Whenever the units received altogether at least part of such manipulation process, they are regarded as pseudo-replicates (see Sect. 1.3.2 for other details and examples)
5. See Sect. 1.3.3 for the definition and examples.
6. Precision relates to slight variation across repeated measurements, while accuracy relates to how close a measure is to the "true" value of the trait being measured. See Sect. 1.1 for details and examples.
7. Replication is discussed in Sect. 1.3.2; the number of replicates in field research usually ranges from 3 (preferably 4) to 5.
8. Randomization is discussed in Sect. 1.3.3.
9. Control is discussed in Sect. 1.3.1.
10. The check is one of the experimental treatments, and it may be included in an experiment as the reference against which all other treatments are evaluated. See Sect. 1.2.2.
11. Mensurative experiments have only one experimental factor with one level (see Sect. 1.2.2). In manipulative experiments, the allocation of treatments to experimental units is typically performed through a manipulation process (see Sect. 1.2.4). Observational experiments consist of observing units that are

A. Onofri, *Field Research Methods in Agriculture*,
https://doi.org/10.1007/978-3-032-08199-5

"naturally" treated (see Sect. 1.2.4), while no manipulation is performed by the researcher to allocate the treatments.

12. The answer can be found in Sect. 1.2.5
13. In (multi)factorial experiments, the levels of two or more factors can be combined in different ways. When all possible combinations of factor levels are included, the design is called a crossed factorial design. In contrast, if the levels of one factor vary depending on the level of another, the design is known as a nested factorial design. See Sect. 1.2.2 for further details and examples.

D.2 Chapter 2

1. The answer can be found in Sect. 2.3.
2. Plants growing along the plot edges are not in the same conditions as those in the middle of each plot, which creates some degree of intra-plot variability. Methods to cope with the border effect are provided in Sect. 2.3.
3. The three types of designs are described in detail in Sects. 2.4.1, 2.4.2, and 2.4.3. CRDs are very rarely used in field research, while they are common in laboratory research, where the degree of environmental homogeneity is rather high. The RCBD is the most common type of design for one-factor factorial field experiments, while the Latin square design is used in the presence of two fertility gradients, when the number of experimental treatments is rather low (4–5, maximum).
4. The answer can be found in Sect. 2.4.4.
5. The answer can be found in Sect. 2.4.4.
6. The answer can be found in Sect. 2.4.4.
7. The experiment may be laid out as a randomized complete block design (RCBD) with four replicates. Each block consists of a long strip with 16 plots, each rectangular, 2.5 meters wide and 10 meters long. The plots stretch along the sowing direction. In total, the experiment covers an area of 10 meters in width and 160 meters in length. Yield is measured at the end of the crop cycle. With this information, the map can be drawn as suggested in Fig. 2.6 (left), *mutatis mutandis*.
8. The experiment follows a two-way crossed factorial design, involving 14 treatments (two sowing dates by seven genotypes). To reduce border effects, the layout may adopt a split-plot design, with sowing dates assigned to main-plots within blocks and genotypes allocated to subplots within each main-plot. A possible field map that fits the available space is shown in Fig. D.1. Among the genotypes, it is appropriate to include a reference genotype, which is widely grown in the nearby farms.
9. A feasible approach is to implement a randomized complete block design (RCBD) on a grid of four rows and eight columns. Each row constitutes a

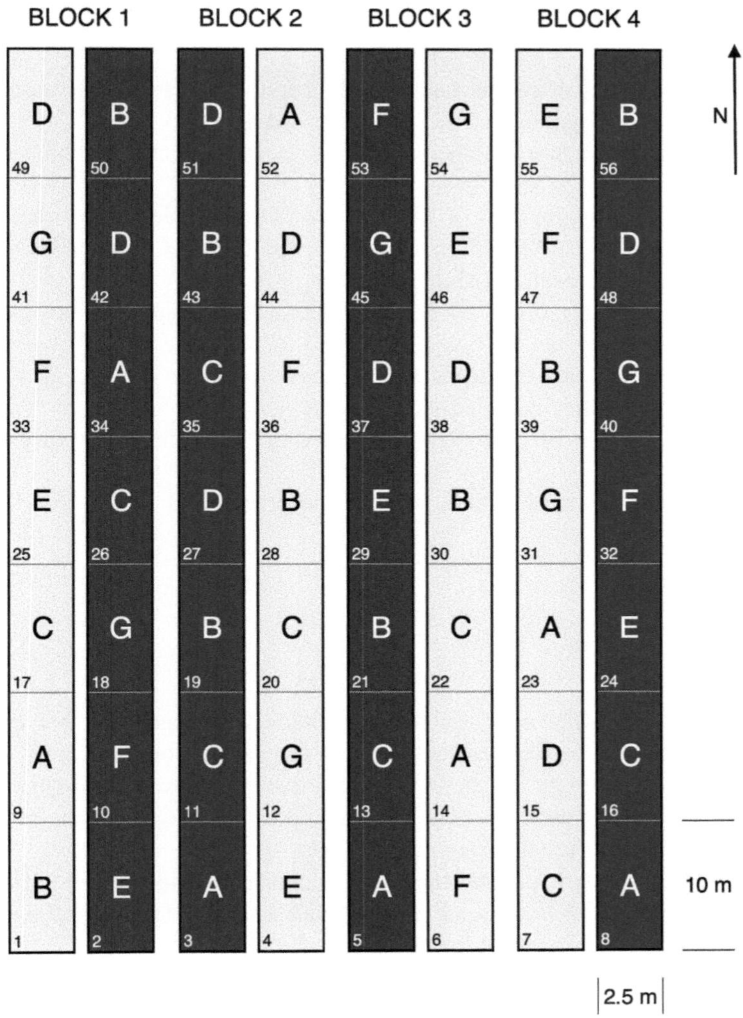

Fig. D.1 A possible field map for Exercise 2.8, representing a split-plot experiment to compare seven faba bean genotypes across two sowing dates. The experiment consists of four blocks, each containing two contiguous main-plots. Sowing dates are randomly allocated to these main-plots within each block (the dark-colored main-plots represent autumn sowing, while the light-colored main-plots represent spring sowing). Within each main-plot, the seven genotypes (labeled A–G using Roman letters) are randomly assigned to subplots

block containing eight plots, each measuring 2 m × 10 m. The eight treatment combinations are randomly assigned to the plots within each block. Because sowing must follow the fertility gradient, a split-plot design is not considered appropriate. The total size of the experiment is 40 m in length and 16 m in width.

D.3 Chapter 3

1. The main statistics of central tendency (location) for quantitative variables are the mean and the median, and they are discussed in Sect. 3.1.
2. The Pearson correlation coefficient is a measure of joint variation, and it is discussed in Sect. 3.5.
3. Mean = 145.33 ng/g; sum of squares = 984.67; mean square = 492.33; standard deviation = 22.19; coefficient of variation = 15.3%. One possible way to present the result is 145.33 ± 22.19 ng/g.
4. The r coefficient is 0.995, which indicates a high degree of positive joint variation.
5. After loading the dataset, means and standard deviations can be calculated by modifying the coding in Code Box 3.3. A barplot can be obtained by modifying the coding in Code Box 3.6. The coefficient of correlation between yield and weed cover is $r = -0.807$.
6. The total yield is 13 ± 0.806, while the average yield is 6.5 ± 0.403 (see Sects. 3.4.1 and 3.4.2).

D.4 Chapter 4

1. Causation occurs when one variable directly causes a change in another, allowing us to distinguish between the cause and the effect. Joint variation, on the other hand, refers to an association between two variables that change together, although we may not necessarily be able to determine which is the cause and which is the effect (see the beginning of Chap. 4).
2. The effect of an experimental treatment is defined as the additive shift in the expected response of treated individuals, relative to either the overall mean or a specified reference treatment level (see Sect. 4.4.3).
3. The ANOVA can be described in several different ways, which can be found in Sect. 4.5.
4. The answer can be found in Sect. 4.7.
5. $F_{\text{herbicide}} = 18.34$ (with 15 DF at the numerator and 45 DF at the denominator).
6. Both the effect of timing and the "timing by genotype" interaction were relevant (respectively, $F_{\text{timing}} = 26.71$ and $F_{\text{interaction}} = 32.49$). Thus, it is reasonable to expect that the best timing changes depending on the genotype.
7. None of the three effects (alcohol, base, and their interaction) is relevant ($F_{\text{alcohol}} = 1.86$, $F_{\text{base}} = 0.18$, and $F_{\text{interaction}} = 0.53$.
8. The ANOVA table is reported below:

```
Response: Yield
                    Df  Sum Sq Mean Sq F value Pr(>F)
Genotype             1 12.5500 12.5500  7.1757 0.0553 .
Fertilizer           1  5.1200  5.1200  2.9274 0.1623
```

```
Genotype:Fertilizer  1  0.3698  0.3698  0.2114 0.6695
Residuals            4  6.9959  1.7490
```

D.5 Chapter 5

1. $P(Y_O > 170) = 0.159$; $P(Y_O < 140) = 0.159$; $P(140 < Y_O < 170) = 0.683$.
2. The expected concentration at 50 days is $Y_E = 3.02$ ng/g. The observed concentration is Gaussian distributed, with a mean of 3.02 and a standard deviation of 0.37. The required probability is is 0.046.
3. The yield/density relationship can be drawn by using the R code `curve(0.8 + 0.8*x - 0.07*x^2, xlim = c(0,10))`. From the graph, we can see that the yield is maximum when the density is, approximately, 6 plants per square meter. If we consider such an optimal density, the expected yield is $Y_E = 3.08$ tons per hectare. The observed yield is Gaussian distributed, with a mean of 3.08 and a standard deviation of 0.604. The required probability is 0.356.
4. $Y_E = 0.845$. $Y_O = 120/150 = 0.8$. The approximate probability $P(Y > 0.8) = 0.748$.
5. The exercise has an infinite number of possible solutions. In order to find one, you can modify the R coding at Code Box 5.7.
6. The exercise has an infinite number of possible solutions. In order to find one, you can modify the R coding at Code Box 5.8 (please note that the experiment is completely randomized).

D.6 Chapter 6

1. The SD is an index of spread for a group of data points in a sample or population. The SE measures the sample-to-sample variability of a sample statistic, such as the mean.
2. A single specific confidence interval does not mean very much. Make sure you are clear with the limitations of the frequentist confidence interval that are described in Sect. 6.6
3. See the solution for Exercise 3.3. The CIs are, respectively, 90.21–200.45 and 18.19–272.48.
4. In order to do the calculations quickly without fitting a model, it is convenient to load the data in a vector of yields and the corresponding genotypes in another index vector. Next, the `tapply()` function can be used to produce the desired results. The confidence intervals for the four genotypes are, respectively, 4.23–6.77, 5.76–6.17, 4.26–5.39, and 6.00–6.69.
5. The CIs are, respectively, 2.14–2.30 and 2.11–2.33.
6. SEs and CIs for model parameters can be obtained from the model object, by using the `summary()` and `confint()` functions.

D.7 Chapter 7

1. P = 0.016
2. P = 0.020
3. P = 0.108
4. P = 0.0048 (Welch test)
5. P = 0.067 (F-test)
6. P = 0.010 (homoscedastic t-test)
7. P = 0.0022 (see Code Box 7.10)
8. P = 0.021 (F-test)
9. P = 0.0072 (paired homoscedastic t-test)
10. F = 48.87; P = 1.06×10^{-9}

D.8 Chapter 8

1. The R coding to check a fitted model object named `mod` can be summarized as follows:

```
plot(mod, which = 1)
plot(mod, which = 2)
boxcox(mod)
leveneTest(mod)
shapiro.test(residuals(mod))
```

   The coding for Levene's test for an experiment with an RCBD needs to be modified as follows:

```
leveneTest(abs(residuals(mod)) ~ FACTOR, data = dataset)
```

   In the previous line of code, "`dataset`" is the dataframe containing the experimental factor named `FACTOR` (see Example 10.1 in Code Box 10.2). None of the datasets for the Exercises from 5 to 7 in Chap. 4 seems to raise concerns relating to the respect of the basic assumptions.

D.9 Chapter 9

1. The results of multiple comparison tests for Exercises 5 and 6 in Chap. 4 are reported below, in accordance with the aims of each experiment. For Exercise 7, the CLD is not reported, as the F-tests in ANOVA were not significant.

```
# Exercise 5 in Chap. 4 ####
Herbicide                      emmean   SE df lower.CL upper.CL .group
Unw.                             21.9 6.32 45     9.13     34.6  A
Al. + terb.                      29.8 6.32 45    17.11     42.6  A
Unw. 2                           35.7 6.32 45    22.99     48.4  A
Metol. + terbu. (pre)            47.0 6.32 45    34.27     59.7  A
Thif.                            51.9 6.32 45    39.19     64.6  AB
Pend. (pre) + rim. (post)        83.0 6.32 45    70.31     95.8   BC
Rim. + thyf.                     84.7 6.32 45    71.94     97.4    C
Rim. (60)                        88.4 6.32 45    75.65    101.1    C
Hand-Weeded                      89.0 6.32 45    76.24    101.7    C
Rim. (50+30 split)               89.2 6.32 45    76.52    102.0    C
Rim. (45)                        91.6 6.32 45    78.84    104.3    C
Rim. + hoeing                    93.9 6.32 45    81.18    106.6    C
Rim. (40)                        95.4 6.32 45    82.67    108.1    C
Pend. (post) + rim. (post)       96.6 6.32 45    83.91    109.4    C
Rim. + Atred                     97.0 6.32 45    84.26    109.7    C
Rim. (50)                        98.0 6.32 45    85.24    110.7    C

# Exercise 6 in Chap. 4 ####
Genotype = A:
Timing emmean   SE df lower.CL upper.CL .group
Early    15.7 4.21 10     6.35     25.1  A
Opt      67.5 4.21 10    58.07     76.8   B
Late     75.3 4.21 10    65.95     84.7   B

Genotype = B:
Timing emmean   SE df lower.CL upper.CL .group
Late     68.6 4.21 10    59.22     78.0  A
Opt      70.6 4.21 10    61.26     80.0  A
Early    72.2 4.21 10    62.79     81.6  A
```

D.10 Chapter 10

For all the Exercises in Chap. 10, the ANOVA table is reported, together with the letter display from multiple comparison testing. Hints are also given about the stabilizing transformation that has been employed, if any. The discussion of results is left to the students.

1. No stabilizing transformation is needed.

```
Response: Yield
          Df Sum Sq Mean Sq F value    Pr(>F)
Variety    4 750.96 187.739  36.076 6.489e-06 ***
Residuals 10  52.04   5.204

Variety emmean   SE df lower.CL upper.CL .group
```

```
D         13.3 1.32 10      10.4      16.2  A
E         23.2 1.32 10      20.3      26.1   B
B         24.5 1.32 10      21.6      27.5   B
C         29.1 1.32 10      26.1      32.0   BC
A         34.7 1.32 10      31.7      37.6    C
```

2. No stabilizing transformation is needed.

```
Response: Growth
          Df  Sum Sq Mean Sq F value    Pr(>F)
Sugar      3 11.8210  3.9403  38.809 1.432e-07 ***
Residuals 16  1.6245  0.1015

Sugar     emmean    SE df lower.CL upper.CL .group
 Fructose   3.60 0.142 16     3.30     3.90  A
 Glucose    3.91 0.142 16     3.61     4.21  AB
 Sucrose    4.35 0.142 16     4.05     4.65   B
 Control    5.62 0.142 16     5.32     5.92    C
```

3. This dataset is affected by heteroscedasticity, and the response variable needs a reciprocal transformation ($\lambda = -1$) or, even better, a transformation into the reciprocal of the square root ($\lambda = -0.5$). Multiple comparison testing is performed on the transformed data, although it is also possible to perform it on the back-transformed data (see Code Box 11.9).

```
Response: Hours_to_failureTr
          Df     Sum Sq    Mean Sq F value    Pr(>F)
Temp       3 5.3974e-06 1.7991e-06  33.083 5.998e-08 ***
Residuals 20 1.0876e-06 5.4380e-08

 Temp response    SE df lower.CL upper.CL .group
  1708      639  38.9 20      567      732  A
  1660      959  87.6 20      806     1185   B
  1620     1726 284.0 20     1285     2626    C
  1520     3128 932.0 20     1930     8258    C
Confidence level used: 0.95
Intervals are back-transformed from the inverse scale
Note: contrasts are still on the reciprocal scale. Consider using
      regrid() if you want contrasts of back-transformed estimates.
P value adjustment: tukey method for comparing a family of 4 estimates
significance level used: alpha = 0.05
```

4. This dataset is affected by heteroscedasticity, and the response variable needs a square root transformation ($\lambda = 0.5$). Multiple comparison testing is performed on the transformed data, although it is also possible to perform it on back-transformed data (see Code Box 11.9).

```
Analysis of Variance Table

Response: sqrt(No_of_eggs)
          Df  Sum Sq Mean Sq F value    Pr(>F)
Substrate  2 1785.54  892.77  153.95 < 2.2e-16 ***
Residuals 42  243.56    5.80

Substrate response    SE df lower.CL upper.CL .group
 C            32.8  7.13 42     20.0     48.8  A
 B           111.3 13.10 42     86.4    139.4   B
 A           434.1 25.90 42    383.3    487.9    C

Confidence level used: 0.95
Intervals are back-transformed from the sqrt scale
Note: contrasts are still on the sqrt scale. Consider using
      regrid() if you want contrasts of back-transformed estimates.
P value adjustment: tukey method for comparing a family of 3 estimates
significance level used: alpha = 0.05
```

5. No significant differences between irrigation methods were found.
6. A logarithmic transformation is advised ($\lambda = 0$). The dataset is unbalanced, and, thus, the use of the Anova() function is advised, to avoid mistakes.

```
Anova Table (Type II tests)

Response: log(P205)
           Sum Sq Df F value    Pr(>F)
Block     0.04951  4  0.7213    0.5906
Fert      1.00100  4 14.5836 4.719e-05 ***
Residuals 0.25740 15

Fert          response    SE df lower.CL upper.CL .group
 Unfertilised     6.02 0.353 15     5.31     6.82  A
 100N             7.42 0.435 15     6.55     8.41  A
 50N              7.47 0.501 15     6.47     8.61  AB
 50N+75P          9.60 0.562 15     8.47    10.87   BC
 100N+75P        10.57 0.619 15     9.33    11.97    C

Results are averaged over the levels of: Block
Confidence level used: 0.95
Intervals are back-transformed from the log scale
P value adjustment: tukey method for comparing a family of 5 estimates
Tests are performed on the log scale
significance level used: alpha = 0.05
```

7. No stabilizing transformation is needed.

```
Analysis of Variance Table

Response: Yield
           Df Sum Sq Mean Sq F value   Pr(>F)
Fertiliser  3 6768.1 2256.02 10.0680 0.009316 **
Row         3 8228.8 2742.95 12.2410 0.005731 **
Column      3  935.6  311.86  1.3918 0.333294
```

```
Residuals   6 1344.5  224.08
 Fertiliser emmean   SE df lower.CL upper.CL .group
 B             165 7.48  6      147      184  A
 C             169 7.48  6      150      187  A
 A             175 7.48  6      157      193  A
 D             216 7.48  6      198      235   B

Results are averaged over the levels of: Row, Column
Confidence level used: 0.95
P value adjustment: tukey method for comparing a family of 4 estimates
significance level used: alpha = 0.05
```

8. A stabilizing transformation is needed, with $\lambda = 0.65$.

```
Analysis of Variance Table

Response: RhizomeWeightTr
              Df Sum Sq Mean Sq F value    Pr(>F)
Length         2  71.03  35.516  8.2472 0.0007489 ***
Timing         5 919.99 183.998 42.7267 < 2.2e-16 ***
Length:Timing 10  42.10   4.210  0.9775 0.4736006
Residuals     54 232.54   4.306

 Timing            response   SE df lower.CL upper.CL .group
 3-4 and 8/9 leaf      3.67 1.45 54     1.20     6.96  A
 4-5 leaf             11.17 2.14 54     7.18    15.75  A
 2-3 leaf             28.99 2.99 54    23.21    35.20   B
 6-7 leaf             38.14 3.30 54    31.74    44.95   BC
 8-9 leaf             43.27 3.45 54    36.56    50.37    C
 Untreated            44.43 3.48 54    37.65    51.59    C

Results are averaged over the levels of: Length
Confidence level used: 0.95
Intervals are back-transformed from the mu^0.65 scale
Note: contrasts are still on the mu^0.65 scale. Consider using
      regrid() if you want contrasts of back-transformed estimates.
P value adjustment: tukey method for comparing a family of 6 estimates
significance level used: alpha = 0.05
```

D.11 Chapter 11

1. $P_{lack} = 0.126$; slope $= -0.021$ (SE $= 0.0024$); average intercept $= 3.567$ (SE $= 0.074$); maximum admissible yield loss $= 0.267$ tons per hectare; minimum admissible yield $= 3.30$ tons per hectar; economic threshold $= 12.98$ (SE $=$ 2.459).
2. Parameter estimates are reported below:

```
Parameter estimates:

                    Estimate Std. Error t-value   p-value
```

```
a:(Intercept) 4.801176   0.643453  7.4616 0.0001418 ***
b:(Intercept) 0.294588   0.029424 10.0118 2.123e-05 ***
```

3. Parameters estimates are reported below. The comparisons among the corresponding parameters for the two curves yield, respectively, the following P-values: $P_b = 0.160$; $P_d = 8.1 \times 10^{-6}$; $P_e = 0.020$.

```
Parameter estimates (weed free):

    Estimate Std. Error t-value   p-value
b   -0.17932    0.03902 -4.5957   0.00035 ***
d 3453.37982  167.64883 20.5989 2.057e-12 ***
e   52.38454    1.58018 33.1511 1.837e-15 ***

Parameter estimates (infested):

    Estimate Std. Error t-value   p-value
b   -0.11876    0.01832  -6.483 1.033e-05 ***
d 2511.95664  127.95600  19.631 4.131e-12 ***
e   58.03099    1.83458  31.632 3.788e-15 ***
```

D.12 Chapter 12

1. The ANOVA table and multiple comparison testing are as follows:

```
Type III Analysis of Variance Table with Satterthwaite's method
                    Sum Sq Mean Sq NumDF DenDF  F value    Pr(>F)
Block               0.9515  0.3172     3    33   3.8396 0.0183587 *
SowingTime         23.6602 23.6602     1    33 286.4169 < 2.2e-16 ***
Genotype            6.4509  1.2902     5    33  15.6182 6.884e-08 ***
SowingTime:Genotype 2.3371  0.4674     5    33   5.6582 0.0007119 ***

SowingTime = autumn:
 Genotype  emmean    SE   df lower.CL upper.CL .group
 Collameno   3.25 0.144 30.9     2.96     3.54  A
 Sicania     3.83 0.144 30.9     3.54     4.12  AB
 Palomb      3.84 0.144 30.9     3.55     4.13  AB
 Chiaro      4.11 0.144 30.9     3.81     4.40   B
 Vesuvio     4.14 0.144 30.9     3.84     4.43   B
 Scuro       4.37 0.144 30.9     4.08     4.66   B

SowingTime = spring:
 Genotype  emmean    SE   df lower.CL upper.CL .group
 Collameno   1.91 0.144 30.9     1.61     2.20  A
 Vesuvio     2.12 0.144 30.9     1.83     2.42  A
 Palomb      2.25 0.144 30.9     1.96     2.54  A
 Chiaro      2.51 0.144 30.9     2.21     2.80  AB
 Scuro       3.05 0.144 30.9     2.76     3.34   BC
```

```
 Sicania     3.27 0.144 30.9     2.98     3.56    C

Results are averaged over the levels of: Block
Degrees-of-freedom method: kenward-roger
Confidence level used: 0.95
P value adjustment: tukey method for comparing a family of 6 estimates
significance level used: alpha = 0.05
```

2. The data need a square root transformation ($\lambda = 0.5$). For each crop, the herbicides are compared to the untreated check, using Dunnett's method.

```
Type III Analysis of Variance Table with Satterthwaite's method
                Sum Sq Mean Sq NumDF DenDF F value    Pr(>F)
Block            17.02   5.672     3     9  1.5168    0.2757
Herbicide       312.05 104.017     3     9 27.8151 6.956e-05 ***
Crop            382.02 127.339     3    36 34.0516 1.301e-10 ***
Herbicide:Crop 440.30  48.922     9    36 13.0821 5.965e-09 ***

Crop = grainsorghum:
 contrast              estimate   SE   df t.ratio p.value
 Imazethapyr - Check    -12.275 1.73 26.7  -7.101  <.0001
 primisulfuron - Check   -1.386 1.73 26.7  -0.802  0.7415
 rimsulfuron - Check      0.949 1.73 26.7   0.549  0.8753

Crop = rape:
 contrast              estimate   SE   df t.ratio p.value
 Imazethapyr - Check     -9.404 1.73 26.7  -5.440  <.0001
 primisulfuron - Check   -9.548 1.73 26.7  -5.523  <.0001
 rimsulfuron - Check      2.064 1.73 26.7   1.194  0.4999

Crop = soyabean:
 contrast              estimate   SE   df t.ratio p.value
 Imazethapyr - Check     -3.509 1.73 26.7  -2.030  0.1327
 primisulfuron - Check   -0.226 1.73 26.7  -0.131  0.9934
 rimsulfuron - Check     -1.630 1.73 26.7  -0.943  0.6559

Crop = sunflower:
 contrast              estimate   SE   df t.ratio p.value
 Imazethapyr - Check    -13.878 1.73 26.7  -8.028  <.0001
 primisulfuron - Check   -0.637 1.73 26.7  -0.368  0.9444
 rimsulfuron - Check      0.128 1.73 26.7   0.074  0.9979

Note: contrasts are still on the sqrt scale
Degrees-of-freedom method: kenward-roger
P value adjustment: dunnettx method for 3 tests
```

3. The ANOVA table and multiple comparisons are reported below:

```
Type III Analysis of Variance Table with Satterthwaite's method
   Sum Sq Mean Sq NumDF DenDF F value    Pr(>F)
B   4675.0   935.0     5    10  5.2800   0.01244 *
V    526.1   263.0     2    10  1.4853   0.27239
N  20020.5  6673.5     3    45 37.6856 2.458e-12 ***
```

```
V:N    321.8    53.6     6    45  0.3028   0.93220

N        emmean   SE   df lower.CL upper.CL .group
0.0cwt     79.4 3.97 30.2     71.3     87.5  A
0.2cwt     98.9 3.97 30.2     90.8    107.0   B
0.4cwt    114.2 3.97 30.2    106.1    122.3    C
0.6cwt    123.4 3.97 30.2    115.3    131.5    C
```

4. A stabilizing transformation is needed, using $\lambda = 0.65$. No significant differences are found.

```
Response: I(Yield^0.65)
           Df  Sum Sq Mean Sq F value  Pr(>F)
Loc        11   2.099 0.19082  0.4655 0.92432
Var        16  10.647 0.66543  1.6233 0.05823 .
Loc:Block  36   4.270 0.11862  0.2894 0.99999
Loc:Var   176  84.864 0.48218  1.1763 0.08496 .
Residuals 576 236.114 0.40992
```

References

Bates D, Mächler M, Bolker B, Walker S (2015) Fitting linear mixed-effects models using lme4. J Stat Softw 67(1):1–48. https://doi.org/10.18637/jss.v067.i01

Covarelli G, Onofri A (1998) Effects of timing of weed removal and emergence in sugarbeet. In: Proceedings 6th EWRS Mediterranean Symposium, Montpellier, 13–15 May 1998. EWRS, pp 65–72

Cristaudo A, Restuccia A, Onofri A, Giudice VL, Gresta F (2015) Species-area relationships and minimum area in citrus grove weed communities. Plant Biosyst 149(2):337–345

Fox J, Weisberg S (2019) An R Companion to Applied Regression, 3rd edn. Sage, Thousand Oaks, CA. https://www.john-fox.ca/Companion/

Graves S, Piepho HP, with help from Sundar Dorai-Raj LS (2024) multcompView: Visualizations of Paired Comparisons. https://CRAN.R-project.org/package=multcompView, r package version 0.1-10

Hothorn T, Bretz F, Westfall P (2008) Simultaneous inference in general parametric models. Biom J 50(3):346–363

Kuehl RO (2000) Design of Experiments: Statistical Principles of Research Design and Analysis. Duxbury Press, Books, Pacific Grove

Kuznetsova A, Brockhoff PB, Christensen RHB (2017) lmerTest package: tests in linear mixed effects models. J Stat Softw 82(13):1–26. https://doi.org/10.18637/jss.v082.i13

Le Clerg EL, Leonard WH, Clark AG (1962) Field Plot Technique. Burgess Publishing Company, Minneapolis

Lenth RV (2024) emmeans: Estimated Marginal Means, aka Least-Squares Means. https://CRAN.R-project.org/package=emmeans. r package version 1.10.4

Ligabue M, Onofri A, Ruozzi F (2009) Le migliori varietà di erba medica da seme. Agricoltura 84:82–84

Monotti M, Onofri A, Gargano E, Selmi C, Tagliaferri A, Craveri L, Severi D, Bruno G, Poli M, Bimbi G, Ginanni M, Moscheni E, Quattrucci M, Tavoletti S, Petrini A, Di Paolo E, Stagnari F, De Mastro G, Carboni G, Pruneddu G, Sarti A, Tonetti L (2009) Azioni di innovazione e ricerca a supporto del piano proteine vegetali: Proteiche da granella. CRPA Editore, Reggio Emilia. http://www.crpa.it/nqcontent.cfm?a_id=7780&tt=crpa_www&sp=crpa

Muller-Dumbois D, Ellenberg H (1974) Community sampling: the relevè method. In: Aims and Methods of Vegetation Ecology. Species/Area curves. Wiley, Hoboken, pp 45–66

Nelson W (1972) A short life test for comparing a sample with previous accelerated test results. Technometrics 14:175–185

Onofri A (2025) statforbiology: Data Analyses in Agriculture and Biology. https://github.com/OnofriAndreaPG/statforbiology, r package version 0.9.9

Onofri A, Ciriciofolo E (2007) Using R to perform the AMMI analysis on agriculture variety trials. R NEWS 7:14–19. https://www.r-project.org

Onofri A, Tei F (1994a) Competitive ability and threshold levels for three broadleaf weed species in sunflower. Weed Res 34:471–479

Onofri A, Tei F (1994b) Influence of application timing on the effectiveness of rimsulfuron against rhizome *Sorghum halepense* (L.) Pers. In: Tei F, Onofri A (eds) Weed Control in Sustainable Agriculture in the Mediterranean Area. Proceedings 5th EWRS Mediterranean Symposium, Università degli Studi di Perugia, Reprints, pp 105–111

Onofri A, Covarelli L, Tei F (1995) Efficacy of rimsulfuron and metribuzin against Solanum nigrum L. at different growth stages in tomato. In: International Meeting on Weed Control. Proceedings 16th COLUMA Conference, Reims, ANPP, reprints, pp 993–1000

Pace R, Benincasa P, Ghanem ME, Quinet M, Lutts S (2012) Germination of untreated and primed seeds in rapeseed (brassica napus var oleifera del.) under salinity and low matric potential. Exp Agric 48(02):238–251. https://doi.org/10.1017/S0014479711001189. http://www.journals.cambridge.org/abstract_S0014479711001189

Pannacci E, Mathiassen S, Kudsk P (2010) The effect of adjuvants on the rainfastness and performance of tribenuron-methyl on broadleaf weeds. Weed Biol Manag 10:126–131

R Core Team (2025) R: A Language and Environment for Statistical Computing. R Foundation for Statistical Computing, Vienna. https://www.R-project.org/

Ritz C, Jensen SM, Gerhard D, Streibig JC (2019) Dose-Response Analysis Using R. CRC Press, Boca Raton

RStudio Team (2020) RStudio: Integrated Development Environment for R. RStudio, Inc., Boston, MA. http://www.rstudio.com/

Stagnari F, Onofri A, Jemison J, Monotti M (2007) Improved multivariate analyses to discriminate the behaviour of faba bean varieties. Agron Sustain Develop 27(4):387–397

Stagnari F, Onofri A, Codianni P, Pisante M (2013) Durum wheat varieties in N-deficient environments and organic farming: a comparison of yield, quality and stability performances. Plant Breeding 132:266–275

Venables WN, Ripley BD (2002) Modern Applied Statistics with S. Statistics and Computing, 4th edn. Springer, New York

Vischetti C, Marini M, Businelli M, Onofri A (1996) The effect of temperature and co-applied herbicides on the degradation rate of phenmedipham, chloridazon and metamitron in a clay loam soil in the laboratory. In: Re AD, Capri E, Evans SP, Trevisan M (eds) The Environmental Fate of Xenobiotics, Proceedings X Symposium on Pesticide Chemistry, Piacenza, La Goliardica Pavese, Piacenza, pp 287–294

Wheeler B (2025) SuppDists: Supplementary Distributions. https://CRAN.R-project.org/package=SuppDists. r package version 1.1-9.9

Wickham H (2016) Ggplot2. Elegant Graphics for Data Analysis. Use R! Springer International Publishing, Cham, https://doi.org/10.1007/978-3-319-24277-4. http://link.springer.com/10.1007/978-3-319-24277-4

Wickham H, Averick M, Bryan J, Chang W, McGowan LD, François R, Grolemund G, Hayes A, Henry L, Hester J, Kuhn M, Pedersen TL, Miller E, Bache SM, Müller K, Ooms J, Robinson D, Seidel DP, Spinu V, Takahashi K, Vaughan D, Wilke C, Woo K, Yutani H (2019) Welcome to the tidyverse. J. Open Source Softw. 4(43):1686. https://doi.org/10.21105/joss.01686

Wickham H, Çetinkaya-Rundel M, Grolemund G (2023) R for Data Science (2e). O'Reilly Media, Santa Rosa

Xie Y (2024) bookdown: Authoring Books and Technical Documents with R Markdown. https://github.com/rstudio/bookdown, r package version 0.40

Xie Y, Hill AP, Thomas A (2017) Blogdown: Creating Websites with R Markdown. Chapman and Hall/CRC, Boca Raton. https://bookdown.org/yihui/blogdown/

Xie Y, Allaire J, Grolemund G (2018) R Markdown: The Definitive Guide. Chapman and Hall/CRC, Boca Raton. https://bookdown.org/yihui/rmarkdown

MIX
Papier aus verantwortungsvollen Quellen
Paper from responsible sources
FSC® C105338

If you have any concerns about our products,
you can contact us on
ProductSafety@springernature.com

In case Publisher is established outside the EU,
the EU authorized representative is:
Springer Nature Customer Service Center GmbH
Europaplatz 3, 69115 Heidelberg, Germany

Printed by Libri Plureos GmbH
in Hamburg, Germany